P9-DDU-622

Contributors

Audrey Knippa, MS, MPH, RN, CNE
Nursing Education Coordinator and
  Content Project Leader

Sheryl Sommer, PhD, MSN, RN, CNE
Director, Nursing Curriculum and
  Education Services

Susan Adcock, MS, RN
Nursing Education Specialist

Brenda Ball, MEd, BSN, RN
Nursing Education Specialist

Lois Churchill, MN, RN
Nursing Education Specialist

Carrie B. Elkins, DHSc, MSN, PHCNS, BC
Nursing Education Specialist

Mary Jane Janowski, MA, BSN, RN
Nursing Resource Specialist

Sharon R. Redding, EdD, RN, CNE
Nursing Education Specialist

Karin Roberts, PhD, MSN, RN, CNE
Nursing Education Coordinator

Mendy G. Wright, DNP, MSN, RN
Nursing Education Specialist

Chris Crawford, BS Journalism
Product Developer and Editorial Project Leader

Derek Prater, MS Journalism
Lead Product Developer

Johanna Barnes, BA Journalism
Product Developer

Joey Berlin, BS Journalism
Product Developer

Hilary E. Groninger, BS Journalism
Product Developer

Megan E. Herre, BS Journalism
Product Developer

Amanda Lehman, BA English
Product Developer

Spring Lenox, BS Journalism
Product Developer

Robin Nelson, BA English
Product Developer

Joanna Shindler, BA Journalism
Product Developer

Morgan Smith, BS Journalism
Media Developer

Brant L. Stacy, BS Journalism, BA English
Product Developer

Mandy Tallmadge, BS Communication
Product Developer

Karen D. Wood, BS Journalism
Product Developer

**Katherine Wood-Raclin, BA English, Mass
Communications**

Consultants

Gale P. Sewell, RN, MSN, CNE

Terri Lemon, MSN, RN

Fleurdeliza T. Cuyco, BSN

INTELLECTUAL PROPERTY NOTICE

IMPORTANT NOTICE TO THE READER

USER'S GUIDE

Welcome to the Assessment Technologies Institute® PN Pharmacology for Nursing Review Module Edition 5.0. The mission of ATI's Content Mastery Series® review modules is to provide user-friendly compendiums of nursing knowledge that will:

- Help you locate important information quickly.

- Assist in your remediation efforts.

- Provide exercises for applying your nursing knowledge.

- Facilitate your entry into the nursing profession as a newly licensed PN.

Organization

This review module is organized into units covering pharmacological principles (Unit 1) and medications affecting the body systems and physiological processes (Units 2 to 12). Chapters within these units conform to one of two organizing principles for presenting the content:

- Basic concepts

- Medications

Basic concepts chapters begin with an overview describing the central concept and its relevance to nursing. Subordinate themes are in outline form to demonstrate relationships and present the information in a clear, succinct manner.

Medications chapters include an overview describing a disorder, group of disorders or specific medication classifications. Sections within the chapters will focus on a prototype or prototype medications. These sections include information about how the medication works, its therapeutic uses, and routes of administration. Next, you will find information about complications, contraindications, and medication and food interactions, as well as nursing interventions and client education to help prevent and/or manage these issues. Finally, the chapter includes information on nursing administration of the medication and evaluation of the medication's effectiveness.

Application Exercises

At the end of each chapter there are questions you can use to practice applying your knowledge. The Application Exercises include both NCLEX-style questions, such as multiple-choice and multiple-select items, and questions that ask you to apply your knowledge in other formats, such as short-answer and matching items. After completing the Application Exercises, go to the Application Exercise Answer Key to check your answers and rationales for correct and incorrect answers.

NCLEX® Connections

To prepare for the NCLEX-PN, it is important for you to understand how the content in this review module is connected to the NCLEX-PN test plan. You can find information on the detailed test plan at the National Council of State Boards of Nursing's Web site: https://www.ncsbn.org/. When reviewing content in this review module, regularly ask yourself, "How does this content fit into the test plan, and what types of questions related to this content should I expect?"

To help you in this process, we've included NCLEX Connections at the beginning of each unit and with each question in the Application Exercises Answer Keys. The NCLEX Connections at the beginning of each unit will point out areas of the detailed test plan that relate to the content within that unit. The NCLEX Connections attached to the Application Exercises Answer Keys will demonstrate how each exercise fits within the detailed content outline.

These NCLEX Connections will help you understand how the detailed content outline is organized, starting with major client needs categories and subcategories and followed by related content areas and tasks. The major client needs categories are:

- Safe and Effective Care Environment
  - Management of Care
  - Safety and Infection Control
- Health Promotion and Maintenance
- Psychosocial Integrity
- Physiological Integrity
  - Basic Care and Comfort
  - Pharmacological Therapies
  - Reduction of Risk Potential
  - Physiological Adaptation

An NCLEX Connection might, for example, alert you that content within a unit is related to:

- Pharmacological Therapies
  - Expected Actions/Outcomes
    - Identify client need for PRN medications.

Icons

Throughout the review module you will see icons that will draw your attention to particular areas. Keep an eye out for these icons:

 This icon indicates an Overview, or introduction, to a particular subject matter. Descriptions and categories will typically be found in an Overview.

 This icon indicates Application Exercises and Application Exercises Answer Keys.

 This icon indicates NCLEX connections.

 This icon indicates gerontological content. When you see this icon, take note of information that is specific to aging or the care of older adult clients.

 This icon indicates content related to safety. When you see this icon, take note of safety concerns or steps that nurses can take to ensure client safety and a safe environment.

 This icon indicates examples of how to apply math concepts, such as in dosage calculation.

 This icon indicates that a media supplement, such as a graphic, an animation, or a video, is available. If you have an electronic copy of the review module, this icon will appear alongside clickable links to media supplements. If you have a hardcopy version of the review module, visit www.atitesting.com for details on how to access these features.

Feedback

ATI welcomes feedback regarding this review module. Please provide comments to: comments@ atitesting.com.

Table of Contents

Unit 5   Medications Affecting the Hematologic System

Unit 6   Medications Affecting the Gastrointestinal System and Nutrition

Unit 7   Medications Affecting the Reproductive System

Unit 11   Medications Affecting the Immune System and for Infectious Diseases

UNIT 1: PHARMACOLOGIC PRINCIPLES

- Pharmacokinetics and Routes of Administration

- Safe Medication Administration and Error Reduction

- Dosage Calculation

- Intravenous Therapy

- Adverse Effects, Interactions, and Contraindications

- Individual Considerations of Medication Administration

NCLEX® CONNECTIONS

When reviewing the chapters in this section, keep in mind the relevant sections of the NCLEX® outline, in particular:

CLIENT NEEDS: SAFETY AND INFECTION CONTROL

Relevant topics/tasks include:
- Accident/Error/Injury Prevention
  - Utilize facility client identification procedures.
- Reporting of Incident/Event/Irregular Occurrence/Variance
  - Identify situations requiring completion of incident/event/irregular occurrence/variance report.

CLIENT NEEDS: PHARMACOLOGICAL THERAPIES

Relevant topics/tasks include:
- Adverse Effects/Contraindications/Side Effects/Interactions
  - Identify potential and actual incompatibilities of client medications.
- Dosage Calculation
  - Perform calculations needed for medication administration.
- Medication Administration
  - Dispose of client unused medications according to facility/agency policy.

UNIT 1	PHARMACOLOGIC PRINCIPLES
Chapter 1	Pharmacokinetics and Routes of Administration

 Overview

- Pharmacokinetics refers to how medications travel through the body. Medications undergo a variety of biochemical processes that result in absorption, distribution, metabolism, and excretion.

Phases of Pharmacokinetics

- Absorption is the transmission of medications from the location of administration (gastrointestinal [GI] tract, muscle, skin, or subcutaneous tissue) to the bloodstream. The most common routes of administration are enteral (through the GI tract) and parenteral (by injection). Each of these routes have a unique pattern of absorption.

  ○ The rate of medication absorption determines how soon the medication will take effect.

  ○ The amount of medication absorbed determines its intensity.

  ○ The route of administration affects the rate and amount of absorption.

ROUTES AND ABSORPTION		
Route	Barriers to Absorption	Absorption Pattern
Oral	Medications must pass through the layer of epithelial cells that line the GI tract.	Varies greatly due to the following variables: • Stability and solubility of the medication • GI pH and emptying time • Presence of food in the stomach or intestines • Other medications currently being administered • Forms of medications (enteric-coated pills, liquids)

Subcutaneous and intramuscular	The capillary wall has large spaces between cells; therefore, there is no significant barrier.	The rate of absorption is determined by:
		• Solubility of the medication in water
		  ○ Highly soluble medications will be absorbed in 10 to 30 min.
		  ○ Poorly soluble medications will be absorbed more slowly.
		• Blood perfusion at the site of injection
		  ○ Sites with high blood perfusion will have rapid absorption.
		  ○ Sites with low blood perfusion will have slow absorption.

Intravenous	There are no barriers.	• Immediate – Administered directly into blood • Complete – All of it reaches the blood

- Distribution is the transportation of medications to sites of action by bodily fluids. Distribution can be influenced by the ability to:

    ○ Travel to the site of action through the bloodstream (peripheral vascular or cardiac disease can delay medication distribution).

    ○ Leave the bloodstream by traveling between the capillaries' cells.

        ▪ Plasma protein binding – Medications compete for protein binding sites within the bloodstream, primarily albumin. The ability of a medication to bind to a protein can affect how much of the medication will leave and travel to target tissues. Two medications can compete for the same binding sites, resulting in toxicity.

        ▪ Barriers – Medications that are lipid soluble or have a transport system that can cross the blood brain barrier or the placenta.

- Metabolism (biotransformation) changes medications into less active or inactive forms by the action of enzymes. This occurs primarily in the liver, but also takes place in the kidneys, lungs, bowel, and blood.

  o Factors influencing the rate of medication metabolism include:

    - Age – Infants have limited medication-metabolizing capacity. The aging process can also influence medication metabolism, but varies by individual. In general, hepatic medication metabolism tends to decline with age.

    - An increase in certain medication-metabolizing enzymes – This can cause that particular medication to be metabolized sooner, requiring an increase in dosage of that medication to maintain a therapeutic level. It can also cause an increase in the metabolism of other medications that are being used concurrently.

    - First-pass effect – Some medications are inactivated on their first pass through the liver and must be given by a nonenteral route because of their high first-pass effect. These medications are usually given by alternate routes, such as SL or IV.

    - Similar metabolic pathways – When two medications are metabolized by the same pathway, this can result in a decrease in metabolism of one or both of the medications. This can lead to medication accumulation.

    - Nutritional status – Malnourished clients may be deficient in the factors that are necessary to produce specific medication-metabolizing enzymes. Consequently, medication metabolism may be impaired.

  o Outcomes of metabolism include:

    - Increased renal excretion of medication

    - Inactivation of medications

    - Increased therapeutic effect

    - Activation of pro-medications into active forms

    - Decreased toxicity when active forms of medications are converted to inactive forms

    - Increased toxicity when inactive forms of medications are converted to active forms

- Excretion is the elimination of medications from the body primarily through the kidneys. Elimination also takes place through the liver, lungs, bowel, and exocrine glands. Renal dysfunction can lead to an increase in duration and intensity of medication response.

- Medication responses – Plasma medication levels can be regulated to control medication responses. Medication dosing attempts to maintain plasma levels between the minimum effective concentration (MEC) and the toxic concentration. A plasma medication level is in the therapeutic range when it is effective and not toxic. Therapeutic levels are well established for many medications, and these levels can be used to monitor a client's response.

- Therapeutic index (TI) – Medications with a high TI have a wide safety margin. Therefore, there is no need for routine serum medication level monitoring. Medications with a low TI should have serum medication levels monitored closely. Monitor peak levels based on the route of administration. For example, an oral medication may have a peak of 1 to 3 hr after administration. If the medication is given intravenously, the peak time might occur within 10 min. (Refer to a drug reference or pharmacist for specific medication peak times.) For trough levels, blood is drawn immediately before the next medication dose regardless of the route of administration.

- Half-life (t½) refers to the period of time needed for a medication to be reduced by 50% in the body. Half-life can be affected by liver and kidney function. It usually takes four half-lives to achieve a steady state of serum concentration (medication intake equals medication metabolism and excretion).

SHORT HALF-LIFE	LONG HALF-LIFE
- Medications leave the body quickly (4 to 8 hr).	- Medications leave the body more slowly (24+ hr). There is a greater risk for medication accumulation and toxicity.
- Short-dosing interval or MEC will drop between doses.	- Medications are given at longer intervals without loss of therapeutic effects. - Medications take a longer time to reach a steady state.

- Pharmacodynamics (mechanism of action) describes the interactions between medications and target cells, organs, and body systems to produce effects. These interactions result in functional changes that are considered the mechanism of action of the medication.

  o An agonist is a medication that can mimic the receptor activity regulated by endogenous compounds. For example, morphine sulfate is classified as an agonist because it activates the receptors that produce analgesia, sedation, constipation, and other effects.

  o An antagonist is a medication that can block normal receptor activity regulated by endogenous compounds or receptor activity caused by other medications. For example, losartan (Cozaar), an angiotensin II receptor blocker, is classified as an antagonist. Losartan works by blocking angiotensin II receptors on blood vessels, which prevents vasoconstriction.

  o Partial agonists can act as an agonist/antagonist and have limited affinity to receptor sites. For example, nalbuphine (Nubain) acts as an antagonist at mu receptors and an agonist at kappa receptors, causing analgesia with minimal respiratory depression at low doses.

Routes of Administration

ROUTE OF ADMINISTRATION	NURSING IMPLICATIONS
Oral or enteral (tablets, capsules, liquids, suspensions, elixirs)	• Contraindications for oral medication administration include vomiting, absence of gag reflex, difficulty swallowing, and decreased level of consciousness. • Have clients sit upright, in Fowler's or semi-Fowler's position, to facilitate swallowing. • Administer irritating medications with small amounts of food. • Do not mix with large amounts of food or beverages in case clients are unable to consume the entire quantity. • Avoid administration with contraindicated foods or beverages, such as grapefruit juice. • In general, administer oral medications on an empty stomach (1 hr before meals, 2 hr after meals). • Follow the manufacturer's directions for crushing, cutting, and diluting medications. A complete list can be found at the Institute for Safe Medication Practice's Web site (http://www.ismp.org). • Have clients swallow coated or time-release medications whole to maintain protective coating and to prevent faster absorption. • Use a liquid form of the medication to facilitate swallowing whenever possible.
Sublingual (under the tongue) and buccal (between the cheek and the gum)	• Instruct clients to keep the medication in place until it is absorbed. • Tell clients not to eat or drink while the tablet is in place.
Liquids, suspensions, elixirs	• Follow directions for dilution and shaking. • When administering the medication, the base of the meniscus (lowest fluid line) is at the level of the desired dose.
Transdermal (medication stored in a skin patch and absorbed through the skin, producing systemic effects)	Instructions to clients should include: • Apply patches as provided to ensure proper dosing. • Wash skin with soap and water, and dry thoroughly before applying a new patch. • Place the patch on a hairless area of the skin and rotate sites to prevent skin irritation.
Topical	• Apply with a glove, tongue blade, or cotton-tipped applicator. • Never apply with a bare hand.

ROUTE OF ADMINISTRATION	NURSING IMPLICATIONS

Instillation (drops, ointments, sprays; generally used for eyes, ears, and nose)	• Eyes
	  ○ Use surgical aseptic technique when instilling medications in eyes.
	  ○ Have clients sit upright or lie supine with the head tilted slightly and looking up at the ceiling.
	  ○ With the radial aspect of your dominant hand resting on the client's forehead, hold the dropper 1 to 2 cm above his conjunctival sac and instill the medication into the center of the sac. Then instruct the client to close his eye gently.
	  ○ Apply gentle pressure with your finger and a clean tissue on the nasolacrimal duct for 30 to 60 seconds to prevent systemic absorption of the medication.
	• Ears
	  ○ Use medical aseptic technique when administering medications into the ears.
	  ○ Have clients sit upright or maintain a side-lying position.
	  ○ Straighten the ear canal by pulling the auricle upward and outward for adults or down and back for children. Hold the dropper 1 cm above the ear canal, instill the medication, and then gently apply pressure to the tragus of the ear with your finger.
	• Nose
	  ○ Use medical aseptic technique when administering medications into the nose.
	  ○ Place clients supine with the head positioned to allow medication to enter the appropriate nasal passage.
	  ○ Use your dominant hand to instill drops, supporting the head with your nondominant hand.
	  ○ Instruct clients to breathe through the mouth, stay in a supine position, and avoid blowing the nose for 5 min after drop insertion.

ROUTE OF ADMINISTRATION	NURSING IMPLICATIONS

Inhalation (medications usually administered through metered dose inhalers [MDI] or dry powder inhalers [DPI])	• For an MDI, instruct clients to:
	  ○ Remove the cap from the inhaler.
	  ○ Shake the inhaler five to six times.
	  ○ Hold the inhaler with the mouthpiece at the bottom.
	  ○ Hold the inhaler with the thumb near the mouthpiece and index and middle fingers at the top.
	  ○ Hold the inhaler approximately 2 to 4 cm (1 to 2 in) away from the front of the mouth.
	  ○ Take a deep breath and then exhale.
	  ○ Tilt the head back slightly, and press the inhaler. While pressing the inhaler, begin a slow, deep breath that should last 3 to 5 seconds to facilitate delivery to the air passages.
	  ○ Hold breath for 10 seconds to allow medication to deposit in the airways.
	  ○ Take the inhaler out of the mouth and slowly exhale through pursed lips.
	  ○ Resume normal breathing.
	• Instruct clients to use a spacer to keep the medication in the device longer, thereby increasing the amount of medication delivered to the lungs and decreasing the amount of the medication in the oropharynx. Instruct clients to:
	  ○ Remove the covers from the mouthpieces of the inhaler and the spacer.
	  ○ Insert the MDI into the end of the spacer.
	  ○ Shake the inhaler five to six times.
	  ○ Exhale completely and then close the mouth around the spacer mouthpiece. Continue as with an MDI.

ROUTE OF ADMINISTRATION	NURSING IMPLICATIONS

Inhalation (medications usually administered through MDI or DPI)	• For a DPI, instruct clients to:
	  ○ Avoid shaking the device.
	  ○ Take the cover off the mouthpiece.
	  ○ Follow the directions of the manufacturer for preparing the medication, such as turning the wheel of the inhaler.
	  ○ Exhale completely.
	  ○ Place the mouthpiece between the lips and take a deep breath through the mouth.
	  ○ Hold breath for 5 to 10 seconds.
	  ○ Take the inhaler out of the mouth and slowly exhale through pursed lips.
	  ○ Resume normal breathing.
	  ○ If more than one puff is ordered, wait the length of time directed before administering the second puff.
	  ○ Remove the canister and rinse the inhaler, cap, and spacer once a day with warm running water and dry completely before using again.

Nasogastric and gastrostomy tubes	• Check for proper tube placement.
	• Use a syringe and allow the medication to flow in by gravity, or push in with the plunger of the syringe.
	• General guidelines
	  ○ Use liquid forms of medications.
	  ○ Do not give sublingual medications.
	  ○ Do not crush specially prepared oral medications (extended/time-release, fluid-filled, enteric coated).
	  ○ Check the compatibility of medications before mixing.
	  ○ Do not mix medications with enteral feedings.
	• To prevent clogging, flush the tubing before and after each medication with 5 to 30 mL of warm water. When administration of medications is complete, flush with 30 to 60 mL of warm water.

ROUTE OF ADMINISTRATION	NURSING IMPLICATIONS
Suppositories	<ul><li>Follow the manufacturer's directions for storage.</li><li>Wear gloves for the procedure.</li><li>Remove the foil wrapper and lubricate the suppository if necessary.</li><li>Rectal suppositories<ul><li>Position clients in left lateral position.</li><li>Insert just beyond the internal sphincter.</li><li>Instruct clients to retain the medication 20 to 30 min for stimulation of defecation and 60 min for systemic absorption.</li></ul></li><li>Vaginal suppositories<ul><li>Position clients supine with knees bent, feet flat on the bed and close to hips (modified lithotomy position).</li><li>Use an applicator for insertion.</li><li>Instruct clients to remain in the position for a prescribed amount of time.</li></ul></li></ul>
Parenteral	General considerations for parenteral medications include:<ul><li>Prepare all medications using sterile technique.</li><li>The vastus lateralis site is usually the recommended site for infants and children less than 2 years of age.</li><li>After age 2, use the ventral gluteal site. Both of these sites can accommodate fluid up to 2 mL. The deltoid site has a smaller muscle mass and can only accommodate up to 1 mL of fluid.</li><li>Use a needle size and length appropriate to the type of injection and client size. Syringe size should approximate the volume of medication.</li><li>Use a tuberculin syringe for solution volume less than 0.5 mL.</li><li>Rotate injection sites to enhance medication absorption, and document each site used.</li><li>Do not use injection sites that are edematous, inflamed, or have moles, birthmarks, or scars.</li><li>If medication is given intravenously, immediately monitor clients for therapeutic and side/adverse effects.</li><li>Discard all sharps (broken ampule bottles, needle) in designated containers. Containers should be leak- and puncture-proof.</li></ul>

ROUTE OF ADMINISTRATION	NURSING IMPLICATIONS
Intradermal	• Use this route for tuberculin testing, checking for medication/allergy sensitivities or some cancer immunotherapy. • Use small amounts of solution (0.01 to 0.1 mL) in a tuberculin syringe with a fine-gauge needle (26 to 27) in lightly pigmented, thin-skinned, hairless sites (inner surface of mid-forearm or scapular area of back) at a 10 to 15° angle.
Subcutaneous	• Use this route for small doses of nonirritating, water-soluble medications (insulin and heparin). • Use a 3/8- to 5/8-inch, 25- to 27-gauge needle, or an insulin syringe of 28- to 31-gauge. Inject no more than 1.5 mL solution. For an average-size client, pinch up skin and inject at a 45 to 90° angle. For an obese client, use a 90° angle. • Select sites by fat-pad size (abdomen, upper hips, lateral upper arms, thighs).
Intramuscular	• Use this route for irritating medications, solutions in oils, and aqueous suspensions. • Use ventrogluteal, dorsogluteal, deltoid, and vastus lateralis (pediatric) muscles. • Use needle size 18 to 27 (usually 22- to 25-gauge), 1 to 1½ inches long, and inject at a 90° angle. For amounts greater than allowable for muscle, divide into two syringes and use two sites.
Z-Track	• Z-track is a type of IM injection that prevents medication from leaking back into subcutaneous tissue. • Use for medications that may cause visible and/or permanent skin stains, such as certain iron preparations.
Intravenous	• Use this route for administration of medications, fluid, and blood products. • Use these IM technique access devices for short-term use (catheters) or long-term use (infusion ports). • Preferred sites for short-term vascular access devices are peripheral veins in the arm or hand.
Epidural	• Use for administration of intravenous opioid analgesia (morphine [Duramorph] or fentanyl [Sublimaze]). • A catheter is advanced through a needle that is inserted into the epidural space at the level of the fourth or fifth vertebrae. • Always use infusion pumps to administer medication.

 View Media Supplement: Sites for Medication Administration (Video)

- Advantages and Disadvantages of Different Routes

ROUTE	ADVANTAGES	DISADVANTAGES
Oral	• The oral route is safe, inexpensive, easy, and convenient.	• Oral medications have a highly variable absorption. • Inactivation can occur by GI tract or first-pass effect. • Clients must be cooperative and conscious. • Contraindications include nausea and vomiting.
Subcutaneous and IM	• Effective for poorly soluble medications. • These routes are appropriate for administering medications that are absorbed slowly for an extended period of time (depot preparations).	• IM injections are associated with a higher cost. • IM injections are inconvenient. • There can be pain with the risk for local tissue damage and nerve damage. • There is a risk for infection at the injection site.
IV	• Onset is rapid, and absorption of the medication into the blood is immediate, which provides an immediate response. • This route allows control over the precise amount of medication given. • This route allows for administration of large volumes of fluid.	• IV injections are associated with an even higher cost. • IV injections are more inconvenient. • Immediate absorption of the medication into the blood can be potentially dangerous if the wrong amount or the wrong medication is given. • There is an increased risk for infection or embolism with IV injections.

Ⓐ APPLICATION EXERCISES

1. Place the phases of pharmacokinetics in the correct order:

    _____ Distribution
    _____ Excretion
    _____ Absorption
    _____ Metabolism

2. Matching: Match the route in column A with the advantage in column B

ROUTE	ADVANTAGE
Oral	A. Provides immediate response
Intramuscular	B. Easy to administer
IV	C. Allows for medication to be administered at site of action
Inhalation	D. Allows for administration of medications poorly soluble in water

3. A nurse is administering eye drops to a client. Which of the following actions should the nurse take? (Select all that apply.)

    _____ Use sterile technique.
    _____ Ask the client to look up at the ceiling before application.
    _____ Place the client in a side-lying position.
    _____ Drop the medication into the conjunctival sac at the inner canthus.
    _____ Instruct the client to close the eye gently after application.

4. A nurse is preparing to administer medications for a client who is receiving intermittent enteral feedings through a gastrostomy tube. Which of the following actions should the nurse take?

    A. Crush extended release tablets.
    B. Administer sublingual tablets under the tongue.
    C. Flush with 10 mL of warm water when completed.
    D. Add medications to enteral feeding.

APPLICATION EXERCISES ANSWER KEY

1. Place the phases of pharmacokinetics in the correct order:

   2 Distribution

   4 Excretion

   1 Absorption

   3 Metabolism

 NCLEX® Connection: Pharmacological Therapies, Expected Actions/Outcomes

2. Matching: Match the route in column A with the advantage in column B

	ROUTE	ADVANTAGE
B	Oral	A. Provides immediate response
D	Intramuscular	B. Easy to administer
A	IV	C. Allows for medication to be administered at site of action
C	Inhalation	D. Allows for administration of medications poorly soluble in water

 NCLEX® Connection: Pharmacological Therapies, Medication Administration

3. A nurse is administering eye drops to a client. Which of the following actions should the nurse take? (Select all that apply.)

   X **Use sterile technique.**

   X **Ask the client to look up at the ceiling before application.**

   _____ Place the client in a side-lying position.

   _____ Drop the medication into the conjunctival sac at the inner canthus.

   X **Instruct the client to close the eye gently after application.**

   The nurse should use sterile technique, and instruct the client to look up at the ceiling before applying the medication and to close the eye gently afterwards. The medication should be dropped into the center of the conjunctival sac. The client should be sitting or in a supine position to facilitate proper administration of eye drops.

 NCLEX® Connection: Pharmacological Therapies, Medication Administration

4. A nurse is preparing to administer medications for a client who is receiving intermittent enteral feedings through a gastrostomy tube. Which of the following actions should the nurse take?

   A. Crush extended release tablets.

   B. Administer sublingual tablets under the tongue.

   C. Flush with 10 mL of warm water when completed.

   D. Add medications to enteral feeding.

   Sublingual tablets should not be given through a gastrostomy tube, but they can be administered under the tongue. Specially formulated medications, such as extended release tablets, should not be crushed. The tube should be flushed with 30 to 60 mL of warm water after all medications have been given. Medications should not be added to the enteral feeding. This may lead to clogging of the tube, and if the client is unable to tolerate the feeding, the entire dose may not be received.

 NCLEX® Connection: Pharmacological Therapies, Medication Administration

UNIT 1	PHARMACOLOGIC PRINCIPLES
Chapter 2	Safe Medication Administration and Error Reduction

 Overview

- The health care providers that are legally permitted to write prescriptions in the United States include physicians, advanced practice nurses, dentists, and physician assistants. These health care providers are responsible for:

    o Obtaining the client's medical history and physical examination

    o Diagnosing

    o Prescribing medications

    o Monitoring the response to therapy

    o Modifying medication orders as necessary

 - Nurses are legally responsible for:

    o Having knowledge of federal, state (nurse practice act), and local laws, and health care facility policies that govern the prescribing, dispensing, and administration of medications

    o Preparing, administering, and evaluating client responses to medications

    o Developing and maintaining an up-to-date knowledge base of medications administered, including uses, mechanisms of action, routes of administration, safe dosage range, side effects, adverse responses, precautions, and contraindications

    o Maintaining acceptable practice and skill competency

    o Determining accuracy of medication orders

    o Reporting all medication errors

    o Safeguarding and storing medications

Medication Category and Classification

- Nomenclature

  - Chemical name is the name of the medication determined by its chemical composition.

  - Generic name is the official or nonproprietary name that is given by the United States Adopted Names Council. Each medication has only one generic name.

  - Trade name is the brand or proprietary name given by the company that manufacturers the medication. One medication may have multiple trade names.

- Prescription medications are administered under the supervision of providers. These medications can be habit-forming, have potential harmful effects, and/or require supervision.

  - Uncontrolled substances require monitoring by a provider, but do not pose risk of abuse and/or addiction. Antibiotics are an example of uncontrolled prescription medications.

  - Controlled substances have a potential for abuse and dependence and are categorized into schedules. Heroin is a Schedule I medication and has no medical use in the United States. Medications categorized in Schedules II through V all have approved applications. Each level has decreasing risk of abuse and dependence. For example, morphine sulfate (Duramorph) is a Schedule II medication that has a greater risk of abuse and dependence than phenobarbital (Luminal), which is a Schedule IV medication.

KNOWLEDGE REQUIRED PRIOR TO MEDICATION ADMINISTRATION	
Medication category/class	Medications can be organized according to pharmacological action, therapeutic use, body system, chemical makeup, and safe use during pregnancy. • For example, lisinopril (Zestril) is classified as an angiotensin-converting enzyme inhibitor (pharmacological action) and an antihypertensive (therapeutic use).
Mechanism of action	This is how the medication produces the desired therapeutic effect. • For example, glipizide (Glucotrol) is an oral hypoglycemic agent that lowers blood glucose levels primarily by stimulating pancreatic islet cells to release insulin.
Therapeutic effect	This is the preferred and expected effect for which the medication is administered to a specific client. One medication may have more than one therapeutic effect. • For example, one client is administered acetaminophen (Tylenol) to lower a fever, whereas another client may be administered this medication to relieve pain.

KNOWLEDGE REQUIRED PRIOR TO MEDICATION ADMINISTRATION	
Side effects	These are usually expected and inevitable when a medication is given at a therapeutic dose. • For example, morphine sulfate given for pain relief usually results in constipation. Side effects are usually identified according to body system.
Adverse effects	These are undesired, inadvertent, and unexpected dangerous effects of the medication. Adverse effects are usually identified according to body system.
Toxic effects	These are effects that occur from an excessive accumulation of the medication. • For example, clients taking digoxin (Lanoxin) should be monitored closely for dysrhythmias, a sign of cardiotoxicity. Hypokalemia places these clients at greater risk for digoxin toxicity.
Medication interactions	These are desired or undesired effects that occur when two or more medications are given concurrently. • For example, using a beta-adrenergic blocker atenolol (Tenormin) concurrently with the calcium channel blocker nifedipine (Procardia) to prevent reflex tachycardia. Take complete medication history and be knowledgeable of clinically significant interactions.
Precautions/ Contraindications	Situations in which nurses use caution when administering medications. • For example, vancomycin (Vancocin) is excreted unchanged in the kidneys and should be used cautiously in clients with renal impairment. Situations in which nurses should not administer medications. • For example, tetracyclines can stain developing teeth and should not be administered to children under 8 years of age.
Preparation, dosage, administration	It is important to know any special considerations for preparation, recommended dosages, and how to administer the medication. • For example, morphine sulfate is available in 10 formulations. Oral doses of morphine are generally higher than parenteral doses due to extensive first-pass effect. Clients who have chronic, severe pain, as seen with cancer, are generally given oral doses of morphine.
Nursing implications	Know how to monitor therapeutic effects, prevent and treat adverse effects, provide for comfort, and instruct clients in the safe use of medications.

Medication Prescriptions

- Each facility has written policies related to medication orders. Policies include which health care providers can write, receive, and transcribe medication orders.

- Types of medication orders include:

  o Routine order/standard order

    ▪ A routine/standard order is an order that identifies medications that are given on a regular schedule. It may or may not have a termination date. Without a specified termination date, the order will be in effect until the provider discontinues it or the client is discharged.

    ▪ Certain medications, such as opioids and antibiotics, must be reordered within a specified amount of time or will automatically be discontinued.

  o Single/one-time order

    ▪ A single/one-time order is to be given once at a specified time or as soon as possible. For example, a one-time order instructs the nurse to give warfarin (Coumadin) 5 mg PO at 1700.

  o Stat order

    ▪ A stat order is only given once, and it is given immediately. For example, a stat order instructs the nurse to give digoxin 0.125 mg PO stat.

  o PRN order

    ▪ A PRN order stipulates at what dosage, what frequency, and under what conditions a medication can be given. The nurse uses clinical judgment to determine the client's need for the medication. For example, a PRN order instructs the nurse to give morphine 10 mg PO q 3 hr PRN for chest pain.

  o Standing orders

    ▪ Standing orders may be written for specific circumstances and/or for specific units. For example, the critical care unit has standing orders to treat a client with asystole.

- Components of a medication order include:

  o The client's name

  o Date and time of order

  o Name of medication (may be generic or brand)

  o Dosage of medication

  o Route of administration

  o Time and frequency of medication administration – Exact times or number of times per day (dictated by facility policy or specific qualities of the medication).

  o Signature of prescribing provider

- Communicating Medication Prescriptions

  ○ Origination of medication prescriptions

    ■ Medication prescriptions are written on the client's medical record by the provider or a nurse who takes a verbal or telephone prescription from a provider. If the nurse writes a medication prescription on the client's medical record, facility policy specifies how much time the provider has in which to sign the prescription (usually 24 hr). Medication prescriptions are transcribed to the medication administration record (MAR) by a nurse or other health care provider.

  ○ Taking a telephone order:

    ■ If possible, have a second nurse listen on an extension.

    ■ Ensure that the prescription is complete and correct by reading back to the provider: the client's name, the name of the medication, the dosage, the time to be given, frequency, and route.

    ■ Remind the provider that the prescription must be signed within the specified amount of time.

    ■ Write the prescription in the client's medical record.

  ○ Medication reconciliation

    ■ The Joint Commission requires policies and procedures for medication reconciliation. Upon admission to a health care facility, nurses should compile a list of the client's current medications, ensuring that all medications are included, with correct dosages, routes, and frequency. Nurses then compare this list with new prescriptions and resolve any discrepancies. Nurses use this as the client's current medication list. This process should take place on admission, when transferring between units or facilities, and at discharge.

Data Collection Prior to Start of Medication Therapy

- The following information should be obtained prior to the initiation of medication therapy, and updated as necessary.

  ○ Health history

    ■ Age

    ■ Diagnosed health problems and current reason for seeking care

    ■ All medications currently being taken (prescription and nonprescription) – Name, dose, route, and frequency of each medication

    ■ Any symptoms possibly related to medication therapy

    ■ Use of herbal or natural products for medicinal purposes

    ■ Use of caffeine, tobacco, alcohol, and/or street drugs

    ■ Client's understanding of the purpose of the medications

    ■ All known medication and food allergies

- o Physical examination

    - ▪ A systemic physical examination provides a baseline to evaluate therapeutic effects of medication therapy and detect possible side and adverse medication effects.

 Six Rights of Safe Medication Administration

- ● Right Client

    - o Verify the client's identification each time a medication is given. The Joint Commission requires nurses to use two client identifiers when administering medications.

        - ▪ Nurses use facility procedures and policies to identify clients. Acceptable identifiers include the client's name, an assigned identification number, telephone number, birth date, or another person-specific identifier.

- ● Right Medication

    - o Correctly interpret the medication order (verify completeness and clarity).

        - ▪ Read the label three times – When the container is selected, when removing the dose from container, and when the container is replaced.

        - ▪ Leave unit-dose medication in its package until administration.

    - o Check for allergies by asking the client, looking for an allergy bracelet, and reviewing the medication administration record.

- ● Right Dose

    - o Calculate the correct medication dose.

    - o Check a medication reference to ensure the dose is within the usual range.

- ● Right Time

    - o Give medication on time to maintain consistent therapeutic blood level.

        - ▪ It is generally acceptable to give the medication ½ hr before or after the scheduled time. However, refer to the medication reference or facility policy for exceptions. Do not give PRN medications sooner than the interval specified by the provider.

- ● Right Route

    - o Select the correct preparation for the ordered route (for example, otic vs ophthalmic topical ointment or drops).

    - o Know how to administer medication safely and correctly.

- ● Right Documentation

    - o Immediately record pertinent information, including the client's response to the medication.

View Media Supplement: Safe Administration of Medications (Video)

Additional Considerations

- Data Collection

  o Collect appropriate data before administering medication (checking apical heart rate before giving digitalis preparations). Observe clients for physical and psychosocial factors that may affect medication response.

- Education

  o Provide accurate information about the medication therapy and its implications (therapeutic response, side/adverse effects). To individualize the teaching, determine what clients already know about the medication, need to know about the medication, and want to know about the medication.

- Evaluation

  o Determine the effectiveness of the medication based on the client's response, as well as the occurrence of side/adverse effects.

- Medication Refusal

  o Clients have the right to refuse to take a medication. Determine the reason for refusal, provide information regarding the risk of refusal, notify the appropriate provider, and document refusal and actions taken.

- Resources for Medication Information

  o Nursing medication handbooks

  o Pharmacology textbooks

  o Professional journals

  o *Physicians' Desk Reference* (PDR)

  o Professional Web sites

 Medication Error Prevention

- Common medication errors include:

  o Wrong medication or IV fluid

  o Incorrect dose or IV rate

  o Wrong client, route, or time

  o Administering a medication to a client who has a known allergy

  o Omission of dose

  o Incorrect discontinuation of medication or IV fluid

- Use the nursing process to prevent medication errors.
  - Data collection
    - Ensure knowledge of the medication to be administered. Use appropriate resources. They include:
      - Health care providers, including nurses, physicians, and pharmacists
      - Poison control centers
      - Sales representatives from medication companies
      - Nursing pharmacology textbooks and medication handbooks
      - *Physicians' Desk Reference*
      - Newsletters including *The Medical Letter on Drugs and Therapeutics* (bimonthly) and *Prescriber's Letter* (monthly)
      - Professional journals
      - Professional Web sites
    - Obtain information about the client's medical diagnoses and conditions related to medication administration, such as ability to swallow; allergies; and heart, liver, and/or kidney disorders.
      - Identify client allergies.
      - Obtain necessary preadministration data (heart rate, blood pressure).
      - Omit or delay doses as indicated by the client's condition.
    - Determine if the medication prescription is complete – Includes name of client, date and time, name of medication, dosage, route of administration, time, frequency, and signature of prescribing provider.
    - Interpret the medication prescription accurately.
      - The Institute for Safe Medication Practices is a nonprofit organization working to educate health care providers and consumers regarding safe medication practices. Tools have been developed to decrease the risk of medication errors. Go to http://www.ismp.org/ for a complete list.
        - Error-Prone Abbreviation List – Abbreviations that have been associated with a high number of medication errors
        - Confused Medication Name List – Soundalike and lookalike medication names
        - High-Alert Medication List – Medications that, if given in error, have a high risk for resulting in significant patient harm
    - Question the provider if the prescription is unclear or seems inappropriate for the client's condition. Do not give a medication if unsafe. Notify the charge nurse or supervisor.
    - Dosage changes are usually made gradually. Question the provider if abrupt and excessive changes in dosages are made.

- ○ Planning
    - Contribute to the care plan by identifying client outcomes for medication administration and setting priorities.
- ○ Implementation
    - Avoid distractions during medication preparation (poor lighting, ringing phones). Interruptions can increase the risk of error.
    - Check the labels for the medication name and concentration. Read labels carefully. Measure doses accurately and double-check high-alert medications, such as insulin and heparin, with a colleague.
    - Question multiple tablets or vials for a single dose. Doses are usually 1 to 2 tablets or one single-dose vial.
    - Follow the Six Rights of Medication Administration consistently. Take the MAR to the bedside.
    - Do not give medications that were prepared by someone else.
    - Encourage clients to become part of the safety net, teaching them about medications and the importance of proper identification before medications are administered. Omit or delay a dose if clients question the size of a dose or appearance of a medication.
    - Follow correct procedures for all routes of administration.
    - Communicate clearly both verbally and in writing.
    - Use verbal orders only for emergencies and follow facility protocol for telephone orders.
    - Omit or delay doses as indicated by the client's condition, and document and report appropriately.
    - Follow all laws and regulations regarding controlled substances when preparing and administering medications. Keep controlled substances in a locked area. Have a licensed nurse witness when discarding an excess of a controlled substances.
    - Only leave medication at the bedside if allowed by facility policy (topical medication).
- ○ Evaluation
    - Evaluate client response to a medication and document and report appropriately.
    - Recognize side/adverse effects and document and report appropriately.
    - Report all errors and implement corrective measures immediately.
        - □ Complete an unusual occurrence report within the specified time frame, usually 24 hr. This report should include:
            - ▸ The client's identification
            - ▸ The time and place of the incident
            - ▸ An accurate account of the event

- ▸ Who was notified
- ▸ What actions were taken
- ▸ The signature of the person completing the report
- ☐ Do not include this report as a part of the client's permanent record and do not reference the report in another part of the record.

APPLICATION EXERCISES

1. A nurse is preparing a client's medications. Which of the following are the nurse's legal responsibilities? (Select all that apply.)

    _____ Evaluating the client's response to the medication

    _____ Determining the accuracy of the medication order

    _____ Choosing the route the medication should be given

    _____ Storing medications safely

    _____ Deciding the dosage of the medication

2. Match the terms with their definitions.

    _____ Contraindications   A. How the medication produces the desired therapeutic effect

    _____ Toxicity   B. Primary action for which the medication is prescribed

    _____ Mechanism of action   C. Indications for why a medication should not be given

    _____ Therapeutic effect   D. A serious adverse effect usually caused by excessive dosing

3. A health care provider prescribes furosemide (Lasix) 40 mg PO now. The nurse should recognize this as which of the following types of order?

    A. Single order

    B. Stat order

    C. Routine order

    D. Standing order

4. A nurse is preparing to administer a client's morning insulin dosage. Which of the following actions should the nurse take first?

    A. Review the client's blood glucose level.

    B. Verify the client's identity.

    C. Ask another nurse to check the amount of insulin drawn into the syringe.

    D. Wash the injection site with soap and water.

APPLICATION EXERCISES ANSWER KEY

1. A nurse is preparing a client's medications. Which of the following are the nurse's legal responsibilities? (Select all that apply.)

   _X_ **Evaluating the client's response to the medication**
   _X_ **Determining the accuracy of the medication order**
   _____ Choosing the route the medication should be given
   _X_ **Storing medications safely**
   _____ Deciding the dosage of the medication

   The nurse is responsible for evaluating the client's response to the medication, determining the accuracy of the medication order, and storing medications safely. If the nurse is unsure of the order, the prescriber should be contacted to verify all components of the order. The prescribing provider is responsible for choosing the route of medication administration and deciding the dosage to be given. In addition, the nurse should obtain information about the client's medical diagnoses and be familiar with why the medications are being given.

 NCLEX® Connection: Pharmacological Therapies, Medication Administration

2. Match the terms with their definitions.

   _C_ Contraindications | A. How the medication produces the desired therapeutic effect
   _D_ Toxicity | B. Primary action for which the medication is prescribed
   _A_ Mechanism of action | C. Indications for why a medication should not be given
   _B_ Therapeutic effect | D. A serious adverse effect usually caused by excessive dosing

 NCLEX® Connection: Pharmacological Therapies, Adverse Effects/Contraindications/Side Effects/Interactions

3. A health care provider prescribes furosemide (Lasix) 40 mg PO now. The nurse should recognize this as which of the following types of order?

   A. Single order

   B. Stat order

   C. Routine order

   D. Standing order

   A stat order is only given once, and it is given immediately. A single order is to be given once at a specified time or as soon as possible. A routine order identifies a medication that should be given on a regular schedule. This medication should be given every day until discontinued. A standing order is written for specific circumstances or a specific unit.

 NCLEX® Connection: Pharmacological Therapies, Medication Administration

4. A nurse is preparing to administer a client's morning insulin dosage. Which of the following actions should the nurse take first?

   A. Review the client's blood glucose level.

   B. Verify the client's identity.

   C. Ask another nurse to check the amount of insulin drawn into the syringe.

   D. Wash the injection site with soap and water.

   Using the nursing process, the first action the nurse should take is collecting data by reviewing the client's blood glucose level to ensure the client is not hypoglycemic prior to receiving insulin. The nurse should then ask another nurse to check the insulin dosage, verify the client's identity, and wash the injection site with soap and water prior to administering the medication.

    NCLEX® Connection: Pharmacological Therapies, Medication Administration

UNIT 1	PHARMACOLOGIC PRINCIPLES
Chapter 3	Dosage Calculation

 Overview

- Basic medication dose conversion and calculation skills are essential to the provision of safe nursing care.

- Nurses are responsible for administering the correct amount of medication by calculating the appropriate amount of medication to give. Types of calculations required include:

  o Solid oral medication

  o Liquid oral medication

  o Injectable medication

  o Correct dose based on the client's weight

  o IV infusion

- Standard conversion factors are as follows:

  o 1 mg = 1,000 mcg

  o 1 g = 1,000 mg

  o 1 kg = 1,000 g

  o 1 oz = 30 mL

  o 1 L = 1,000 mL

  o 1 tsp = 5 mL

  o 1 tbsp = 15 mL

  o 1 tbsp = 3 tsp

  o 1 kg = 2.2 lb

  o 1 gr = 60 mg

- General Rounding Guidelines

  o If the number to the right of the desired place is equal to or greater than 5, round up by adding 1 to the number in the desired place.

  o If the number to the right of the desired place is less than 5, round down by dropping the number to the right of the desired place.

- ○ For dosages less than 1.0, round to the nearest hundredth.

  - For example: The calculated dose is 0.746 mL. Look at the number in the thousandths place (6). Six is greater than 5. Therefore, to round to the nearest hundredths place, add 1 to 4 and drop the 6. The rounded dose is 0.75 mL.

  - For example: The calculated dose is 0.523. Look at the number in the thousandths place (3). Three is less than 5. Therefore, to round to the nearest hundredths place, drop the 3. The rounded dose is 0.52.

- ○ For dosages greater than 1.0, round to the nearest tenth.

  - For example: The calculated dose is 2.76. Look at the number in the hundredths place (6). Six is greater than 5. Therefore, to round to the nearest tenths place, add 1 to 7 and drop the 6. The rounded dose is 2.8.

  - For example: The calculated dose is 3.72. Look at the number in the hundredths place (2). Two is less than 5. Therefore, to round to the nearest tenths place, drop the 2. The rounded dose is 3.7.

- ○ Follow these examples when rounding to the nearest whole number:

  - For example: The calculated dose is 16.7. Look at the number to the right of the desired place (7). Seven is greater than 5. Therefore, to round to the nearest whole number, add 1 to 6 and drop the 7. The rounded dose is 17.

  - For example: The calculated dose is 15.2. Look at the number to the right of the desired place (2). Two is less than 5. Therefore, to round to the nearest whole number, drop the 2. The rounded dose is 15.

DOSAGE CALCULATIONS USING RATIO AND PROPORTION

- Process for calculating solid, liquid, and injectable dosage using ratio and proportion

  STEP 1: What is the dose needed? Dose needed = Desired

  STEP 2: What is the dose available? Dose available = Have

  STEP 3: Do the units of measurement need to be converted? Convert the unit of measurement of what is desired to the unit of measurement of what is available.

  STEP 4: Determine the quantity of the dose available. This refers to how the medication is provided, such as 2 mL or 3 tablets.

  STEP 5: Set up an equation using knowledge about basic equivalents and solve for X.

  $$\frac{\text{Have}}{\text{Quantity}} = \frac{\text{Desire}}{\text{X}}$$

  STEP 6: Reassess to determine if the amount to be given makes sense.

Solid dosage

 Example: A provider prescribes phenytoin (Dilantin) 0.2 g PO, TID. The amount available is 200 mg/capsule. How many capsules should the nurse give? Round to the nearest whole number.

- Follow the steps:

    STEP 1: What is the dose needed? Dose needed = Desired

    0.2 g

    STEP 2: What is the dose available? Dose available = Have

    200 mg

    STEP 3: Do the units of measurement need to be converted?

    Yes (g ≠ mg)

    Convert the unit of measurement of what is desired to the unit of measurement of what is available.

    Desire: g

    Have: mg

    0.2 g = X mg

    Equivalents:

    1 g = 1,000 mg (1 • 1,000)

    Therefore:

    0.2 g = 200 mg (0.2 • 1,000)

    STEP 4: What is the quantity of the dose available?

    1 capsule

STEP 5: Set up an equation and solve:

$$\frac{\text{Have}}{\text{Quantity}} = \frac{\text{Desire}}{\text{X}}$$

$$\frac{200 \text{ mg}}{1 \text{ capsule}} = \frac{200 \text{ mg}}{\text{X}}$$

Cross multiply and solve for X:

200X = 200

Isolate X by dividing both sides by 200:

$$\frac{200X}{200} = \frac{200}{200}$$

X = 1 capsule

STEP 6: Reassess to determine if the amount to be given makes sense. If there are 200 mg/capsule and the prescribed amount is 0.2 g or 200 mg, it makes sense to give 1 capsule.

The nurse should administer phenytoin 1 capsule PO 3 times per day.

Liquid dosage

Example: A provider prescribes erythromycin (E-Mycin) oral suspension 0.25 g, PO, TID. The amount available is erythromycin oral suspension, 250 mg/mL. How many mL should the nurse administer with each dose? Round to the nearest tenth.

- Follow the steps:

    STEP 1: What is the dose needed? Dose needed = Desired

    0.25 g

    STEP 2: What is the dose available? Dose available = Have

    250 mg

STEP 3: Do the units of measurement need to be converted?

Yes (g ≠ mg)

Convert the unit of measurement of what is desired to the unit of measurement of what is available.

Desire: g

Have: mg

0.25 g = X mg

Equivalents

1 g = 1,000 mg (1 • 1,000)

Therefore:

0.25 g = 250 mg (0.25 • 1,000)

STEP 4: What is the quantity of the dose available?

1 mL

STEP 5: Set up an equation and solve:

$$\frac{\text{Have}}{\text{Quantity}} = \frac{\text{Desire}}{\text{X}}$$

$$\frac{250 \text{ mg}}{1 \text{ mL}} = \frac{250 \text{ mg}}{\text{X}}$$

Cross multiply and solve for X:

250X = 250

Isolate X by dividing both sides by 250:

$$\frac{250X}{250} = \frac{250}{250}$$

X = 1 mL

STEP 6: Reassess to determine if the amount to be given makes sense. If there are 250 mg/mL and the prescribed amount is 0.25 g, it makes sense to give 1 mL.

The nurse should administer erythromycin 1 mL PO 3 times a day.

Injectable Dosage

 Example: A provider prescribes heparin 8,000 units subcutaneously, Q12 hr. The amount available is 5,000 units/mL. How many mL should the nurse administer? Round to the nearest tenth.

- Follow the steps:

    STEP 1: What is the dose needed? Dose needed = Desired

    8,000 units

    STEP 2: What is the dose available? Dose available = Have

    5,000 units

    STEP 3: Do the units of measurement need to be converted?

    No (units = units)

    STEP 4: What is the quantity of the dose available?

    1 mL

    STEP 5: Set up an equation and solve:

    $$\frac{\text{Have}}{\text{Quantity}} = \frac{\text{Desire}}{\text{X}}$$

    $$\frac{5,000 \text{ units}}{1 \text{ mL}} = \frac{8,000 \text{ units}}{\text{X}}$$

Cross multiply and solve for X:

    5,000X = 8,000

Isolate X by dividing both sides by 5,000.

    $$\frac{5,000\text{X}}{5,000} = \frac{8,000}{5,000}$$

    X = 1.6 mL

    STEP 6: Reassess to determine if the amount to be given makes sense. If there are 5,000 units/mL and the prescribed amount is 8,000 units, it makes sense to give 1.6 mL.

The nurse should administer heparin 1.6 mL subcutaneously every 12 hr.

read up

Dosages by Weight

- Process for calculating dosage by weight using ratio and proportion

- Medications may be prescribed in daily amounts per kg of body weight, such as "5 mg/kg/day," which is then divided into doses given throughout the day. Use the same process as calculating oral dosages, but first determine the client's weight in kg, then the total daily dose, and then the amount per dose.

 Example: A provider prescribes cefixime (Suprax) 8 mg/kg/day PO to be given in 2 divided doses. The client weighs 22 lb. The amount available is 100 mg/5 mL suspension. How many mL should the nurse administer per dose? Round to the nearest tenth.

STEP 1: What is the client's weight in kg?

2.2 lb = 1 kg

Client's weight in lb = X kg

Set up an equation:

$$\frac{2.2 \text{ lb}}{1 \text{ kg}} = \frac{\text{Client's weight in lb}}{\text{X kg}}$$

$$\frac{2.2 \text{ lb}}{1 \text{ kg}} = \frac{22 \text{ lb}}{\text{X kg}}$$

Cross multiply and solve for X:

2.2X = 22

X = 10 kg

STEP 2: What is the total daily dose?

Amount prescribed • kg weight (mg • kg) = total daily dose

8 mg/kg • 10 kg = 80 mg

STEP 3: What is the amount per dose?

$$\frac{\text{Total daily dose}}{\text{Number of doses prescribed per day}} = \text{Amount per dose}$$

$$\frac{80 \text{ mg}}{2 \text{ doses}} = 40 \text{ mg/dose}$$

STEP 4: What is the dose needed? Dose needed = Desired

Desired = 40 mg

STEP 5: What is the dose available? Dose available = Have

Have = 100 mg

STEP 6: Do the units of measurement need to be converted?

No (mg = mg)

STEP 7: What is the quantity of the dose available?

Quantity = 5 mL

STEP 8: Set up an equation using knowledge about basic equivalents.

$$\frac{\text{Have}}{\text{Quantity}} = \frac{\text{Desire}}{X}$$

$$\frac{100 \text{ mg}}{5 \text{ mL}} = \frac{40 \text{ mg}}{X}$$

Cross multiply and solve for X:

100X = 200

Isolate X by dividing each side by 100.

$$\frac{100X}{100} = \frac{200}{100}$$

X = 2 mL

STEP 9: Reassess to determine if the amount to be given makes sense. If there are 100 mg/5 mL and the prescribed dose is 40 mg, it makes sense for the nurse to give 2 mL.

The nurse should administer cefixime 2 mL PO with each dose.

IV flow rates

- Calculate IV flow rates for either:

  ○ Electronic IV pumps

    ▪ Flow rates on IV infusion pumps are set in whole mL/hr. The pump regulates the number of gtt/min based on this mL/hr setting.

    ▪ While IV infusion pumps are usually programmed for whole numbers, most pumps are able to accept decimal flow rates. Use of decimal flow rates occurs most often in the critical care setting or for pediatric clients where precise dosing is essential.

- Manual IV infusions
    - Base the flow rate for manual IV infusions on drops per minute.
        - Drops per minute is expressed as gtt/min.
    - Calculate flow rates using "drop factors" found on each manufacturer's IV tubing.
        - The drop factor is the number of drops per mL of liquid that an IV tubing set will drip into its drip chamber. Express drops per mL as gtt/mL.
- Rounding
    - If a calculation results in a remaining decimal, round to the nearest whole number.
        - If the remaining decimal is less than 0.5, round down to the nearest whole number.
            - For example: Round 16.3 mL/hr to 16 mL/hr.
        - If the remaining decimal is 0.5 or greater, round up to the nearest whole number.
            - For example: Round 16.6 mL/hr to 17 mL/hr.
- When the time in hr is known, use the following formula:

$$\frac{\text{Volume (mL)}}{\text{Time (hr)}} = \text{IV flow rate (mL/hr)}$$

Example: A provider prescribes dextrose 5% in water 500 mL IV to infuse over the next 4 hr. The nurse should set the IV infusion pump to deliver how many mL/hr? Round to the nearest whole number.

STEP 1: What is the volume to be infused? Volume to be infused = Volume (mL)

500 mL

STEP 2: What is the time for the infusion? Time of infusion = Time (hr)

4 hr

STEP 3: Set up an equation and solve:

$$\frac{\text{Volume (mL)}}{\text{Time (hr)}} = \text{IV flow rate (mL/hr)}$$

$$\frac{500 \text{ mL}}{4 \text{ hr}} = 125 \text{ mL/hr}$$

STEP 4: Reassess to determine if the IV flow rate makes sense. If 500 mL are to be infused in 4 hr, it makes sense to administer 125 mL/hr.

The nurse should set the IV pump to deliver 125 mL/hr.

- When the time in minutes is known, use ratio and proportion to find the flow rate (mL/hr):

    STEP 1: What is the volume to be infused? Volume to be infused = Volume (mL)

    STEP 2: What is the time for the infusion? Time of infusion = Time (min)

    STEP 3: Set up an equation and solve:

    $$\frac{\text{Volume (mL)}}{\text{Time (min)}} = \frac{\text{X mL}}{60 \text{ min}}$$

    Cross multiply and solve for X:

    Time (min) • X mL = Volume (mL) • 60 min

    STEP 4: Reassess to determine if the IV flow rate makes sense.

 Example: A provider prescribes cefotaxime (Claforan) 1 g by intermittent IV bolus. The amount available is cefotaxime 1 g in 100 mL of 0.9% sodium chloride, to infuse over 45 min. The nurse should set the IV infusion pump to deliver how many mL/hr? Round to the nearest whole number.

- Follow these steps:

    STEP 1: What is the volume to be infused? Volume to be infused = Volume (mL)

    100 mL

    STEP 2: What is the time for the infusion? Time of infusion = Time (min)

    45 min

    STEP 3: Set up an equation and solve:

    $$\frac{\text{Volume (mL)}}{\text{Time (min)}} = \frac{\text{X mL}}{60 \text{ min}}$$

    $$\frac{100 \text{ mL}}{45 \text{ min}} = \frac{\text{X mL}}{60 \text{ min}}$$

    Cross multiply and solve for X:

    45X = 6,000

    X = 133.3 or 133

    STEP 4: Reassess to determine if the IV flow rate makes sense. If 100 mL are to be infused in 45 min, it makes sense to administer 133 mL/hr.

The nurse should set the IV pump to deliver 133 mL/hr.

- Calculate flow rates for manual IV infusions by using this simple formula:

$$\frac{\text{Volume to be infused}}{\text{Time (min)}} \cdot \text{Drop factor (gtt/mL)} = \text{IV flow rate (gtt/min)}$$

STEP 1: What is the volume to be infused? Volume to be infused = Volume (mL)

STEP 2: What is the time for the infusion? Time of infusion = Time (min)

Convert hr to min:

$$\frac{1 \text{ hr}}{60 \text{ min}} = \frac{\text{Prescribed hr}}{\text{X min}}$$

STEP 3: What is the drop factor on the IV tubing?

STEP 4: Set up an equation and solve:

$$\frac{\text{Volume to be infused}}{\text{Time (min)}} \cdot \text{Drop factor (gtt/mL)} = \text{IV flow rate (gtt/min)}$$

STEP 5: Reassess to determine if the IV flow rate makes sense.

 Example: A provider prescribes lactated Ringer's IV 250 mL to infuse at 75 mL/hr. The drop factor on the manual IV tubing is 20 gtt/mL. The nurse should set the IV flow rate to deliver how many gtt/min? Round to the nearest whole number.

- Follow these steps:

STEP 1: What is the volume to be infused? Volume to be infused = Volume (mL)

75 mL

STEP 2: What is the time for the infusion? Time of infusion = Time (min)

Convert hr to min:

$$\frac{1 \text{ hr}}{60 \text{ min}} = \frac{\text{Prescribed hr}}{\text{X min}}$$

1 hr = 60 min

STEP 3: What is the drop factor on the IV tubing?

20 gtt/mL

STEP 4: Set up an equation.

$$\frac{\text{Volume to be infused}}{\text{Time (min)}} \cdot \text{Drop factor (gtt/mL)} = \text{IV flow rate (gtt/min)}$$

$$\frac{75 \text{ mL}}{60 \text{ min}} \cdot 20 \text{ gtt/mL} = \frac{1,500 \text{ gtt}}{60 \text{ min}} = 25 \text{ gtt/min}$$

STEP 5: Reassess to determine if the IV flow rate makes sense.

The nurse should set the manual IV flow rate at 25 gtt/min.

 Example: A provider prescribes ranitidine (Zantac) 150 mg by intermittent IV bolus. The amount available is ranitidine 150 mg dextrose 5% in water 100 mL to infuse over 30 min. The drop factor on the manual IV tubing is 10 gtt/mL. The nurse should set the IV flow rate to deliver how many gtt/min? Round to the nearest whole number.

- Follow these steps:

    STEP 1: What is the volume to be infused? Volume to be infused = Volume (mL)

    100 mL

    STEP 2: What is the time for the infusion? Time of infusion = Time (min)

    30 min

    STEP 3: What is the drop factor on the IV tubing?

    10 gtt/mL

    STEP 4: Set up an equation.

$$\frac{\text{Volume to be infused}}{\text{Time (min)}} \cdot \text{Drop factor (gtt/mL)} = \text{IV flow rate (gtt/min)}$$

$$\frac{100 \text{ mL}}{30 \text{ min}} \cdot 10 \text{ gtt/mL} = \frac{1,000 \text{ gtt}}{30 \text{ min}} = 33.3 \text{ or } 33 \text{ gtt/min}$$

    STEP 5: Reassess to determine if the IV flow rate makes sense.

The nurse should set the manual IV flow rate at 33 gtt/min.

DOSAGE CALCULATIONS USING THE DESIRED OVER HAVE METHOD

- Process of calculating solid, liquid, and injectable dosage using the desired over have method

    STEP 1: What is the dose needed? Dose needed = Desired

    STEP 2: What is the dose available? Dose available = Have

STEP 3: Do the units of measurement need to be converted? Convert the unit of measurement of what is desired to the unit of measurement of what is available.

STEP 4: Determine the quantity of the dose available. Quantity of the available dose refers to how the medication is provided, such as 2 mL or 3 tablets.

STEP 5: Set up an equation and solve:

$$\frac{\text{Desired} \cdot \text{Quantity}}{\text{Have}} = \text{Amount to be given}$$

STEP 6: Reassess to determine if the amount to be given makes sense.

Solid Dosages

 Example: A provider prescribes phenytoin (Dilantin) 0.2 g PO, TID. The amount available is 200 mg/capsule. How many capsules should the nurse give? Round to the nearest whole number.

- Follow the steps:

    STEP 1: What is the dose needed? Dose needed = Desired

    0.2 g

    STEP 2: What is the dose available? Dose available = Have

    200 mg

    STEP 3: Do the units of measurement need to be converted?

    Yes (g ≠ mg)

    Convert the unit of measurement of what is desired to the unit of measurement of what is available.

    Desire: g

    Have: mg

    0.2 g = X mg

    Equivalents:

    1 g = 1,000 mg (1 • 1,000)

    Therefore:

    0.2 g = 200 mg (0.2 • 1,000)

    STEP 4: What is the quantity of the dose available?

    1 capsule

STEP 5: Set up an equation and solve:

$$\frac{\text{Desired} \cdot \text{Quantity}}{\text{Have}} = \text{Amount to be given}$$

$$\frac{200 \text{ mg} \cdot 1 \text{ capsule}}{200 \text{ mg}} = \text{X capsules}$$

$$\frac{200 \cdot 1}{200} = \frac{200}{200} = \text{X capsules}$$

X = 1 capsule

STEP 6: Reassess to determine if the amount to be given makes sense. If there are 200 mg/capsule and the prescribed amount is 0.2 g or 200 mg, it makes sense to give 1 capsule.

The nurse should administer phenytoin 1 capsule PO 3 times per day.

Liquid dosage

Example: A provider prescribes erythromycin (E-Mycin) oral suspension 0.25 g, PO, TID. The amount available is erythromycin oral suspension, 250 mg/mL. How many mL should the nurse administer with each dose? Round to the nearest tenth.

- Follow these steps

  STEP 1: What is the dose needed? Dose needed = Desired

  0.25 g

  STEP 2: What is the dose available? Dose available = Have

  250 mg

  STEP 3: Do the units of measurement need to be converted?

  Yes (g ≠ mg)

  Convert the unit of measurement of what is desired to the unit of measurement of what is available.

  Desire: g

  Have: mg

  0.25 g = X mg

  Equivalents

  1 g = 1,000 mg (1 · 1,000)

Therefore:

0.25 g = 250 mg (0.25 • 1,000)

STEP 4: What is the quantity of the dose available?

1 mL

STEP 5: Set up an equation and solve:

$$\frac{\text{Desired} \bullet \text{Quantity}}{\text{Have}} = \text{Amount to be given}$$

$$\frac{250 \text{ mg} \bullet 1 \text{ mL}}{250 \text{ mg}} = X \text{ mL}$$

$$\frac{250 \bullet 1}{250} = \frac{250}{250} = X \text{ mL}$$

X = 1 mL

STEP 6: Reassess to determine if the amount to be given makes sense. If there are 250 mg/mL and the prescribed amount is 250 mg, it makes sense to give 1 mL.

The nurse should administer erythromycin 1 mL PO 3 times a day.

Injectable Dosage

 Example: A provider prescribes heparin 8,000 units subcutaneously, every 12 hr. The amount available is 5,000 units/mL. How many mL should the nurse administer? Round to the nearest tenth.

- Follow the steps:

    STEP 1: What is the dose needed? Dose needed = Desired

    8,000 units

    STEP 2: What is the dose available? Dose available = Have

    5,000 units

    STEP 3: Do the units of measurement need to be converted?

    No (units = units)

    STEP 4: What is the quantity of the dose available?

    1 mL

STEP 5: Set up an equation and solve:

$$\frac{\text{Desired} \cdot \text{Quantity}}{\text{Have}} = \text{Amount to be given}$$

$$\frac{8,000 \text{ units} \cdot 1 \text{ mL}}{5,000 \text{ units}} = X \text{ mL}$$

$$\frac{8,000 \cdot 1}{5,000} = \frac{8,000}{5,000} = X \text{ mL}$$

$$X = 1.6 \text{ mL}$$

STEP 6: Reassess to determine if the amount to be given makes sense. If there are 5,000 units/mL and the prescribed amount is 8,000 units, it makes sense to give 1.6 mL.

The nurse should administer heparin 1.6 mL subcutaneously every 12 hr.

Dosages by Weight

- Process for calculating dosage by weight using the desired over have method

  o Medications may be prescribed in daily amounts per kg of body weight, such as "5 mg/kg/day," which is then divided into doses given throughout the day. Use the same process as calculating oral dosages, but first determine the client's weight in kg, then the total daily dose, and then the amount per dose.

 Example: A provider prescribes cefixime (Suprax) 8 mg/kg/day PO to be given in 2 divided doses. The client weighs 22 lb. The amount available is 100 mg/5 mL suspension. How many mL should the nurse administer per dose? Round to the nearest tenth.

STEP 1: What is the client's weight in kg?

2.2 lb = 1 kg

Client's weight in lb = X kg

Set up an equation:

$$\frac{2.2 \text{ lb}}{1 \text{ kg}} = \frac{\text{Client's weight in lb}}{X \text{ kg}}$$

$$\frac{2.2 \text{ lb}}{1 \text{ kg}} = \frac{22 \text{ lb}}{X}$$

Cross multiply and solve for X:

2.2X = 22

X = 10 kg

STEP 2: What is the total daily dose?

Amount prescribed • kg weight (mg • kg) = total daily dose

8 mg/kg • 10 kg = 80 mg

STEP 3: What is the amount per dose?

$$\frac{\text{Total daily dose}}{\text{Number of doses prescribed per day}} = \text{Amount per dose}$$

$$\frac{80 \text{ mg}}{2 \text{ doses}} = 40 \text{ mg/dose}$$

STEP 4: What is the dose needed? Dose needed = Desired

Desired = 40 mg

STEP 5: What is the dose available? Dose available = Have

Have = 100 mg

STEP 6: Do the units of measurement need to be converted?

No (mg = mg)

STEP 7: What is the quantity of the dose available?

Quantity = 5 mL

STEP 8: Set up an equation:

$$\frac{\text{Desired} \cdot \text{Quantity}}{\text{Have}} = \text{Amount to be given}$$

$$\frac{40 \text{ mg} \cdot 5 \text{ mL}}{100 \text{ mg}} = X \text{ mL}$$

$$\frac{40 \cdot 5}{100 \text{ mg}} = X \text{ mL}$$

$$\frac{40 \cdot 5}{100} = \frac{200}{100} = X \text{ mL}$$

X = 2 mL

STEP 9: Reassess to determine if the amount to be given makes sense. If there are 100 mg/5 mL and the prescribed dose is 40 mg, it makes sense for the nurse to give 2 mL.

The nurse should administer cefixime 2 mL PO with each dose.

DOSAGE CALCULATIONS USING DIMENSIONAL ANALYSIS

- Dimensional analysis is a method of calculation in which a series of ratios or factors, organized in the form of fractions, are multiplied.

  - Factors are two quantities that are related, such as 30 mg in 2 mL.

  - Express factors as fractions.

  - Express 30 mg in 2 mL as:

$$\frac{30 \text{ mg}}{2 \text{ mL}} \text{ or } \frac{2 \text{ mL}}{30 \text{ mg}}$$

- Convert one unit of measurement to another unit of measurement by means of conversion factors or unit equivalence. A conversion factor is a unit equivalence, such as 2.2 lb = 1 kg or 1,000 mcg = 1 mg.

  - Conversion factors link units of measurement of what is desired with units of measurement of what is available.

  - Arrange conversion factors in the form of a fraction.

  - 1,000 mcg = 1 mg can be expressed as:

$$\frac{1,000 \text{ mcg}}{1 \text{ mg}} \text{ or } \frac{1 \text{ mg}}{1,000 \text{ mcg}}$$

- To create an equation using dimensional analysis:

  - Start with the unit of measurement that is to be calculated:

    - For example, when converting mcg to mg, mg are desired, start with:

      mg =

  - Find the quantity with the same unit of measurement or the conversion factor with the same unit of measurement as what is desired (1 mg = 1,000 mcg) and place this (mg) in the numerator.

$$mg = \frac{1 \text{ mg}}{1,000 \text{ mcg}}$$

    - Remember, fractions are set up as the numerator over the denominator:

      $$\frac{\text{numerator}}{\text{denominator}}$$

    o   The fractions are arranged so that unwanted units cancel out and desired units remain.

        ■   Arrange single quantity not associated with a related quantity as a fraction by placing it in the numerator and placing 1 in the denominator.

$$\frac{X \text{ mcg}}{1}$$

    o   If mcg are available and mg are desired, arrange the conversion factor so that mcg may be canceled out to leave mg remaining:

$$mg = \frac{1 \text{ mg}}{1,000 \text{ mcg}} \cdot \frac{X \text{ mcg}}{1}$$

Cross out the identical units that are across and diagonal:

$$mg = \frac{1 \text{ mg}}{1,000 \, \cancel{\text{mcg}}} \cdot \frac{X \, \cancel{\text{mcg}}}{1}$$

    o   When using dimensional analysis, multiply fractions. To multiply fractions, first multiply across the numerator, and then multiply across the denominator. Finally, divide the numerator by the denominator.

    o   Arrange equations involving multiple factors so that the unit of measurement in the denominator of one factor is placed in the numerator of the following factor and so on. Cancel unwanted units.

        ■   Remember:

            □   Express a single quantity not associated with a related quantity as a fraction by placing it in the numerator and placing 1 in the denominator.

            □   Factors are two quantities that are related. Arrange related quantities as fractions.

●   Process of calculating dosage using dimensional analysis:

    STEP 1: What is to be calculated?

        What is the unit of measurement that is to be calculated?

    STEP 2: What quantities are needed? Needed – desired

        The quantity needed may be the prescribed dosage.

    STEP 3: What quantities are available? Available = have

    STEP 4: Are conversion factors needed to find the units that are to be calculated?

        Conversion factors link units of measurement of what is available with units of measurement of what is to be calculated.

    STEP 5: Set up an equation of factors using needed and available quantities and the conversion factors.

STEP 6: Multiply the numerator.

Multiply the denominator.

Divide the numerator by the denominator.

STEP 7: Reassess to determine if the amount makes sense.

Solid dosages

 Example: A provider prescribes phenytoin (Dilantin) 0.2 g PO, TID. The amount available is 200 mg/capsule. How many capsules should the nurse give? Round to the nearest whole number.

- Follow the steps:

  STEP 1: What is to be calculated?

  What is the unit of measurement that is to be calculated?

  capsule

  STEP 2: What quantities are needed? Needed = desired

  The quantity needed may be the prescribed dosage.

  0.2 g/1

  STEP 3: What quantities are available? Available = have

  200 mg/capsule

  STEP 4: Are conversion factors needed to find what is desired?

  Conversion factors link units of measurement of what is available with units of measurement of what is desired.

  1,000 mg = 1 g

  STEP 5: Set up an equation of factors using needed and available quantities and the conversion factors.

  $$\text{capsule} = \frac{1 \text{ capsule}}{200 \text{ mg}} \cdot \frac{1{,}000 \text{ mg}}{1 \text{ g}} \cdot \frac{0.2 \text{ g}}{1}$$

  Cancel out identical units:

  $$\text{capsule} = \frac{1 \text{ capsule}}{200 \, \cancel{\text{mg}}} \cdot \frac{1{,}000 \, \cancel{\text{mg}}}{1 \, \cancel{\text{g}}} \cdot \frac{0.2 \, \cancel{\text{g}}}{1}$$

STEP 6: Multiply the numerator.

Multiply the denominator.

Divide the numerator by the denominator.

$$\text{capsule} = \frac{200 \text{ capsule}}{200} = 1 \text{ capsule}$$

STEP 7: Reassess to determine if the amount to be given makes sense. If there are 200 mg/capsule and the prescribed amount is 0.2 g or 200 mg, it makes sense to give 1 capsule.

The nurse should administer phenytoin 1 capsule PO 3 times per day.

Liquid dosage

 Example: A provider prescribes erythromycin (E-Mycin) oral suspension 0.25 g, PO, TID. The amount available is erythromycin oral suspension, 250 mg/mL. How many mL should the nurse administer with each dose? Round to the nearest tenth.

- Follow the steps:

STEP 1: What is to be calculated?

What is the unit of measurement that is to be calculated?

mL

STEP 2: What quantities are needed? Needed = desired

The quantity needed may be the prescribed dosage.

0.25g/1

STEP 3: What quantities are available? Available = have

250 mg/mL

STEP 4: Are conversion factors needed to find what is desired?

Conversion factors link units of measurement of what is available with units of measurement of what is desired.

1 g = 1,000 mg

STEP 5: Set up an equation of factors using needed and available quantities and the conversion factors.

$$mL = \frac{1\ mL}{250\ mg} \cdot \frac{1{,}000\ mg}{1\ g} \cdot \frac{0.25\ g}{1}$$

Cancel out identical units:

$$mL = \frac{1\ mL}{250\ \cancel{mg}} \cdot \frac{1{,}000\ \cancel{mg}}{1\ \cancel{g}} \cdot \frac{0.25\ \cancel{g}}{1}$$

STEP 6: Multiply the numerator.

Multiply the denominator.

Divide the numerator by the denominator.

$$mL = \frac{250\ mL}{250} = 1\ mL$$

STEP 7: Reassess to determine if the amount to be given makes sense. If there are 250 mg/mL and the prescribed amount is 250 mg, it makes sense to give 1 mL.

The nurse should administer erythromycin 1 mL PO 3 times a day.

Injectable Dosage

 Example: A provider prescribes heparin 8,000 units subcutaneously, every 12 hr. The amount available is 5,000 units/mL. How many mL should the nurse administer? Round to the nearest tenth.

- Follow the steps:

    STEP 1: What is to be calculated?

    What is the unit of measurement that is to be calculated?

    mL

    STEP 2: What quantities are needed? Needed = desired

    The quantity needed may be the prescribed dosage.

    8,000 units/1

    STEP 3: What quantities are available? Available = have

    5,000 units /mL

STEP 4: Are conversion factors needed to find what is desired?

Conversion factors link units of measurement of what is available with units of measurement of what is desired.

No

STEP 5: Set up an equation of factors using needed and available quantities and the conversion factors.

$$mL = \frac{1\ mL}{5{,}000\ units} \cdot \frac{8{,}000\ units}{1}$$

Cancel out identical units:

$$mL = \frac{1\ mL}{5{,}000\ \cancel{units}} \cdot \frac{8{,}000\ \cancel{units}}{1}$$

STEP 6: Multiply the numerator.

Multiply the denominator.

Divide the numerator by the denominator.

$$mL = \frac{8{,}000\ mL}{5{,}000} = 1.6\ mL$$

STEP 7: Reassess to determine if the amount to be given makes sense. If there are 5,000 units in 1 mL and the prescribed amount is 8,000 units, it makes sense to give 1.6 mL.

The nurse should administer heparin 1.6 mL subcutaneously every 12 hr.

Dosages by Weight

- Process for calculating dosage by weight using dimensional analysis

    o Medications may be prescribed in daily amounts per kg of body weight, such as "5 mg/kg/day," which is then divided into doses given throughout the day. Use the same process as for calculating oral dosages.

 Example: A provider prescribes cefixime (Suprax) 8 mg/kg/day PO to be given in 2 divided doses. The client weighs 22 lb. The amount available is 100 mg/5 mL suspension. How many mL should the nurse administer per dose? Round to the nearest tenth.

- Follow these steps:

    STEP 1: What is to be calculated?

    What is the unit of measurement that is to be calculated?

    mL/dose

STEP 2: What quantities are needed? Needed = desired

The quantity needed may be the prescribed dosage.

8 mg/kg/day

STEP 3: What quantities are available? Available = have

2 doses/day

22 lb/1

100 mg/5 mL

STEP 4: Are conversion factors needed to find the units that are wanted?

Conversion factors link units of measurement of what is available with units of measurement of what is to be calculated.

2.2 lb = 1 kg

STEP 5: Set up an equation of factors using needed and available quantities and the conversion factors.

$$mL/dose = \frac{5\ mL}{100\ mg} \cdot \frac{8\ mg}{kg/day} \cdot \frac{1\ kg}{2.2\ lb} \cdot \frac{22\ lb}{1} \cdot \frac{1\ day}{2\ doses}$$

Cancel out identical units:

$$mL/dose = \frac{5\ mL}{100\ \cancel{mg}} \cdot \frac{8\ \cancel{mg}}{\cancel{kg/day}} \cdot \frac{1\ kg}{2.2\ \cancel{lb}} \cdot \frac{22\ \cancel{lb}}{1} \cdot \frac{1\ \cancel{day}}{2\ doses}$$

STEP 6: Multiply the numerator.

Multiply the denominator.

Divide the numerator by the denominator.

$$mL/dose = \frac{5\ mL \cdot 8 \cdot 22}{100 \cdot 2.2 \cdot 2\ dose} \cdot \frac{880\ mL}{440\ dose} = 2\ mL/dose$$

STEP 7: Reassess to determine if the amount to be given makes sense.

The nurse should administer cefixime 2 mL PO with each dose.

IV Flow Rates

- To determine mL/hr when administering fluid via an IV pump, the process is the same as the ratio and proportion/desired over have methods.

- When calculating gtt/min, follow these steps:

    STEP 1: What is to be calculated?

    What is the unit of measurement that is to be calculated?

    gtt/min

    STEP 2: What quantities are needed? Needed = desired

    The quantity needed may be the prescribed dosage.

    Volume (mL)/infusion time (min or hr)

    STEP 3: What quantities are available? Available = have

    Drop factor (gtt/mL)

    STEP 4: Are conversion factors needed to find what is desired?

    Conversion factors link units of measurement of what is available with units of measurement of what is desired.

    60 min = 1 hr

    STEP 5: Set up an equation of factors using needed and available quantities and the conversion factors.

- If minutes are available, the process is the same as the ratio and proportion/desired over have methods.

- If hours are available:

$$\text{IV flow rate (gtt/min)} \ = \ \frac{\text{gtt}}{\text{mL}} \cdot \frac{\text{Volume (mL)}}{\text{Time (hr)}} \cdot \frac{\text{1 hr}}{\text{60 min}}$$

    Cancel out identical units:

$$\text{IV flow rate (gtt/min)} \ = \ \frac{\text{gtt}}{\cancel{\text{mL}}} \cdot \frac{\text{Volume (}\cancel{\text{mL}}\text{)}}{\text{Time (}\cancel{\text{hr}}\text{)}} \cdot \frac{\text{1 }\cancel{\text{hr}}}{\text{60 min}}$$

STEP 6: Multiply the numerator.

Multiply the denominator.

Divide the numerator by the denominator.

STEP 7: Reassess to determine if the amount makes sense.

 Example: A provider prescribes lactated Ringer's 250 mL to infuse at 75 mL/hr. The drop factor on the manual IV tubing is 20 gtt/mL. The nurse should set the IV flow rate to deliver how many gtt/min? Round to the nearest whole number.

STEP 1: What is to be calculated?

What is the unit of measurement that is to be calculated?

gtt/min

STEP 2: What quantities are needed? Needed = desired

The quantity needed may be the prescribed dosage.

75 mL/hr

STEP 3: What quantities are available? Available = have

20 gtt/mL

STEP 4: Are conversion factors needed to find what is desired?

Conversion factors link units of measurement of what is available with units of measurement of what is desired.

60 min = 1 hr

STEP 5: Set up an equation of factors using needed and available quantities and the conversion factors.

o   Hours are available:

$$\text{IV flow rate (gtt/min)} = \frac{20 \text{ gtt}}{1 \text{ mL}} \cdot \frac{75 \text{ mL}}{1 \text{ hr}} \cdot \frac{1 \text{ hr}}{60 \text{ min}}$$

Cancel out identical units:

$$\text{IV flow rate (gtt/min)} = \frac{20 \text{ gtt}}{1 \text{ mL}} \cdot \frac{75 \text{ mL}}{1 \text{ hr}} \cdot \frac{1 \text{ hr}}{60 \text{ min}}$$

STEP 6: Multiply the numerator.

Multiply the denominator.

Divide the numerator by the denominator.

$$\text{IV flow rate (gtt/min)} = \frac{1,500 \text{ gtt}}{60 \text{ min}} = 25 \text{ gtt/min}$$

STEP 7: Reassess to determine if the amount makes sense.

The nurse should set the manual IV flow rate at 25 gtt/min.

APPLICATION EXERCISES

Directions: Solve each problem using ratio and proportion.

1. A provider prescribes phenytoin 5 mg/kg/day PO to be given in 2 divided doses. The client weighs 33 lb. The amount available is phenytoin 125 mg/5 mL. How many mL should the nurse administer per dose? Round to the nearest tenth.

2. A provider prescribes heparin 9,000 units subcutaneous Q12 hr. The amount available is 5,000 units/mL. How many mL should the nurse administer Q12 hr? Round to the nearest tenth.

3. A provider prescribes 0.9% sodium chloride 1 L IV to infuse at 100 mL/hr. The drop factor on the manual IV tubing is 15 gtt/mL. The nurse should set the IV flow rate to deliver how many gtt/min? Round to the nearest whole number.

Directions: Solve each problem using the desired over have method.

4. A provider prescribes furosemide (Lasix) oral solution 40 mg PO daily. The amount available is furosemide 10 mg/mL. How many mL should the nurse administer? Round to the nearest whole number.

5. A provider prescribes dextrose 5% in water 500 mL IV to infuse over 4 hr. The nurse should set the IV pump to deliver how many mL/hr? Round to the nearest whole number.

Directions: Solve each problem using dimensional analysis.

6. A provider prescribes haloperidol (Haldol) 3 mg, PO TID. The amount available is 2 mg/tablet. How many tablets should the nurse administer with each dose? Round to the nearest tenth.

7. A provider prescribes amoxicillin (Amoxil) 30 mg/kg/day PO to be given in 3 divided doses. The client weighs 44 lb. The amount available is amoxicillin 250 mg/5 mL. How many mL should the nurse administer per dose? Round to the nearest tenth.

APPLICATION EXERCISES ANSWER KEY

Directions: Solve each problem using ratio and proportion.

1. A provider prescribes phenytoin 5 mg/kg/day PO to be given in 2 divided doses. The client weighs 33 lb. The amount available is phenytoin 125 mg/5 mL. How many mL should the nurse administer per dose? Round to the nearest tenth.

   STEP 1: What is the client's weight in kg?

$$\frac{2.2\ lb}{1\ kg} = \frac{Client\ weight\ in\ lb}{X\ kg}$$

$$\frac{2.2\ lb}{1\ kg} = \frac{33\ lb}{X\ kg}$$

   Cross multiply and solve for X:

   X = 15 kg

   STEP 2: What is the total daily dose?

   5 mg x 15 kg = 75 mg

   STEP 3: What is the amount per dose?

   75 mg ÷ 2 doses = 37.5 mg

   STEP 4: What is the dose needed? Dose needed = Desired

   37.5 mg

   STEP 5: What is the dose available? Dose available = Have

   125 mg

   STEP 6: Do the units of measurement need to be converted?

   No (mg = mg)

   STEP 7: What is the quantity of the dose available?

   5 mL

STEP 8: Set up an equation and solve:

$$\frac{\text{Have}}{\text{Quantity}} = \frac{\text{Desire}}{X}$$

$$\frac{125 \text{ mg}}{5 \text{ mL}} = \frac{37.5 \text{ mg}}{X}$$

Cross multiply and solve for X:

$125X = 187.5$

Isolate X by dividing both sides by 125.

$$\frac{125X}{125} = \frac{187.5}{125}$$

$X = 1.5 \text{ mL}$

STEP 9: Reassess to determine if the amount to be given makes sense. If there are 125 mg in 5 mL and the prescribed dose is 37.5 mg, it makes sense to give 1.5 mL.

The nurse should administer phenytoin 1.5 mL PO per dose.

 NCLEX® Connection: Pharmacological Therapies, Parenteral/Intravenous Therapy

2. A provider prescribes heparin 9,000 units subcutaneous Q12 hr. The amount available is 5,000 units/mL. How many mL should the nurse administer Q12 hr? Round to the nearest tenth.

STEP 1: What is the dose needed? Dose needed = Desired

9,000 units

STEP 2: What is the dose available? Dose available = Have

5,000 units

STEP 3: Do the units of measurement need to be converted?

No (units = units)

STEP 4: What is the quantity of the dose available?

1 mL

STEP 5: Set up an equation and solve.

$$\frac{\text{Have}}{\text{Quantity}} = \frac{\text{Desire}}{X}$$

$$\frac{5{,}000 \text{ units}}{1 \text{ mL}} = \frac{9{,}000 \text{ units}}{X \text{ mL}}$$

Cross multiply and solve for X:

$5{,}000X = 9{,}000$

Isolate X by dividing both sides by 5,000.

$$\frac{5{,}000X}{5{,}000} = \frac{9{,}000}{5{,}000}$$

Simplify:

$$\frac{9}{5} = X \text{ mL}$$

$X = 1.8 \text{ mL}$

STEP 6: Reassess to determine if the amount to be given makes sense. If there are 5,000 units in 1 mL and the prescribed amount is 9,000 units, it makes sense to give 1.8 mL.

The nurse should administer 1.8 mL heparin subcutaneously every 12 hr.

 NCLEX® Connection: Pharmacological Therapies, Parenteral/Intravenous Therapy

3. A provider prescribes 0.9% sodium chloride 1 L IV to infuse at 100 mL/hr. The drop factor on the manual IV tubing is 15 gtt/mL. The nurse should set the IV flow rate to deliver how many gtt/min? Round to the nearest whole number.

STEP 1: What is the volume to be infused? Volume to be infused = Volume (mL)

100 mL

STEP 2: What is the time for the infusion? Time of infusion = Time (min)

Convert hr to min:

$$\frac{60 \text{ min}}{1 \text{ hr}} = \frac{X \text{ min}}{\text{prescribed hr}}$$

60 min = 1 hr

STEP 3: What is the drop factor on the IV tubing?

15 gtt/mL

STEP 4: Set up an equation.

$$\frac{\text{Volume to be infused}}{\text{Time (min)}} \cdot \text{Drop factor (gtt/mL)} = \text{IV flow rate (gtt/min)}$$

$$\frac{100 \text{ mL}}{60 \text{ min}} \cdot 15 \text{ gtt/mL} = \frac{1,500 \text{ gtt}}{60 \text{ min}} = 25 \text{ gtt/min}$$

STEP 5: Reassess to determine if the IV flow rate makes sense.

The nurse should set the manual IV flow rate at 25 gtt/min.

 NCLEX® Connection: Pharmacological Therapies, Parenteral/Intravenous Therapy

Directions: Solve each problem using the desired over have method.

4. A provider prescribes furosemide (Lasix) oral solution 40 mg PO daily. The amount available is furosemide 10 mg/mL. How many mL should the nurse administer? Round to the nearest whole number.

STEP 1: What is the dose needed? Dose needed = Desired

40 mg

STEP 2: What is the dose available? Dose available = Have

10 mg

STEP 3: Do the units of measurement need to be converted?

No (mg = mg)

STEP 4: What is the quantity of the dose available?

1 mL

STEP 5: Set up an equation and solve:

$$\frac{\text{Desired} \cdot \text{Quantity}}{\text{Have}} = \text{Amount to be given}$$

$$\frac{40 \text{ mg} \cdot 1 \text{ mL}}{10 \text{ mg}} = \text{X mL}$$

$$\frac{40 \cdot 1}{10} = \frac{40}{10} = \text{X mL}$$

X = 4 mL

STEP 6: Reassess to determine if the amount to be given makes sense. If there are 10 mg/mL and the prescribed amount is 40 mg, it makes sense to give 4 mL.

The nurse should administer furosemide 4 mL PO daily.

 NCLEX® Connection: Pharmacological Therapies, Dosage Calculation

5. A provider prescribes dextrose 5% in water 500 mL IV to infuse over 4 hr. The nurse should set the IV pump to deliver how many mL/hr? Round to the nearest whole number.

STEP 1: What is the volume to be infused? Volume to be infused = Volume (mL)

500 mL

STEP 2: What is the time for the infusion? Time of infusion = Time (hr)

4 hr

STEP 3: Set up an equation and solve:

$$\frac{\text{Volume (mL)}}{\text{Time (hr)}} = \text{IV flow rate (mL/hr)}$$

$$\frac{500 \text{ mL}}{4 \text{ hr}} = 125 \text{ mL/hr}$$

STEP 4: Reassess to determine if the IV flow rate makes sense. If 500 mL are to be infused in 4 hr, it makes sense to administer 125 mL/hr.

The nurse should set the IV pump to deliver 125 mL/hr.

 NCLEX® Connection: Pharmacological Therapies, Dosage Calculation

Directions: Solve each problem using dimensional analysis.

6. A provider prescribes haloperidol (Haldol) 3 mg, PO TID. The amount available is 2 mg/tablet. How many tablets should the nurse administer with each dose? Round to the nearest tenth.

STEP 1: What is to be calculated?

What is the unit of measurement that is to be calculated?

tablets

STEP 2: What quantities are needed? Needed = desired

The quantity needed may be the prescribed dosage.

3 mg/1

STEP 3: What quantities are available? Available = have

2 mg/tablet

STEP 4: Are conversion factors needed to find what is desired?

Conversion factors link units of measurement of what is available with units of measurement of what is desired.

No

STEP 5: Set up an equation of factors using needed and available quantities and the conversion factors.

$$\text{tablet} = \frac{1 \text{ tablet}}{2 \text{ mg}} \cdot \frac{3 \text{ mg}}{1}$$

Cancel out identical units:

$$\text{tablet} = \frac{1 \text{ tablet}}{2 \text{ mg}} \cdot \frac{3 \text{ mg}}{1}$$

STEP 6: Multiply the numerator.

Multiply the denominator.

Divide the numerator by the denominator.

$$\text{tablet} = \frac{1 \cdot 3}{2} = 1.5 \text{ tablets}$$

STEP 7: Reassess to determine if the amount to be given makes sense. If there are 2 mg/tablet and the prescribed amount is 3 mg, it makes sense to give 1.5 tablets.

The nurse should administer haloperidol 1.5 tablets PO 2 times per day.

 NCLEX® Connection: Pharmacological Therapies, Dosage Calculation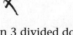

7. A provider prescribes amoxicillin (Amoxil) 30 mg/kg/day PO to be given in 3 divided doses. The client weighs 44 lb. The amount available is amoxicillin 250 mg/5 mL. How many mL should the nurse administer per dose? Round to the nearest tenth.

STEP 1: What is to be calculated?

What is the unit of measurement that is to be calculated?

mL/dose

STEP 2: What quantities are needed? Needed = desired

The quantity needed may be the prescribed dosage.

30 mg/kg/day

STEP 3: What quantities are available? Available = have

3 doses/day

44 lb/1

250 mg/5 mL

STEP 4: Are conversion factors needed to find what is desired?

Conversion factors link units of measurement of what is available with units of measurement of what is desired.

2.2 lb = 1 kg

STEP 5: Set up an equation of factors using needed and available quantities and the conversion factors.

$$\text{mL/dose} = \frac{5\ \text{mL}}{250\ \text{mg}} \cdot \frac{30\ \text{mg}}{\text{kg/day}} \cdot \frac{1\ \text{kg}}{2.2\ \text{lb}} \cdot \frac{44\ \text{lb}}{1} \cdot \frac{1\ \text{day}}{3\ \text{doses}}$$

Cancel out identical units:

$$\text{mL/dose} = \frac{5\ \text{mL}}{250\ \cancel{\text{mg}}} \cdot \frac{30\ \cancel{\text{mg}}}{\cancel{\text{kg/day}}} \cdot \frac{1\ \cancel{\text{kg}}}{2.2\ \cancel{\text{lb}}} \cdot \frac{44\ \cancel{\text{lb}}}{1} \cdot \frac{1\ \cancel{\text{day}}}{3\text{doses}}$$

STEP 6: Multiply the numerator.

Multiply the denominator.

Divide the numerator by the denominator.

$$\text{mL/dose} = \frac{5\ \text{mL} \cdot 30 \cdot 44}{250 \cdot 2.2 \cdot 3 \cdot \text{dose}} \cdot \frac{6,600\ \text{mL}}{1,650\ \text{dose}} = 4\ \text{mL/dose}$$

STEP 7: Reassess to determine if the amount to be given makes sense.

The nurse should administer amoxicillin 4 mL PO with each dose.

 NCLEX® Connection: Pharmacological Therapies, Dosage Calculation

| UNIT 1 | PHARMACOLOGIC PRINCIPLES |
| Chapter 4 | Intravenous Therapy |

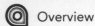 Overview

- IV therapy involves administering fluids via an IV catheter for the purpose of providing medications, supplementing fluid intake, or giving fluid replacement, electrolytes, or nutrients.

- Large-volume IV infusions are administered as continuous infusions.

- An IV medication may be mixed in a large volume of fluid and given as a continuous IV infusion, mixed in a small amount of solution and given intermittently (intermittent IV bolus), or given in a small amount of solution, concentrated or diluted, and injected over a short time (1 to 2 min) (IV bolus dose).

Indications and Risk Factors

- Advantages and Disadvantages of IV Therapy

ADVANTAGES	DISADVANTAGES
• Fast absorption and onset of action • Less discomfort after initial insertion • Maintains constant therapeutic blood levels • Less irritation to subcutaneous and muscle tissue	• Circulatory fluid overload is possible if the infusion is large and/or too rapid. • Immediate absorption leaves no time to correct errors. • IV administration can cause irritation to the lining of the vein. • Failure to maintain surgical asepsis can lead to local infection and septicemia.

Description of Procedure

- The provider prescribes the type of IV fluid, volume to be infused, and either the rate at which the IV fluid should be infused or the total amount of time it should take for the fluid to be infused. The nurse regulates the IV infusion to ensure the appropriate amount is administered. This can be done with an IV pump or manually.

- Large-volume IV infusions are administered on a continuous basis, such as 0.9% sodium chloride IV to infuse at 100 mL/hr or 0.9% sodium chloride 1,000 mL to be given IV over 3 hr.

- A fluid bolus is a large amount of IV fluid given in a short period of time, usually less than an hour. It is given to rapidly replace fluid loss that could be caused by dehydration, shock, hemorrhage, burns, or trauma.

  o Use a large-gauge angiocatheter (18 gauge or larger) to maintain the rapid rate necessary to give a fluid bolus to an adult.

- Methods to administer IV medication infusions:

  o Mix medication in a large volume of fluid (500 to 1,000 mL) and administer as continuous IV infusion. Administer potassium chloride this way.

  o Use premixed solution bags or solutions that have been prepared by the pharmacist.

  o Intermittent IV bolus administration

    ■ Some medications, such as antibiotics, are given intermittently in a small amount of solution (25 to 250 mL) through a continuous IV system, or with saline or heparin lock systems.

    ■ The medications infuse for short periods of time and are given on a scheduled basis.

    ■ These infusions can be administered by a piggyback IV bag or bottle or tandem setup, volume-control administration set, or mini-infusion pump.

  o IV bolus dose administration

    ■ The medications are typically in small amounts of solution, concentrated or diluted, that can be injected over a short time (1 to 2 min) in emergent and nonemergent situations.

    ■ Some medications, such as pain medications, are given directly into the peripheral IV or access port to achieve an immediate medication level in the bloodstream.

    ■ Make sure medications are prepared according to recommended concentration and administered according to the safe recommended rate.

    ■ Use extreme caution and observe for signs and symptoms of complications (redness, burning, or increasing pain).

- Types of IV Access

  o IV access can be via a peripheral or central vein (central venous access device).

  o Central venous access devices can be peripherally inserted or directly inserted into the jugular or subclavian vein.

Guidelines for Safe IV Medication Administration

- Certain medications, such as potassium chloride, can cause serious adverse reactions and should be infused with an IV pump for accurate dosage control and never given by IV bolus.

- Add medication to a new IV fluid container, not to an IV container that is already hanging.

- Never administer IV medication through tubing that is infusing blood, blood products, or parenteral nutritional solutions.

- Verify compatibility of medications before infusing a medication through tubing that is infusing another medication.

- Needlestick Prevention

  o Be familiar with IV insertion equipment.

  o Avoid using needles when needleless systems are available.

  o Use protective safety devices when available.

  o Dispose of needles immediately in designated puncture-resistant receptacles.

  o Do not break, bend, or recap needles.

- Special Considerations

  o Older adult clients, clients taking anticoagulants, or clients with fragile veins:

    ▪ Avoid tourniquets.

    ▪ Use a blood pressure cuff instead.

    ▪ Do not slap the extremity to visualize veins.

  o Edema in extremities:

    ▪ Apply digital pressure over the selected vein to displace edema.

    ▪ Apply pressure with an alcohol pad.

    ▪ Perform cannulation quickly.

  o Obese clients may require the use of anatomical landmarks to find veins.

- Preventing IV Infections

  o Use standard precautions.

  o Have IV sites changed according to facility/agency policy (usually 72 hr).

  o Remove catheters as soon as they are no longer clinically indicated.

  o Use a sterile needle/catheter for each insertion attempt.

  o Avoid writing on IV bags with pens or markers, because ink could contaminate the solution.

  o Change tubing immediately if contamination is known or suspected.

  o Fluids should not hang more than 24 hr unless it is a closed system (pressure bags for hemodynamic monitoring).

  o Wipe all ports with alcohol or an antiseptic swab before connecting IV lines or inserting a syringe to prevent the introduction of micro-organisms into the system.

  o Never disconnect tubing for convenience or to position the client.

  o Do not allow ports to remain exposed to air.

  o Perform hand hygiene before and after handling the IV system.

Preprocedure

- Equipment
  - Correct size catheter:
    - 16 gauge for trauma clients, rapid fluid volume
    - 18 gauge for surgical clients, rapid blood administration
    - 22 to 24 gauge all other clients (adults)
  - Correct tubing
  - Infusion pump, if indicated
  - Clean gloves
  - Scissors or electric shaver for hair removal
  - Tourniquet or blood pressure cuff
  - IV dressing supplies
- Nursing Actions
  - Check the provider's order (solution, rate).
  - Check clients for allergies to products used in initiating and maintaining IV therapy (latex, tape, iodine).
  - Follow the Six Rights of medication administration (including compatibilities of all IV solutions).
  - Perform hand hygiene.
  - Examine the solution to be infused for clarity, leaks, and expiration date.
  - Prime tubing as indicated.
  - Don clean gloves before insertion.
  - Observe extremities and veins. If hair removal is needed, clip it with scissors or shave it with an electric shaver.
- Client Education
  - Identify clients and explain the procedure
  - Place clients in a comfortable position.

Intraprocedure

- Nursing Actions
  - Use a clean tourniquet or blood pressure cuff (especially for older adults), 10.16 to 15.24 cm (4 to 6 in) above the selected site to compress only venous blood flow.

- ○ Select vein by choosing:
  - ▪ Distal veins first on the nondominant hand
  - ▪ A site that is not painful or bruised and will not interfere with activity
  - ▪ A vein that is resilient with a soft, bouncy feeling
  - ▪ Additional methods to enhance venous access include:
    - ▫ Gravity, fist clenching, friction with alcohol, and heat
    - ▫ Percussion with gentle tapping
  - ▪ Avoid:
    - ▫ Varicosed veins that are permanently dilated and tortuous
    - ▫ Veins in the inner wrist with bifurcations, in flexion areas, near valves (appearing as bumps), in lower extremities, and in the antecubital fossa (except for emergency access)
    - ▫ Veins that are sclerosed or hard
    - ▫ Veins in an extremity with impaired sensitivity (scar tissue, paralysis), lymph nodes removed, recent infiltration, or arteriovenous fistula/graft
- ○ Untie the tourniquet or deflate the BP cuff.
- ○ Cleanse the area at the site using friction in a circular motion from the middle and outward with alcohol, iodine preparation, or chlorhexidine. Allow to air dry for 1 to 2 min.
- ○ Remove cover from catheter, grasp plastic hub, and examine device for smooth edges.
- ○ Retie the tourniquet, or reinflate the BP cuff.
- ○ Anchor the vein below the site of insertion.
- ○ Pull skin taut and hold it.
- ○ Warn clients of a sharp, quick stick.
- ○ Insert the catheter into the skin with bevel up at an angle of 10 to 30° using steady, smooth motion.
- ○ Advance the catheter through the skin and into the vein, maintaining a 10 to 30° angle. Flashback of blood will confirm placement in vein.
- ○ Lower the hub of the catheter close to the skin to prepare for threading into the vein, approximately 0.64 cm (0.25 in).
- ○ Loosen the needle from the catheter and pull back slightly on the needle so that it no longer extends past the tip of the catheter.
- ○ Use the thumb and index finger to advance the catheter into the vein until the hub rests against the insertion site.
- ○ Stabilize the IV catheter with one hand and release the tourniquet, or deflate the BP cuff, with the other.

- o Apply pressure approximately 3 cm (1.25 in) above the insertion site with the middle finger and stabilize the catheter with the index finger.

- o Remove the needle and activate the safety device.

- o Maintain pressure above the IV site and connect the appropriate equipment to the hub of the IV catheter.

- o Apply dressing per facility protocol. The dressing is usually left in place until the catheter is removed, unless it becomes damp, loose, or soiled.

- o Avoid encircling the entire extremity with tape, and taping under the sterile dressing.

- o If continuous IV infusion is prescribed, regulate IV infusion rate according to the provider's order.

- o Dispose of used equipment properly.

- o Document in chart:

  - ■ Date and time of insertion

  - ■ Insertion site and appearance

  - ■ Catheter size

  - ■ Type of dressing

  - ■ IV fluid and rate (if applicable)

  - ■ Number, locations, and conditions of site-attempted cannulations

  - ■ Client response

  - ■ Sample documentation: 1/1/2011, 1635, #22-gauge IV catheter inserted into left wrist cephalic vein (1 attempt) with sterile occlusive dressing applied. IV D$_5$LR infusing at 100 mL/hr per infusion pump without redness or edema at the site. Tolerated without complications. J. Doe, RN

Postprocedure

- • Nursing Actions

  - o Maintaining patency of IV access

    - ■ Do not stop a continuous infusion or allow blood to back up into the catheter for any length of time. Clots can form at the tip of the needle or catheter and can be lodged against the vein wall, blocking the flow of fluid.

    - ■ Instruct clients not to manipulate flow rate device, change settings on IV pump, or lie on the tubing.

    - ■ Make sure the IV insertion site dressing is not too tight.

    - ■ Flush intermittent IV catheters with appropriate solution after every medication administration or every 8 to 12 hr when not in use.

    - ■ Monitor site and infusion rate at least every hour.

- ○ Discontinuing IV therapy
  - Check order/prepare equipment.
  - Perform hand hygiene.
  - Don clean gloves.
  - Remove tape and dressing, stabilizing IV catheter.
  - Clamp IV tubing.
  - Apply sterile gauze pad over the site without putting pressure on the vein. Do not use alcohol.
  - Using the other hand, withdraw the catheter by pulling straight back from the site.
  - Elevate and apply pressure for 2 min.
  - Observe the site.
  - Apply tape over gauze.
  - Use pressure dressing, if needed.
  - Observe the catheter for intactness.
  - Document.

Complications

- Complications require notification of the provider and complete documentation. Remove IV catheter and restart with new tubing and catheter.

COMPLICATIONS	FINDINGS	TREATMENT	PREVENTION
Infiltration	Pallor, local swelling at the site, decreased skin temperature around the site, damp dressing, slowed infusion	• Stop the infusion and remove the catheter. • Elevate the extremity. • Encourage active range of motion. • Apply warm compresses three to four times/day. • Restart the infusion proximal to the site or in another extremity.	• Carefully select site and catheter. • Secure the catheter.

COMPLICATIONS	FINDINGS	TREATMENT	PREVENTION
Phlebitis/ thrombophlebitis	Edema; throbbing, burning, or pain at the site; increased skin temperature; erythema; a red line up the arm with a palpable band at the vein site; slowed infusion	• Promptly discontinue the infusion and remove the catheter. • Elevate the extremity. • Apply warm compresses three to four times/day. • Restart the infusion proximal to the site or in another extremity. • Culture the site and catheter if drainage is present.	• Ensure sites are rotated at least every 72 hr. • Avoid the lower extremities. • Use hand hygiene. • Use surgical aseptic technique.
Hematoma	Ecchymosis at site	• Do not apply alcohol. • Apply pressure after IV catheter removal. • Use warm compress and elevation after bleeding stops.	• Minimize tourniquet time. • Remove the tourniquet before starting IV infusion. • Maintain pressure after IV catheter removal.
Cellulitis	Pain; warmth; edema; induration; red streaking; fever, chills, and malaise	• Promptly discontinue the infusion and remove catheter. • Elevate the extremity. • Apply warm compresses three to four times/day. • Culture the site and cannula if drainage is present. • Administer ○ Antibiotics ○ Analgesics ○ Antipyretics	• Ensure sites are rotated at least every 72 hr. • Avoid the lower extremities. • Use hand hygiene. • Use surgical aseptic technique.

COMPLICATIONS	FINDINGS	TREATMENT	PREVENTION
Fluid overload	Distended neck veins; increased blood pressure; tachycardia; shortness of breath; crackles in the lungs; edema	• Stop infusion. • Raise the head of the bed. • Check vital signs. • Adjust rate as prescribed. • Administer diuretics if prescribed.	• Use an infusion pump. • Monitor I&O.
Catheter embolus	Missing catheter tip when discontinued; severe pain at the site with migration, or no symptoms if no migration	• Place the tourniquet high on the extremity to limit venous flow. • Prepare for removal under x-ray or via surgery. • Save the catheter after removal to determine the cause.	• Do not reinsert the stylet into the catheter.

Ⓐ APPLICATION EXERCISES

1. A nurse is caring for a client with a continuous IV infusion. Which of the following findings indicates the IV site is infiltrated? (Select all that apply.)

   _____ Damp dressing

   _____ A decreased rate of infusion

   _____ Palpable, hard mass or band above the insertion site

   _____ Cool, pale skin surrounding the insertion site

   _____ Ecchymosis at insertion site

2. A nurse is caring for a client receiving dextrose 5% in water IV at 100 mL/hr. Which of the following may indicate fluid overload?

   A. Decreased blood pressure

   B. Bradycardia

   C. Flattened neck veins

   D. Crackles heard in lungs

3. A nurse is preparing to discontinue a saline lock after checking the provider's order and performing hygiene. Place the next steps in the correct order:

   _____ Elevate and apply pressure for 2 min.

   _____ Remove tape and dressing, stabilizing IV catheter.

   _____ Use nondominant hand to apply sterile gauze pad over site without putting pressure on vein.

   _____ Assess site.

   _____ Document.

   _____ Don clean gloves.

   _____ Use dominant hand to withdraw catheter by pulling straight back from the site.

   _____ Assess catheter for intactness.

   _____ Apply tape over gauze.

4. The nurse checks for patency of an IV saline lock by

   A. assessing the site for redness.

   B. flushing the IV saline lock with 0.9% sodium chloride.

   C. asking the client if the site is painful.

   D. checking the date of insertion.

APPLICATION EXERCISES ANSWER KEY

1. A nurse is caring for a client with a continuous IV infusion. Which of the following findings indicates the IV site is infiltrated? (Select all that apply.)

   <u> X </u> **Damp dressing**

   <u> X </u> **A decreased rate of infusion**

   <u>   </u> Palpable, hard mass or band above the insertion site

   <u> X </u> **Cool, pale skin surrounding the insertion site**

   <u>   </u> Ecchymosis at insertion site

   A damp dressing, decreased rate of infusion, and cool, pale skin surrounding the insertion site are findings consistent with an IV infiltration. A palpable, hardened band above the insertion site and ecchymosis at the insertion site are findings consistent with phlebitis.

 NCLEX® Connection: Pharmacological Therapies, Parenteral/Intravenous Therapy

2. A nurse is caring for a client receiving dextrose 5% in water IV at 100 mL/hr. Which of the following may indicate fluid overload?

   A. Decreased blood pressure

   B. Bradycardia

   C. Flattened neck veins

   D. Crackles heard in lungs

   Findings of fluid overload include: increased blood pressure, tachycardia, crackles heard in the lungs, and distended neck veins.

 NCLEX® Connection: Pharmacological Therapies, Adverse Effects/Contraindications/Side Effects/Interactions

3. A nurse is preparing to discontinue a saline lock after checking the provider's order and performing hygiene. Place the next steps in the correct order:

   <u> 6 </u> Elevate and apply pressure for 2 min.

   <u> 2 </u> Remove tape and dressing, stabilizing IV catheter.

   <u> 3 </u> Use nondominant hand to apply sterile gauze pad over site without putting pressure on vein.

   <u> 7 </u> Assess site.

   <u> 9 </u> Document.

   <u> 1 </u> Don clean gloves.

   <u> 4 </u> Use dominant hand to withdraw catheter by pulling straight back from the site.

   <u> 5 </u> Assess catheter for intactness.

   <u> 8 </u> Apply tape over gauze.

 NCLEX® Connection: Pharmacological Therapies, Parenteral/Intravenous Therapy

4. The nurse checks for patency of an IV saline lock by

    A. assessing the site for redness.

    B. flushing the IV saline lock with 0.9% sodium chloride.

    C. asking the client if the site is painful.

    D. checking the date of insertion.

Free flow of solution through the IV indicates patency. Absence of redness and reports of pain are not positive indicators of IV patency. The date of insertion will identify when the IV catheter should be changed, but will not determine if it is still patent.

 NCLEX® Connection: Pharmacological Therapies, Parenteral/Intravenous Therapy

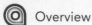

UNIT 1   PHARMACOLOGIC PRINCIPLES

Chapter 5   Adverse Effects, Interactions, and Contraindications

Overview

- To ensure safe medication administration and to prevent errors, nurses must know why a medication is prescribed and its intended therapeutic effect. In addition, nurses must be aware of potential side/adverse effects, interactions, contraindications, and precautions.

- Every medication has the potential to cause side effects and/or adverse effects. Side effects are usually expected when a medication is given at a therapeutic dose. Adverse effects are undesired, inadvertent, and unexpected dangerous effects of the medication. Adverse effects can occur at both therapeutic and higher than therapeutic doses.

- Medications are chemicals that affect the body. When more than one medication is given, there is a potential for an interaction. In addition, medications can interact with foods.

- Contraindications and precautions of specific medications refer to client conditions that make it unsafe or potentially harmful to administer these medications.

Side/Adverse Medication Effects

- These effects can be classified according to body systems.

SIDE/ADVERSE MEDICATION EFFECTS	NURSING INTERVENTIONS/CLIENT EDUCATION
Central nervous system (CNS) effects may result from either CNS stimulation (excitement) or CNS depression.	• If CNS stimulation is expected, clients may be at risk for seizures, and precautions should be taken. • If CNS depression is likely, advise clients not to drive or participate in other activities that can be dangerous.
Extrapyramidal symptoms (EPS) (abnormal body movements) can include involuntary fine motor tremors, rigidity, uncontrollable restlessness, and acute dystonias (spastic movements and/or muscle rigidity affecting the head, neck, eyes, facial area, and limbs). These may occur within a few hours or may take months to develop.	• EPS are more often associated with medications affecting the CNS, such as those used to treat mental health disorders. • Instruct clients to report symptoms to provider.

SIDE/ADVERSE MEDICATION EFFECTS	NURSING INTERVENTIONS/CLIENT EDUCATION
Anticholinergic effects are side effects that are a result of muscarinic receptor blockade. Most effects are seen in the eyes, smooth muscle, exocrine glands, and the heart.	• Advise clients to relieve dry mouth by sipping on liquids; manage photophobia by use of sunglasses; and reduce urinary retention by urinating before taking the medication.
Cardiovascular effects can involve blood vessels and the heart.	• For example, antihypertensives can cause orthostatic hypotension. • Instruct clients about signs of orthostatic hypotension (lightheadedness, dizziness). Advise clients to change positions slowly, and if feeling light-headed or dizzy, to sit or lie down. Orthostatic hypotension can be minimized by getting up and changing position slowly.
Gastrointestinal (GI) effects can result from local irritation of the GI tract. Stimulation of the vomiting center also results in adverse effects.	• NSAIDs can cause GI upset. Advise clients to take these medications with food.
Hematologic effects are relatively common and potentially life-threatening with some groups of medications.	• Bone marrow depression/suppression is generally associated with anticancer medications and hemorrhagic disorders with anticoagulants and thrombolytics. Educate clients about signs and symptoms of bleeding (bruising, discolored urine/stool, petechiae, bleeding gums). Tell clients to notify the provider if these effects occur.
Hepatotoxicity can occur with many medications. Because most medications are metabolized in the liver, the liver is particularly vulnerable to drug-induced injury. Damage to liver cells can impair metabolism of many medications, causing medication accumulation in the body and producing adverse effects. Many medications can alter normal values of liver function tests with no obvious clinical signs of liver dysfunction.	• When two or more medications that are hepatotoxic are combined, the risk for liver damage is increased. • Clients starting a medication known to be hepatotoxic should have baseline liver function tests performed and periodically thereafter.
Nephrotoxicity can occur with a number of medications, but is primarily the result of certain antimicrobial agents and NSAIDs. Damage to the kidneys can interfere with medication excretion leading to medication accumulation and adverse effects.	• Aminoglycosides can cause renal damage. Monitor serum creatinine and BUN levels of clients taking an aminoglycoside.

SIDE/ADVERSE MEDICATION EFFECTS	NURSING INTERVENTIONS/CLIENT EDUCATION
Toxicity is an adverse medication effect that is considered severe and can be life-threatening. It can be caused by an excessive dose, but can also occur at therapeutic dose levels.	• Liver damage will occur with an acetaminophen (Tylenol) overdose. There is a greater risk of liver damage with chronic alcohol use. Use the antidote acetylcysteine (Mucomyst) to minimize liver damage.
Allergic reactions occur when an individual develops an immune response to a medication. The individual has been previously exposed to the medication and has developed antibodies. Allergic reactions range from minor to serious.	• Treat rashes and hives with diphenhydramine (Benadryl). • Before administering any medications, take a complete medication history.
Anaphylactic reaction is a life-threatening, immediate allergic reaction that causes respiratory distress, severe bronchospasm, and cardiovascular collapse.	• Treat with epinephrine, bronchodilators, and antihistamines. Provide respiratory support and inform the provider.
Immunosuppression is decreased or absent immune response.	• Glucocorticoids depress the immune response and increase the risk for infection. • Monitor clients taking a glucocorticoid for signs and symptoms of infection.

Drug-Drug Interactions

CONSEQUENCES OF DRUG-DRUG INTERACTIONS	
TYPE OF INTERACTION	EXAMPLES/NURSING IMPLICATIONS
Increase therapeutic effects	• Some medications can be given together to increase therapeutic effects. Instruct clients who have asthma to use albuterol (Proventil), a beta-adrenergic agonist inhaler, 5 min prior to using triamcinolone acetonide (Azmacort), a glucocorticoid inhaler, to increase the absorption of triamcinolone acetonide.
Increase side/adverse effects	• Clients may take two medications that have the same side/adverse effect. Taking these two medications together increases the risk of these effects. Diazepam (Valium) and hydrocodone 5 mg/acetaminophen 500 mg (Vicodin) both have CNS depressant effects. When these medications are used together, the client has an increased risk for CNS depression.
Decrease therapeutic effects	• One medication can increase the metabolism of a second medication, and therefore decrease the serum level and effectiveness of the second medication. Phenytoin (Dilantin) increases hepatic medication-metabolizing enzymes that affect warfarin (Coumadin), and thereby decreases the serum level and the effect of warfarin.

CONSEQUENCES OF DRUG-DRUG INTERACTIONS	
TYPE OF INTERACTION	EXAMPLES/NURSING IMPLICATIONS
Decrease side/ adverse effects	• One medication can be given to counteract the side/adverse effects of another medication. Administer ondansetron (Zofran), an antiemetic, to counteract the side effects of nausea and vomiting for a client receiving chemotherapy.
Increase serum levels, leading to toxicity	• One medication can decrease the metabolism of a second medication, and therefore increase the serum level of the second medication. This can lead to toxicity. Fluconazole (Diflucan) inhibits hepatic medication-metabolizing enzymes that affect aripiprazole (Abilify), and thereby increases serum levels of this medication.

OVER-THE-COUNTER (OTC) MEDICATIONS	
INTERACTIONS	NURSING INTERVENTIONS/CLIENT EDUCATION
Ingredients in OTC medications can interact with other OTC or prescription medications.	• Obtain a complete medication history. • Instruct clients to follow the manufacturer's recommendation for dosage.
Inactive ingredients such as dyes, alcohol, or preservatives can cause adverse reactions.	
Potential for overdose exists because of the use of several preparations (including prescription medications) with similar ingredients.	
Interactions of certain prescription and OTC medications can interfere with therapeutic effects.	• Advise clients to use caution and to check with their provider before using any OTC preparations such as antacids, laxatives, decongestants, or cough syrups.

Medication-Food Interactions

- Food can alter medication absorption and/or can contain substances that react with certain medications.

- Examples include:

  o Consuming foods with tyramine while taking monoamine oxidase inhibitors (MAOIs) can lead to hypertensive crisis. Clients taking MAOIs should be aware of such foods and avoid them.

  o Vitamin K can decrease the therapeutic effects of warfarin (Coumadin) and place clients at risk for developing blood clots. Clients taking warfarin should consume a consistent amount of vitamin K in their diet.

  o Tetracycline can interact with a chelating agent such as milk, and form an insoluble, unabsorbable compound. Instruct clients not to take tetracycline within 2 hr of consuming any dairy products.

    ○   Grapefruit juice seems to act by inhibiting presystemic medication metabolism in the small bowel, thus increasing absorption of certain oral medications. The risk of toxicity to these medications is increased by consuming grapefruit juice. Instruct clients not to drink grapefruit juice if they are taking such a medication.

Ⓢ Contraindications and Precautions

- A specific medication can be contraindicated for a client based on the client's condition. For example, penicillins are contraindicated for clients who have an allergy to this medication.

- Take precautions for clients who are more likely to have an adverse reaction than other clients. Morphine depresses respiratory function, so use with caution for clients who have asthma or impaired respiratory function.

- The U.S. Food and Drug Administration places medications in categories based on risk to a fetus.

    ○   Category A – There is no evidence of risk to fetus during pregnancy based on adequate and well-controlled studies.

    ○   Category B – There is no evidence of risk to animal fetus based on studies, but there are no adequate and well-controlled studies in pregnant women.

    ○   Category C – Adverse effects have been demonstrated on animal fetuses. There are no adequate and well-controlled studies in pregnant women, but use of the medication during pregnancy may be warranted based on the potential benefits.

    ○   Category D – Adverse effects have been demonstrated on human fetuses based on data from investigational or marketing experience, but use of the medication during pregnancy may be warranted based on the potential benefits.

    ○   Category X – Adverse effects have been demonstrated on animal and human fetuses based on studies and data from investigational or marketing experience. The use of the medication is contraindicated during pregnancy because the risks outweigh the potential benefits.

APPLICATION EXERCISES

1. A nurse is obtaining a medication history from a client who is to start a new prescription for warfarin (Coumadin). Which of the following over-the-counter medications should the nurse instruct the client to avoid?

    A. Ranitidine (Zantac)

    B. Docusate sodium (Colace)

    C. Acetaminophen

    D. Aspirin

2. A nurse is ready to administer the first dose of a new oral penicillin prescription to a client. The client states she took penicillin 3 years ago and developed a rash. What action should the nurse take?

3. A nursing responsibility for a client receiving an antihypertensive medication is to

    A. decrease the dose if the client experiences tachycardia.

    B. teach the client to change positions slowly to avoid dizziness or fainting.

    C. instruct the client to check his blood pressure every 8 hr.

    D. discontinue the client's medication if blood pressure decreases.

4. Do drug-drug interactions produce increased or decreased medication effects? Explain.

APPLICATION EXERCISES ANSWER KEY

1. A nurse is obtaining a medication history from a client who is to start a new prescription for warfarin (Coumadin). Which of the following over-the-counter medications should the nurse instruct the client to avoid?

    A. Ranitidine (Zantac)

    B. Docusate sodium (Colace)

    C. Acetaminophen

    D. Aspirin

    Aspirin decreases platelet aggregation. Warfarin suppresses coagulation. Concurrent use increases the risk for bleeding. Therefore, instruct the client to avoid aspirin use. There are no contraindications for taking ranitidine, docusate sodium, or acetaminophen concurrently with warfarin.

     NCLEX® Connection: Pharmacological Therapies, Adverse Effects/Contraindications/Side Effects/Interactions

2. A nurse is ready to administer the first dose of a new oral penicillin prescription to a client. The client states she took penicillin 3 years ago and developed a rash. What action should the nurse take?

    The nurse should withhold the medication and notify the provider of the client's previous reaction. The client was exposed to penicillin 3 years ago and is now sensitized to the medication. Re-exposure to this medication can cause an allergic reaction, ranging from mild to life-threatening. Therefore, it is important for the provider to be informed of the client's prior sensitization. The provider may choose to use a different medication.

     NCLEX® Connection: Pharmacological Therapies, Adverse Effects/Contraindications/Side Effects/Interactions

3. A nursing responsibility for a client receiving an antihypertensive medication is to

    A. decrease the dose if the client experiences tachycardia.

    B. teach the client to change positions slowly to avoid dizziness or fainting.

    C. instruct the client to check his blood pressure every 8 hr.

    D. discontinue the client's medication if blood pressure decreases.

    Orthostatic hypotension is a common side effect of antihypertensives. By changing positions slowly, it allows the body to adjust to the change and prevents dizziness or fainting. It is not within the scope of practice for the nurse to change the dose or discontinue the medication. It is not necessary for the client to check his blood pressure every 8 hr.

     NCLEX® Connection: Pharmacological Therapies, Medication Administration

4. Do drug-drug interactions produce increased or decreased medication effects? Explain.

   Drug-drug interactions can produce increased or decreased medication effects. These effects can be beneficial or detrimental to the client.

 NCLEX® Connection: Pharmacological Therapies, Adverse Effects/Contraindications/Side Effects/Interactions

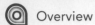

| UNIT 1 | PHARMACOLOGIC PRINCIPLES |
| Chapter 6 | Individual Considerations of Medication Administration |

 Overview

- Various factors may affect how clients respond to medications. It is important for nurses to recognize these factors in order to individualize nursing care when administering medications.

Factors Affecting Medication Dosages and Responses

- Body weight – Because medications are absorbed and distributed in body tissue, individuals with a greater body mass may require larger doses.

- Age – Young children with immature liver and kidney function, and older adults, often with reduced liver and kidney function, may require proportionately smaller medication doses.

- Gender – Females may respond differently to medications than males due to a higher proportion of body fat and the effects of female hormones.

- Genetics – Genetic factors such as missing enzymes can alter the metabolism of certain medications, thus enhancing or reducing medication action.

- Biorhythmic cycles – Responses to certain medications vary with the biologic rhythms of the body. For example, hypnotic medications work better when given at the usual sleep time than at other times.

- Tolerance – Reduced responsiveness to a medication may be either congenital (genetic factors) or acquired (stimulation of liver enzymes or other physiologic variations). Cross-tolerance may occur with other chemically similar medications.

- Accumulation – Medication concentration in the body can be increased by the inability to metabolize or excrete a medication rapidly enough, resulting in a toxic medication effect. For older adults, decreased renal function is the major cause of medication accumulation leading to toxicity.

- Psychological factors – Emotional state and expectations can influence the effects of a medication. Positive medication effects influenced by psychological factors result in the placebo effect.

- Medical Disorders

    o Inadequate gastric acid inhibits the absorption of medications that require an acid medium to dissolve.

    o Diarrhea causes oral medications to pass too quickly through the gastrointestinal (GI) tract to be absorbed.

    o Vascular insufficiency prevents distribution of a medication to affected tissue.

    o Liver disease/failure impairs medication metabolism, which may cause toxicity.

    o Kidney disease/failure prevents or delays medication excretion, which may cause toxicity.

Pharmacology and Children

- While most medications administered to adults are useful for children, the dosages are different. Pediatric dosages are based on body weight or body surface area (BSA). Neonates (less than 1 month old) and infants (1 month to 1 year old) have immature liver and kidney function, alkaline gastric juices, and an immature blood-brain barrier.

- Additional pharmacokinetic factors specific to children include:

    o Decreased gastric acid production and slower gastric emptying time

    o Decreased first-pass medication metabolism

    o Increased absorption of topical medications (proportionately greater body surface area and thinner skin)

    o Lower blood pressure (more blood flow to the liver and brain and less blood flow to the kidneys)

    o Higher body water content (dilutes water-soluble medications)

    o Decreased serum protein-binding sites (until age 1). There may be an increase in serum medication level of protein-binding medications

- Be particularly alert when administering medications to children due to the risk for medication errors.

    o Dosages are usually based on weight or BSA.

    o Most medications are not tested on children.

    o Adult medication forms and concentrations may require dilution, calculation, preparation, and administration of very small doses.

    o Limited sites exist for IV medication administration.

- Nursing interventions for children

    o Check dosage calculation with another nurse

    o Question dosages that seem too large

- o Ensure medication is being given to the right child. A parent or guardian should verify identity for young children.

- o Consider the oral route as the preferred route for children and milliliters (mL) as the preferred measurement (5 mL = 1 tsp, 30 mL = 1 oz).

- o Use plastic, needleless syringes for measurement and administration of small doses of medications.

- o Use only a small amount of liquid or soft food when mixing medications to ensure the total dose is given.

- o Use age-appropriate strategies to obtain cooperation.

 Pharmacology and Older Adults (65+ Years)

- Physiologic changes associated with aging that impact pharmacokinetics include:

  - o Increased gastric pH (alkaline)

  - o Decreased GI motility and gastric emptying time

  - o Decreased blood flow through cardiovascular system, liver, and kidneys

  - o Decreased hepatic enzyme function

  - o Decreased kidney function and glomerular filtration rate

  - o Decreased protein-binding sites

  - o Decreased body water, increased body fat, and decreased lean body mass

- Other factors affecting medication therapy for older adults may include:

  - o Impaired memory or altered mental state

  - o Changes in vision and hearing

  - o Decreased mobility and dexterity

  - o Poor adherence

  - o Reduced financial resources

  - o Polypharmacy

    - ▪ The practice of taking several medications simultaneously (prescribed and/or over-the-counter [OTC]) together with diminished bodily functions and certain medical disorders can contribute to the potential for medication toxicity.

- Nursing interventions for older adults:

  - o Decrease the risk of adverse medication effects.

    - ▪ Obtain a complete medication history and include all OTC medications.

    - ▪ Make sure medication therapy starts at the lowest possible dose.

    - ▪ Monitor for therapeutic and adverse effects.

    - ▪ Monitor for drug-drug and drug-food interactions.

- Document findings.
- Notify the provider of adverse effects.

○ Promote adherence

- Give clear and concise instructions, verbally and in writing.
- Ensure that the dosage form is appropriate. Administer liquid forms to clients who have difficulty swallowing tablets or capsules.
- Provide clearly marked containers that are easy to open.
- Assist clients to set up a daily calendar with the use of pill containers.
- Suggest that clients obtain assistance from a friend, neighbor, or relative.

ⓢ Pharmacology and Pregnancy/Lactation

- Pregnancy – Any medication ingested by a woman who is pregnant will be distributed to the fetus, as well.

  ○ Medications are classified according to potential harm to the fetus. In general, most medications are potentially harmful to the fetus; therefore, benefits of maternal medication administration must be weighed against possible fetal risk.

  ○ Medications are most commonly used during pregnancy as nutritional supplements (iron, vitamins, minerals) and for the treatment of nausea, vomiting, gastric acidity, and mild discomforts.

  ○ Chronic medical disorders such as diabetes or hypertension must be managed with careful maternal-fetal monitoring. Live virus vaccines (e.g., measles, mumps, polio, rubella, yellow fever) are contraindicated due to possible teratogenic effects.

- Lactation – Most medications taken by lactating women are secreted in breast milk. Medications that have an extended half-life or medications that are known to be harmful to infants should be avoided. For medications that are safe, give the medication immediately after breastfeeding to minimize medication concentration in the next feeding.

APPLICATION EXERCISES

1. When giving a medication that is highly protein-bound to an infant, will there be more or less free medication available? Will medication effects be increased or decreased? Explain.

2. A nurse is preparing to administer a small amount of liquid oral medication to a toddler. Which of the following interventions should the nurse use in order to prevent medication error? (Select all that apply.)

    _____ Stir measured medication into a glass of the child's preferred beverage.

    _____ Verify identity of the child with the child's parents.

    _____ Calculate medication amount in either teaspoons or ounces before administering.

    _____ Check dosage calculations with another nurse.

    _____ Administer medication using a plastic needleless syringe

3. A nurse is reinforcing discharge teaching for an older adult client who states she has difficulty remembering to take her daily medications. Describe a nursing intervention that could be used to promote medication adherence for this client.

APPLICATION EXERCISES ANSWER KEY

1. When giving a medication that is highly protein-bound to an infant, will there be more or less free medication available? Will medication effects be increased or decreased? Explain.

   More free medication will be available due to fewer protein-binding sites. Medication effects will be increased with greater potential for toxicity.

 NCLEX® Connection: Pharmacological Therapies, Expected Actions/Outcomes

2. A nurse is preparing to administer a small amount of liquid oral medication to a toddler. Which of the following interventions should the nurse use in order to prevent medication error? (Select all that apply.)

   _____ Stir measured medication into a glass of the child's preferred beverage.

   __X__ **Verify identity of the child with the child's parents.**

   _____ Calculate medication amount in either teaspoons or ounces before administering.

   __X__ **Check dosage calculations with another nurse.**

   __X__ **Administer medication using a plastic needleless syringe**

   The nurse should verify the child's identity with the child's parents, check pediatric dosage calculations with another nurse, and use a plastic needleless syringe to administer a small amount of medication. Do not stir medication into a glass of the child's beverage because the child might not finish the entire beverage and may then refuse the beverage if the medication has given it an unacceptable taste. Calculate medications in mL to ensure accuracy, rather than in teaspoons or ounces.

 NCLEX® Connection: Pharmacological Therapies, Medication Administration

3. A nurse is reinforcing discharge teaching for an older adult client who states she has difficulty remembering to take her daily medications. Describe a nursing intervention that could be used to promote medication adherence for this client.

   The nurse could help set up a daily medication calendar or medication containers clearly marked for each day.

 NCLEX® Connection: Pharmacological Therapies, Medication Administration

UNIT 2: MEDICATIONS AFFECTING THE NERVOUS SYSTEM

- Anxiety Disorders

- Depression

- Bipolar Disorders

- Psychoses

- Behavioral Disorders

- Substance Abuse

- Chronic Neurological Disorders

- Eye and Ear Disorders

- Miscellaneous Central Nervous System Medications

- Sedative-Hypnotics

NCLEX® CONNECTIONS

When reviewing the chapters in this section, keep in mind the relevant sections of the NCLEX® outline, in particular:

CLIENT NEEDS: PHARMACOLOGICAL THERAPIES

Relevant topics/tasks include:
- Adverse Effects/Contraindications/Side Effects/Interactions
  - Identify a contraindication to the administration of prescribed over-the-counter medication to the client.
- Expected Actions/Outcomes
  - Identify client expected response to medication.
- Medication Administration
  - Identify client need for PRN medications.

UNIT 2	MEDICATIONS AFFECTING THE NERVOUS SYSTEM
Chapter 7	Anxiety Disorders

 Overview

- The major medications used to treat anxiety disorders include:

    o Benzodiazepine sedative hypnotic anxiolytics such as diazepam (Valium)

    o Atypical anxiolytic/nonbarbiturate anxiolytics such as buspirone (BuSpar)

    o Selective Serotonin Reuptake Inhibitors (SSRI antidepressants) such as paroxetine (Paxil)

- Other classifications include:

    o Antidepressants, such as

        ▪ Amitriptyline (Elavil), a tricyclic antidepressant (TCA)

        ▪ Phenelzine (Nardil), a monoamine oxidase inhibitor (MAOI)

        ▪ Venlafaxine (Effexor) or duloxetine (Cymbalta), are both serotonin-norepinephrine reuptake inhibitors

        ▪ Sertraline (Zoloft), an SSRI

    o CNS stimulants, such as methylphenidate (Ritalin, Concerta)

    o Antihistamines, such as hydroxyzine (Vistaril)

    o Beta-adrenergic blockers, such as propranolol (Inderal)

    o Anticonvulsants, such as gabapentin (Neurontin)

MEDICATION CLASSIFICATION: SEDATIVE HYPNOTIC ANXIOLYTIC – BENZODIAZEPINE

- Select Prototype Medication – Diazepam

- Other Medications:

    o Alprazolam (Xanax)

    o Lorazepam (Ativan)

    o Chlordiazepoxide (Librium)

    o Clorazepate (Tranxene)

    o Oxazepam (Serax)

    o Clonazepam (Klonopin)

Purpose

- Expected Pharmacological Action

  ○ Diazepam enhances the inhibitory effects of gamma-aminobutyric acid in the CNS. Relief from anxiety occurs rapidly following administration.

- Therapeutic Uses

  ○ Generalized anxiety disorder (GAD) and panic disorder

  ○ Other uses for benzodiazepines include:

    ▪ Seizure disorders

    ▪ Insomnia

    ▪ Muscle spasm

    ▪ Alcohol withdrawal (for prevention and treatment of acute symptoms)

    ▪ Induction of anesthesia

Complications

SIDE/ADVERSE EFFECTS	NURSING INTERVENTIONS/CLIENT EDUCATION
CNS depression (sedation, light-headedness, ataxia, decreased cognitive function)	• Advise clients to observe for symptoms and to notify the provider if symptoms occur. • Advise clients to avoid hazardous activities (driving, operating heavy equipment/machinery).
Anterograde amnesia (difficulty recalling events that occur after dosing)	• Advise clients to observe for symptoms and to notify the provider if symptoms occur. Advise clients to stop the medication if symptoms occur.
Acute oral toxicity (drowsiness, lethargy, confusion)	• Advise clients to watch for manifestations of overdose and to notify the provider if these occur. • Use gastric lavage followed by the administration of activated charcoal or saline cathartics for oral toxicity. • Monitor clients receiving flumazenil (Romazicon) IV to counteract sedation and reverse side effects. • Assist with emergency care as necessary.
Paradoxical response (insomnia, excitation, euphoria, anxiety, rage)	• Advise clients to observe for symptoms. Instruct clients to notify the provider and stop the medication if symptoms occur.
Withdrawal symptoms, which occur infrequently with short-term use (anxiety, insomnia, diaphoresis, tremors, light-headedness)	• Advise clients that, after a long period of use, the medication will be tapered slowly to avoid withdrawal symptoms.

Contraindications/Precautions

- Diazepam is a Pregnancy Risk Category D medication.

- Benzodiazepines are classified under Schedule IV of the Controlled Substances Act.

- Diazepam is contraindicated in clients with sleep apnea and/or respiratory depression.

- Use diazepam cautiously in clients with substance abuse and liver disease.

Interactions

MEDICATION/FOOD INTERACTIONS	NURSING INTERVENTIONS/CLIENT EDUCATION
CNS depressants (alcohol, barbiturates, opioids) may result in respiratory depression.	• Advise clients to observe for symptoms and to notify the provider if symptoms occur. • Advise clients to avoid hazardous activities (driving, operating heavy equipment/ machinery).

Nursing Administration

- Advise clients to take the medication as prescribed and to avoid abrupt discontinuation of long-term treatment to prevent withdrawal symptoms. Instruct clients to taper the dose over several weeks when the medication has been discontinued.

- Advise clients to administer the medication with meals or snacks if gastrointestinal (GI) upset occurs.

- Advise clients to swallow sustained-release tablets and to avoid chewing or crushing the tablets.

- Inform clients about the possible development of dependency during and after treatment and to notify the provider if symptoms occur.

MEDICATION CLASSIFICATION: ATYPICAL ANXIOLYTIC/NONBARBITURATE ANXIOLYTIC

- Select Prototype Medication – Buspirone

Purpose

- Expected Pharmacological Action

  ○ The exact antianxiety mechanism of this medication is unknown. This medication binds to serotonin and dopamine receptors. Abuse is much less likely than with other anxiolytics, and use of buspirone does not result in sedation or potentiate the effects of other CNS depressants.

- Therapeutic Uses

  o Panic disorder, obsessive-compulsive disorder, social anxiety disorder, and post-traumatic stress disorder

Complications

SIDE/ADVERSE EFFECTS	NURSING INTERVENTIONS/CLIENT EDUCATION
Dizziness, nausea, headache, light-headedness, agitation	• Advise clients to take with food to decrease nausea. • Instruct clients that most side effects are self-limiting.

 Contraindications/Precautions

- Buspirone is Pregnancy Risk Category B.

- Buspirone is not recommended for use by nursing mothers.

 • Use buspirone cautiously in older adult clients and clients with liver and/or renal dysfunction.

- Buspirone is contraindicated for concurrent use with MAOI antidepressants or for 14 days after MAOIs are discontinued. Hypertensive crisis may result.

Interactions

MEDICATION/FOOD INTERACTIONS	NURSING INTERVENTIONS/CLIENT EDUCATION
Erythromycin, ketoconazole, and grapefruit juice may increase the effects of buspirone.	• Avoid concurrent use. • Advise clients to avoid drinking grapefruit juice.

Nursing Administration

- Advise clients to take the medication with meals to prevent gastric irritation.

- Advise clients that effects do not occur immediately. It may take a week to notice the first therapeutic effects and several more weeks for the full benefit. Tell clients to take medication on a regular basis and not PRN.

- Instruct clients that tolerance, dependence, or withdrawal symptoms should not occur with this medication.

MEDICATION CLASSIFICATION: SELECTIVE SEROTONIN REUPTAKE INHIBITORS (SSRI ANTIDEPRESSANTS)

- Select Prototype Medication – Paroxetine
- Other Medications:
  - Sertraline (Zoloft)
  - Escitalopram (Lexapro)
  - Fluoxetine (Prozac)
  - Fluvoxamine (Luvox)

Purpose

- Expected Pharmacological Action
  - Paroxetine selectively inhibits serotonin reuptake, allowing more serotonin to stay at the junction of the neurons.
  - It does not block uptake of dopamine or norepinephrine.
  - Paroxetine produces CNS stimulation, which can cause insomnia.
  - The medication has a long effective half-life. A timeframe of about 4 weeks is necessary to produce therapeutic medication levels.
- Therapeutic Uses
  - Paroxetine
    - GAD
    - Panic disorder
      - Decreases both the frequency and intensity of panic attacks and also prevents anticipatory anxiety about attacks
    - Obsessive-compulsive disorder (OCD)
      - Reduces symptoms by increasing serotonin
    - Social anxiety disorder
    - Posttraumatic stress disorder (PTSD)
    - Depressive disorders

MEDICATION	INDICATION
Sertraline	Panic disorder, OCD, social anxiety disorder, and PTSD
Escitalopram	GAD and OCD
Fluoxetine	Panic disorder and OCD
Fluvoxamine	OCD and social anxiety disorder

Complications

SIDE/ADVERSE EFFECTS	NURSING INTERVENTIONS/CLIENT EDUCATION
Early adverse effects (first few days/weeks): nausea, diaphoresis, tremor, fatigue, drowsiness	• Advise clients that these effects should soon subside. • Instruct clients to take the medication as prescribed.
Later adverse effects (after 5 to 6 weeks of therapy): sexual dysfunction (impotence, delayed or absent orgasm, delayed or absent ejaculation, decreased sexual interest)	• Instruct clients to report problems with sexual function (may be managed with dose reduction, medication holiday, changing medications).
Weight gain	• Advise clients to follow a well-balanced diet and exercise regularly.
Gastrointestinal bleeding	• Advise clients to report signs of bleeding such as dark stool or coffee ground emesis.
Hyponatremia (more likely in older adult clients taking diuretics)	• Obtain baseline serum sodium, and monitor level periodically throughout treatment.
Serotonin syndrome • Agitation, confusion, disorientation, difficulty concentrating, anxiety, hallucinations, hyperreflexia, incoordination, tremors, fever, diaphoresis • Usually begins 2 to 72 hr after initiation of treatment • Resolves when the medication is discontinued	• Watch for and advise clients to report any of these symptoms, which could indicate a lethal problem.

Bruxism: grinding and clenching of teeth, usually during sleep	• Instruct clients to report to the provider, who may:
	  ○ Switch clients to another class of medication.
	  ○ Treat bruxism with low-dose buspirone.
	  ○ Advise clients to use a mouth guard during sleep.

Withdrawal syndrome • Nausea, sensory disturbances, anxiety, tremor, malaise, unease	• Advise clients not to discontinue use abruptly. • Reinforce to clients how to slowly taper the medication dosage after a long period of use to avoid withdrawal symptoms.

 Contraindications/Precautions

- Paroxetine is a Pregnancy Risk Category D medication.

- Paroxetine is contraindicated in clients taking MAOIs or a TCA.

- Clients taking paroxetine should avoid alcohol.

- Use paroxetine cautiously in clients with liver and renal dysfunction, seizure disorders, a history of GI bleeding, or those taking NSAIDs or anticoagulants.

Interactions

MEDICATION/FOOD INTERACTIONS	NURSING INTERVENTIONS/CLIENT EDUCATION
Use of MAOI antidepressants or TCAs can cause serotonin syndrome.	Educate clients about this combination. Avoid concurrent use.

Nursing Administration

- Advise clients that medications may be taken with food. Sleep disturbances may be minimized by taking medication in the morning.

- Instruct clients to take the medication on a daily basis to establish therapeutic plasma levels.

- Assist with medication regimen adherence by informing clients that therapeutic effects may not be experienced for 1 to 3 weeks.

Nursing Evaluation of Medication Effectiveness

- Depending on therapeutic intent, effectiveness may be evidenced by:

  o Maintaining normal sleep pattern

  o Verbalizing feeling less anxious and more relaxed

  o Greater ability to participate in social and occupational interactions

APPLICATION EXERCISES

1. A client should receive a dose of flumazenil (Romazicon) to treat symptoms of which of the following?

    A. obsessive-compulsive disorder (OCD).

    B. benzodiazepine overdose.

    C. panic disorder.

    D. serotonin syndrome.

2. A nurse is reinforcing teaching to a client who is prescribed diazepam (Valium) for anxiety. Which of the following statements indicates the client understands the teaching?

    A. "I should not take this medication at bedtime."

    B. "I should not take this medication if I am taking acetaminophen."

    C. "I will tell my doctor before I stop taking this medication."

    D. "I will need to take this medication for the rest of my life."

3. For what reason might a client be prescribed buspirone (BuSpar) instead of diazepam (Valium)?

4. A client who has been taking paroxetine (Paxil) for several weeks to treat an anxiety disorder suddenly develops bruxism. What is bruxism, and what treatment should the nurse expect to be prescribed for this adverse reaction to paroxetine?

APPLICATION EXERCISES ANSWER KEY

1. A client should receive a dose of flumazenil (Romazicon) to treat symptoms of

    A. obsessive-compulsive disorder (OCD).

    B. benzodiazepine overdose.

    C. panic disorder.

    D. serotonin syndrome.

    Flumazenil reverses the sedative effects of benzodiazepines and is used as an antidote to treat benzodiazepine overdose. It is not indicated to treat OCD, panic disorder, or serotonin syndrome.

 NCLEX® Connection: Pharmacological Therapies, Expected Actions/Outcomes

2. A nurse is reinforcing teaching to a client who is prescribed diazepam (Valium) for anxiety. Which of the following statements indicates the client understands the teaching?

    A. "I should not take this medication at bedtime."

    B. "I should not take this medication if I am taking acetaminophen."

    C. "I will tell my doctor before I stop taking this medication."

    D. "I will need to take this medication for the rest of my life."

    Abrupt discontinuation of diazepam, a benzodiazepine, may cause withdrawal symptoms. The medication may need to be tapered for several weeks before discontinuing. Taking the medication at bedtime can promote sleep. There is no indication the medication cannot be taken while taking acetaminophen. A short-term course of diazepam may resolve the client's anxiety. Life-long therapy is not always necessary.

 NCLEX® Connection: Pharmacological Therapies, Medication Administration

3. For what reason might a client be prescribed buspirone (BuSpar) instead of diazepam (Valium)?

    Buspirone is not a benzodiazepine and does not depress the central nervous system. Therefore, a client taking buspirone is not at risk to experience severe sedation or manifestations of physical or psychologic dependence which may occur with diazepam and other benzodiazepines.

 NCLEX® Connection: Pharmacological Therapies, Adverse Effects/Contraindications/Side Effects/Interactions

4. A client who has been taking paroxetine (Paxil) for several weeks to treat an anxiety disorder suddenly develops bruxism. What is bruxism, and what treatment should the nurse expect to be prescribed for this adverse reaction to paroxetine?

   Bruxism, grinding of the teeth, can be treated by changing the client to another type of antianxiety medication, prescribing buspirone (BuSpar) along with the paroxetine, and/or by having the client wear a mouth guard while sleeping.

 NCLEX® Connection: Pharmacological Therapies, Adverse Effects/Contraindications/Side Effects/Interactions

UNIT 2	MEDICATIONS AFFECTING THE NERVOUS SYSTEM
Chapter 8	Depression

 Overview

- Depression is a mood (affective) disorder and is a widespread problem, ranking high among causes of disability.

- Advise clients starting antidepressant medication therapy for depression that symptom relief can take 1 to 3 weeks and possibly 2 to 3 months for full benefits to be achieved. Encourage continued adherence.

- Clients with major depression may require hospitalization with close observation and suicide precautions until the antidepressant medications reach their peak effect.

- Antidepressant mediations are classified into four main groups:

    o Tricyclic antidepressants (TCAs)

    o Selective serotonin reuptake inhibitors (SSRIs)

    o Monoamine oxidase inhibitors (MAOIs)

    o Atypical antidepressants

MEDICATION CLASSIFICATION: TRICYCLIC ANTIDEPRESSANTS (TCAs)

- Select Prototype Medication – Amitriptyline (Elavil)

- Other Medications

    o Imipramine (Tofranil)

    o Doxepin (Sinequan)

    o Nortriptyline (Aventyl)

    o Trimipramine (Surmontil)

Purpose

- Expected Pharmacological Action

    o These medications block reuptake of norepinephrine and serotonin in the synaptic space, thereby intensifying the effects of these neurotransmitters.

- Therapeutic Uses

  ○ Depression

  ○ Depressive episodes of bipolar disorders

  ○ Other Uses

    ▪ Chronic pain

    ▪ Enuresis

Complications

SIDE/ADVERSE EFFECTS	NURSING INTERVENTIONS/CLIENT EDUCATION
Orthostatic hypotension	• Instruct clients about the signs of orthostatic hypotension (lightheadedness, dizziness). If these occur, advise clients to sit or lie down. Advise clients to change positions slowly and to sit or lie down if symptoms occur. • Monitor blood pressure (BP) and heart rate for clients in the hospital for orthostatic changes before administration and 1 hr after. If a significant decrease in blood pressure and/or increase in heart rate are noted, do not administer the medication, and notify the provider.

Anticholinergic effects
• Dry mouth
• Blurred vision
• Photophobia
• Urinary hesitancy or retention
• Constipation
• Tachycardia
	• Instruct clients on ways to minimize anticholinergic effects. These include:
	  ○ Chewing sugarless gum
	  ○ Sipping on water
	  ○ Wearing sunglasses when outdoors
	  ○ Eating foods high in fiber
	  ○ Participating in regular exercise
	  ○ Increasing fluid intake to at least 2 to 3 L/day from beverages and food sources
	  ○ Voiding just before taking medication
	• Advise clients to notify the provider if symptoms persist.

Sedation	• Advise clients that this effect usually diminishes over time. • Advise clients to avoid hazardous activities such as driving if sedation is excessive. • Advise clients to take medication at bedtime to minimize daytime sleepiness and to promote sleep.

SIDE/ADVERSE EFFECTS	NURSING INTERVENTIONS/CLIENT EDUCATION
Toxicity resulting in cholinergic blockade and cardiac toxicity evidenced by dysrhythmias, mental confusion, and agitation, followed by seizures, coma, and possible death	• Give a 1-week supply of medication to clients who are acutely ill. • Obtain the client's baseline ECG. • Monitor vital signs frequently. • Monitor clients for signs of toxicity. • Notify the provider if signs of toxicity occur.
Decreased seizure threshold	• Monitor clients who have seizure disorders.
Excessive sweating	• Inform clients of side effect. Assist clients with frequent linen changes.

 Contraindications/Precautions

- TCAs are Pregnancy Risk Category C.

- These medications are contraindicated in clients who have seizure disorders

- Use cautiously in clients who have coronary artery disease; diabetes, liver, kidney and respiratory disorders; urinary retention and obstruction; angle-closure glaucoma; benign prostatic hypertrophy; and hyperthyroidism.

Interactions

MEDICATION/FOOD INTERACTIONS	NURSING INTERVENTIONS/CLIENT EDUCATION
Concurrent use of MAOIs and St. John's wort may lead to serotonin syndrome.	• Avoid concurrent use.
Antihistamines and other anticholinergic agents have additive anticholinergic effects.	
Increased effects of epinephrine, dopamine (direct-acting sympathomimetics) occur because uptake into the nerve terminals is blocked by TCAs and they remain for a longer amount of time in the synaptic space.	
TCAs decrease the effects of ephedrine, amphetamine (indirect-acting sympathomimetics), because uptake into the nerve terminals is blocked and they are unable to reach their site of action.	
Alcohol, benzodiazepines, opioids, and antihistamines cause additive CNS depression when used concurrently.	• Advise clients to avoid other CNS depressants.

MEDICATION CLASSIFICATION: SELECTIVE SEROTONIN REUPTAKE INHIBITORS (SSRIs)

- Select Prototype Medication – Fluoxetine (Prozac)
- Other Medications
  - Citalopram (Celexa)
  - Escitalopram (Lexapro)
  - Paroxetine (Paxil)
  - Sertraline (Zoloft)

Purpose

- Expected pharmacological action
  - SSRIs selectively block reuptake of the monoamine neurotransmitter serotonin in the synaptic space, thereby intensifying the effects of serotonin.
- Therapeutic Uses
  - Major depression
  - Obsessive compulsive disorders
  - Bulimia nervosa
  - Premenstrual dysphoric disorders
  - Panic disorders
  - Posttraumatic disorder

Complications

SIDE/ADVERSE EFFECTS	NURSING INTERVENTIONS/CLIENT EDUCATION
Sexual dysfunction (no orgasm, impotence, decreased libido)	• Warn clients of possible side effects and to notify the provider if intolerable. • Instruct clients to report problems with sexual function (may be managed with dose reduction, medication holiday, changing medications). Bupropion (Wellbutrin) and nefazodone (Serzone) may be indicated.
CNS stimulation (inability to sleep, agitation, anxiety)	• Advise clients to notify the provider. Tell clients the provider may decrease dosage. • Advise clients to take dose in the morning. • Advise clients to avoid caffeinated beverages. • Instruct clients to practice relaxation techniques to promote sleep.

SIDE/ADVERSE EFFECTS	NURSING INTERVENTIONS/CLIENT EDUCATION
Weight loss early in therapy, may be followed by weight gain with long-term treatment	• Monitor the client's weight. • Encourage clients to participate in regular exercise and to follow a healthy, well-balanced diet.
Serotonin syndrome may begin 2 to 72 hr after starting treatment and may be lethal. Manifestations include: • Mental confusion, difficulty concentrating • Fever • Agitation • Anxiety • Hallucinations • Incoordination, hyperreflexia • Diaphoresis • Tremors	• Advise clients to observe for symptoms and to notify the provider and stop the medication.
Withdrawal syndrome resulting in headache, nausea, visual disturbances, anxiety, dizziness, and tremors	• Advise clients not to discontinue use abruptly. • Reinforce to clients how to slowly taper the medication dosage after a long period of use to avoid withdrawal symptoms.
Hyponatremia (more likely in older adult clients taking diuretics)	• Obtain baseline serum sodium, and monitor level periodically throughout treatment.
Rash	• Advise clients to treat a rash with an antihistamine or withdrawal of medication.
Sleepiness, faintness, lightheadedness	• Advise clients that these side effects are not common, but can occur. • Advise clients to avoid driving if these side effects occur.
Gastrointestinal bleeding	• Use caution in clients with history of gastrointestinal (GI) bleeding, ulcers, and those taking NSAIDs or anticoagulants.

Bruxism	• Advise clients to report to the provider. who may:
	  ○ Switch clients to another class of medication
	  ○ Treat bruxism with low-dose buspirone
	• Advise clients to use a mouth guard during sleep

Contraindications/Precautions

- Fluoxetine is a Pregnancy Risk Category C.

  o Fluoxetine and paroxetine may increase the risk of birth defects. The provider may prescribe other SSRIs. Late in pregnancy, use of SSRIs may increase the risk of withdrawal symptoms or pulmonary hypertension in the newborn.

- SSRIs are contraindicated in clients taking MAOIs or TCAs.

- Use cautiously in clients with liver and renal dysfunction, cardiac disease, seizure disorders, diabetes, ulcers, a history of GI bleeding, and those taking NSAIDs or anticoagulants.

Interactions

MEDICATION/FOOD INTERACTIONS	NURSING INTERVENTIONS/CLIENT EDUCATION
MAOIs and St. John's wort increase the risk of serotonin syndrome.	• MAOIs should be discontinued for 14 days prior to starting an SSRI. If already taking fluoxetine, clients should wait 5 weeks before starting an MAOI. • Advise clients against concurrent use of SSRIs and St. John's wort.
Fluoxetine can displace warfarin (Coumadin) from bound protein and result in increased warfarin levels.	• Monitor the client's PT and INR levels. • Monitor clients for signs of bleeding and the need for dosage adjustment.
Fluoxetine can increase the levels of tricyclic antidepressants and lithium.	• Avoid concurrent use.
Fluoxetine suppresses platelet aggregation and thus increases the risk of bleeding when used concurrently with NSAIDs and anticoagulants.	• Advise clients to monitor for signs of bleeding (bruising, hematuria) and to notify the provider if they occur.

MEDICATION CLASSIFICATION: MONOAMINE OXIDASE INHIBITORS (MAOIs)

- Select Prototype Medication – Phenelzine (Nardil)

- Other Medications:

  o Isocarboxazid (Marplan)

  o Tranylcypromine (Parnate)

  o Selegiline (Emsam) – Transdermal MAOI

Purpose

- Expected Pharmacological Action

  o These medications block MAO-A in the brain, thereby increasing the amount of norepinephrine, dopamine, and serotonin available for transmission of impulses. An increased amount of these neurotransmitters at nerve endings intensifies responses and relieves depression.

- Therapeutic Uses

  o Atypical depression

  o Bulimia nervosa

  o Obsessive compulsive disorders (OCD)

Complications

SIDE/ADVERSE EFFECTS	NURSING INTERVENTIONS/CLIENT EDUCATION
CNS stimulation (anxiety, agitation, mania, or hypomania)	• Advise clients to observe for symptoms and notify the provider if they occur.
Orthostatic hypotension	• Monitor the client's BP and heart rate for orthostatic changes. Hold medication and notify the provider for significant changes. Instruct clients to change positions slowly.
Hypertensive crisis resulting from intake of dietary tyramine • Severe hypertension occurs as a result of intensive vasoconstriction and stimulation of the heart • Clients will most likely experience headache, nausea, increased heart rate and blood pressure	• Assist with emergency care.
Local rash may occur with transdermal preparation.	• Instruct clients to choose a clean, dry area for each application. • Instruct clients to apply a topical glucocorticoid on the affected area.

(S) Contraindications/Precautions

- MAOIs are Pregnancy Risk Category C.

- These medications are contraindicated in clients taking SSRIs and in those with pheochromocytoma, cardiovascular and cerebral vascular disease, and severe renal insufficiency.

- Use cautiously in clients with diabetes and seizure disorders or those taking TCAs.

- Transdermal selegiline is contraindicated for clients taking carbamazepine (Tegretol) or oxcarbazepine (Trileptal), which may increase blood levels of the MAOI.

Interactions

MEDICATION/FOOD INTERACTIONS	NURSING INTERVENTIONS/CLIENT EDUCATION
Indirect-acting sympathomimetic medications (ephedrine, amphetamine) promote the release of norepinephrine and can lead to hypertensive crisis	• Instruct clients to avoid over-the-counter decongestants and cold remedies, which frequently contain medications with sympathomimetic action.
Use of tricyclic antidepressants (TCAs) and MAOIs can lead to hypertensive crisis.	• Avoid concurrent use.
Use with SSRIs can lead to serotonin syndrome.	• Avoid concurrent use.
Antihypertensives have an additive hypotensive effect.	• Monitor the client's BP. • Notify the provider if there is a significant drop in the client's BP. The provider may reduce the dosage.
Use with meperidine (Demerol) can lead to hyperpyrexia	• Use an alternative analgesic.
Tyramine-rich foods can lead to hypertensive crisis. Clients will most likely experience headache, nausea, increased HR and increased BP.	• Monitor clients for ability to follow strict adherence to dietary restrictions. • Give written information regarding tyramine-rich foods to include aged cheese, pepperoni, salami, avocados, figs, bananas, smoked fish, protein dietary supplements, soups, soy sauce, some beers, and red wine. • Inform clients of symptoms and to notify the provider if they occur. • Advise clients to avoid taking any medications without approval of the provider.
Concurrent use of vasopressors (phenylethylamine, caffeine) may result in hypertension	• Advise clients to avoid foods that contain these agents (caffeinated beverages, chocolate, fava beans, ginseng).

MEDICATION CLASSIFICATION: ATYPICAL ANTIDEPRESSANTS

- Select Prototype Medication – Bupropion HCl (Wellbutrin)

Purpose

- Expected Pharmacological Action

  o This medication acts by inhibiting dopamine uptake.

- Therapeutic Uses

  o Treatment of depression

  o Alternative to SSRIs for clients unable to tolerate sexual dysfunction side effects of SSRIs

  o Aid to quit smoking

  o Prevention of SAD (seasonal affective disorder)

Complications

SIDE/ADVERSE EFFECTS	NURSING INTERVENTIONS/CLIENT EDUCATION
Headache, dry mouth, GI distress, constipation, increased heart rate, nausea, restlessness, and insomnia	• Advise clients to observe for symptoms and to notify the provider if intolerable. • Recommend that clients treat headache with mild analgesic. • Advise clients to sip on fluids to treat dry mouth and to increase dietary fiber to prevent constipation.
Suppresses appetite and often causes weight loss	• Monitor client's weight and food intake.
Seizures	• Avoid use with clients at risk for seizures, such as clients with a head injury. • Monitor clients for seizures and treat accordingly.

 Contraindications/Precautions

- Bupropion HCl is a Pregnancy Risk Category B.

- This medication is contraindicated in clients taking MAOIs.

- Use cautiously in clients who have seizure disorders.

Interactions

MEDICATION/FOOD INTERACTIONS	NURSING INTERVENTIONS/CLIENT EDUCATION
MAOIs such as phenelzine increase the risk of toxicity.	• Discontinue MAOIs 2 weeks prior to beginning treatment with bupropion.

OTHER ATYPICAL ANTIDEPRESSANTS

AGENT	PHARMACOLOGICAL ACTION	NURSING INTERVENTIONS/CLIENT EDUCATION
Venlafaxine (Effexor), duloxetine (Cymbalta) (SNRIs)	These medications inhibit serotonin and norepinephrine reuptake, thereby increasing the amount of these neurotransmitters available in the brain for impulse transmission. There is also a minimal amount of dopamine blockade.	• Inform clients that side effects include headache, nausea, agitation, anxiety, and sleep disturbances. • Monitor for hyponatremia, especially in older adult clients. • Monitor clients for weight loss. • Monitor clients for increase in diastolic pressure. • Discuss ways to manage interference with sexual functioning. • Advise clients not to stop medication abruptly.
Mirtazapine (Remeron)	This medication increases the release of serotonin and norepinephrine and thereby increases the amount of neurotransmitters available for impulse transmission.	• Inform clients that therapeutic effects may occur sooner with less sexual dysfunction than with SSRIs. • Inform clients that mirtazapine is generally well-tolerated, but they may experience sleepiness that can be exacerbated by other CNS depressants (alcohol, benzodiazepines), weight gain, and elevated cholesterol
Reboxetine (Edronax)	This medication selectively inhibits the reuptake of norepinephrine, thereby increasing the amount of neurotransmitters available for impulse transmission.	• Inform clients that reboxetine is generally well-tolerated, but clients may experience dry mouth, decreased BP, constipation, sexual dysfunction, and urinary hesitancy or retention.
Trazodone (Desyrel)	This medication has moderate selective blockade of serotonin receptors, which allows more serotonin to be available for impulse transmission.	• Inform clients that priapism may be an adverse effect and they should seek medical attention immediately if this occurs. • Sedation may be a problem; therefore, clients taking an SSRI may benefit from its use.

Nursing Administration

- Monitor clients for suicidal thoughts during the first few weeks of therapy, as the client's energy may increase without relieving symptoms, thereby placing clients at risk for suicide.

- Instruct clients to take these medications as prescribed on a daily basis to establish therapeutic plasma levels.

- Assist with medication regimen adherence by informing clients that therapeutic effects may not be experienced for 1 to 3 weeks. Full therapeutic effects may take 2 to 3 months.

- Instruct clients to continue therapy after improvement in symptoms. Sudden discontinuation of medication can result in relapse.

- Advise clients that therapy usually continues for 6 months after resolution of symptoms and may continue for a year or longer.

 • Facilitate suicide prevention by recommending that the provider prescribe only a week's worth of medication for an acutely ill client, and then only prescribing 1 month's worth of medication at a time, especially with TCAs.

- For SSRIs:

  o Advise clients to take medication in the morning to minimize sleep disturbances

  o Advise clients to take medications with food to minimize GI disturbances.

 o Obtain baseline sodium levels for older adult clients taking diuretics and monitor periodically.

- For MAOIs:

  o Give clients a list of tyramine-rich foods to avoid to prevent a hypertensive crisis.

  o Advise clients to avoid taking any other prescription or nonprescription medications unless approved by the provider.

- For bupropion HCL:

  o Advise clients with SAD to take medication beginning in the autumn each year and gradually taper dose and discontinue by spring.

Nursing Evaluation of Medication Effectiveness

- Depending on therapeutic intent, effectiveness may be evidenced by:

  o Verbalizing improvement in mood

  o Ability to perform ADLs

  o Improved sleeping and eating habits

  o Increased interaction with peers

APPLICATION EXERCISES

1. A client who has depression has just begun a new prescription for bupropion (Wellbutrin). For which of the following adverse effects should the nurse plan to monitor this client?

   A. Excessive sleepiness

   B. Seizures

   C. Increased blood glucose

   D. Bleeding

2. A nurse is reinforcing teaching to a client who is starting amitriptyline (Elavil) for treatment of depression. Which of the following should the nurse include? (Select all that apply.)

   _____ Expect effects to occur within 12 hr.

   _____ Stop taking the medication after a week of improved mood.

   _____ Change positions slowly to minimize dizziness.

   _____ Decrease dietary fiber intake to control diarrhea.

   _____ Chew sugarless gum to prevent dry mouth.

3. A nurse is caring for a hospitalized client who takes an MAOI antidepressant. The client was discovered eating food which contains tyramine. List the physical manifestations for which the nurse should monitor this client.

4. A nurse is caring for an older adult client who is prescribed fluoxetine (Prozac). Which of the following laboratory values should the nurse plan to monitor for this client?

   A. White blood count (WBC)

   B. Blood urea nitrogen (BUN)

   C. Serum potassium

   D. Serum sodium

5. A nurse is caring for a client who has depression and has been taking paroxetine (Paxil) for two days. The client suddenly develops a high fever, hallucinations, and anxiety. Which of the following adverse reactions is the client likely to be experiencing?

   A. Bruxism

   B. Serotonin syndrome

   C. Anticholinergic effects

   D. Hypernatremia

APPLICATION EXERCISES ANSWER KEY

1. A client who has depression has just begun a new prescription for bupropion (Wellbutrin). For which of the following adverse effects should the nurse plan to monitor this client?

   A. Excessive sleepiness

   B. Seizures

   C. Increased blood glucose

   D. Bleeding

   Bupropion increases the risk for seizures, and the nurse should monitor the client for this potential adverse effect. Excessive sleepiness, increased blood glucose, and bleeding are not adverse effects the nurse should expect to see in a client taking bupropion.

    NCLEX® Connection: Pharmacological Therapies, Adverse Effects/Contraindications/Side Effects/Interactions

2. A nurse is reinforcing teaching to a client who is starting amitriptyline (Elavil) for treatment of depression. Which of the following should the nurse include? (Select all that apply.)

   _____ Expect effects to occur within 12 hr.

   _____ Stop taking the medication after a week of improved mood.

   __X__ **Change positions slowly to minimize dizziness.**

   _____ Decrease dietary fiber intake to control diarrhea.

   __X__ **Chew sugarless gum to prevent dry mouth.**

   Advise clients to change positions slowly to minimize effects of orthostatic hypotension, such as dizziness and lightheadedness. Advise clients to chew sugarless gum to minimize dry mouth. Therapeutic effects may take several weeks to be achieved. Medication should not be stopped abruptly, and therapy will most likely last 6 to 12 months to prevent relapse. Clients should increase dietary fiber to prevent constipation.

    NCLEX® Connection: Pharmacological Therapies, Adverse Effects/Contraindications/Side Effects/Interactions

3. A nurse is caring for a hospitalized client who takes an MAOI antidepressant. The client was discovered eating food which contains tyramine. List the physical manifestations for which the nurse should monitor this client.

   The nurse should monitor this client for signs of hypertensive crisis, which can include headache, nausea, increased heart rate, and increased blood pressure.

    NCLEX® Connection: Pharmacological Therapies, Adverse Effects/Contraindications/Side Effects/Interactions

4. A nurse is caring for an older adult client who is prescribed fluoxetine (Prozac). Which of the following laboratory values should the nurse plan to monitor for this client?

   A. White blood count (WBC)

   B. Blood urea nitrogen (BUN)

   C. Serum potassium

   D. Serum sodium

   Fluoxetine can cause hyponatremia, particularly in older adult clients, and especially in those who also take thiazine diuretics. The nurse should monitor the client's serum sodium. WBC counts, BUN, and serum potassium level should not be affected by fluoxetine.

    NCLEX® Connection: Pharmacological Therapies, Adverse Effects/Contraindications/Side Effects/Interactions

5. A nurse is caring for a client who has depression and has been taking paroxetine (Paxil) for two days. The client suddenly develops a high fever, hallucinations, and anxiety. Which of the following adverse reactions is the client likely to be experiencing?

   A. Bruxism

   B. Serotonin syndrome

   C. Anticholinergic effects

   D. Hypernatremia

   This client is likely to be experiencing serotonin syndrome, which may occur within 72 hours of beginning a prescription of an SSRI antidepressant, such as paroxetine (Paxil). The manifestations of serotonin syndrome do not resemble those of bruxism, anticholinergic effects, or hypernatremia.

    NCLEX® Connection: Pharmacological Therapies, Adverse Effects/Contraindications/Side Effects/Interactions

UNIT 2	MEDICATIONS AFFECTING THE NERVOUS SYSTEM
Chapter 9	Bipolar Disorders

 Overview

- Bipolar disorders are primarily managed with a mood-stabilizing medication such as lithium carbonate (Lithane, Eskalith, Lithobid).

- Classifications include:

    o Antiepileptic medications – carbamazepine (Tegretol), valproic acid (Depakote), lamotrigine (Lamictal)

    o Atypical antipsychotics – These can be useful in early treatment to promote sleep and to decrease anxiety and agitation. These medications also demonstrate mood-stabilizing properties.

    o Anxiolytics – Clonazepam (Klonopin) and lorazepam (Ativan) can be useful in treating acute mania and managing the psychomotor agitation often seen in mania.

MEDICATION CLASSIFICATION: MOOD STABILIZER

- Select Prototype Medication – Lithium carbonate

Purpose

- Expected Pharmacological Action

    o Lithium carbonate produces neurochemical changes in the brain, including serotonin receptor blockade.

    o There is evidence that the use of lithium carbonate can cause a decrease in neuronal atrophy and/or an increase in neuronal growth.

- Therapeutic Uses

    o Controls episodes of acute mania, helps prevent the return of mania or depression, and decreases the incidence of suicide. It is especially used for euphoric mania.

    o Other uses:

        ▪ Alcoholism

        ▪ Bulimia

        ▪ Schizophrenia

Complications

- Effects with therapeutic lithium carbonate levels (some effects will resolve within a few weeks)

SIDE/ADVERSE EFFECTS	NURSING INTERVENTIONS/CLIENT EDUCATION
Gastrointestinal (GI) distress (nausea, diarrhea, abdominal pain)	<ul><li>Advise clients that symptoms are usually transient.</li><li>Suggest clients take medication with meals or milk.</li></ul>
Fine hand tremors that can interfere with purposeful motor skills and can be exacerbated by factors such as stress and caffeine	<ul><li>Use a beta-adrenergic blocking agent such as propranolol (Inderal) to control tremors.</li><li>Administer the lowest effective dose.</li><li>Advise clients to report an increase in tremors.</li></ul>
Polyuria, mild thirst	<ul><li>Instruct clients to maintain adequate fluid intake by consuming at least 2 to 3 L of fluid from beverages and food sources.</li></ul>
Weight gain	<ul><li>Assist clients to follow a healthy diet and regular exercise regimen.</li></ul>
Renal toxicity	<ul><li>Monitor the client's I&O.</li><li>Monitor baseline kidney function and monitor kidney function periodically.</li></ul>
Goiter and hypothyroidism with long-term treatment	<ul><li>Obtain the client's baseline T_3, T_4, and TSH levels prior to starting treatment, and then annually.</li><li>Advise clients to monitor for signs of hypothyroidism (cold, dry skin; decreased heart rate; weight gain).</li><li>Use levothyroxine (Synthroid) to manage hypothyroid symptoms.</li></ul>
Bradydysrhythmia, hypotension, and electrolyte imbalances	<ul><li>Encourage clients to maintain adequate fluid intake.</li></ul>

- Signs and symptoms of toxicity

SIGNS AND SYMPTOMS OF TOXICITY			
Early signs	Less than 1.5 mEq/L	Diarrhea, nausea, vomiting, thirst, polyuria, muscle weakness, and slurred speech	• Advise clients to discontinue medication and notify the provider. • Administer new dosage based on serum lithium levels.
Advanced signs	1.5 to 2.0 mEq/L	Ongoing GI distress including nausea, vomiting, and diarrhea, mental confusion, and poor coordination and coarse tremors	• Advise clients to discontinue medication and notify the provider. • Administer new dosage based on serum lithium carbonate levels.
Severe toxicity	Greater than 2.0 to 2.5 mEq/L	Extreme polyuria of dilute urine, tinnitus, blurred vision, ataxia, seizures, severe hypotension leading to coma and possibly death from respiratory complications	• Give alert clients an emetic. • Assist with clients undergoing gastric lavage. • Assist with clients who are receiving medications to increase the rate of excretion.
	Greater than 2.5 mEq/L	Rapid progression of symptoms leading to coma and death	Hemodialysis may be indicated.

 Contraindications/Precautions

- Lithium carbonate is Pregnancy Risk Category D. This medication is teratogenic, especially during the first trimester.

- Discuss alternatives to breastfeeding if lithium carbonate therapy is necessary.

- Use cautiously in clients with renal dysfunction, heart disease, sodium depletion, and dehydration.

Interactions

MEDICATION/FOOD INTERACTIONS	NURSING INTERVENTIONS/CLIENT EDUCATION
Sodium is excreted with the use of diuretics. Reduced serum sodium decreases lithium carbonate excretion, which can lead to toxicity.	• Monitor clients for signs of toxicity. • Advise clients to observe for symptoms and to notify the provider. • Encourage clients to maintain a diet adequate in sodium, and to drink 2,000 to 3,000 mL of water each day from food and beverage sources.
Concurrent use of NSAIDs (ibuprofen [Motrin] and celecoxib [Celebrex]) will increase renal reabsorption of lithium carbonate, leading to toxicity.	• Encourage clients to avoid use of these NSAIDs and to use aspirin as a mild analgesic.
Anticholinergics (antihistamines, tricyclic antidepressants) can induce urinary retention and polyuria, leading to abdominal discomfort.	• Advise clients to avoid medications with anticholinergic effects.

Nursing Administration

- Monitor serum lithium carbonate levels while undergoing treatment. At initiation of treatment, monitor levels every 2 to 3 days and then every 1 to 3 months. Obtain lithium carbonate blood levels in the morning, usually 12 hr after the last dose.

  ○ During initial treatment of a manic episode, levels should be between 0.8 and 1.4 mEq/L.

  ○ Maintenance level range is between 0.4 and 1.0 mEq/L.

  ○ Plasma levels greater than 1.5 mEq/L can result in toxicity.

- Care for clients who have a toxic serum lithium carbonate level in an inpatient setting and provide supportive measures. Hemodialysis may be indicated.

- Advise clients that effects begin within 7 to 14 days.

- Advise clients to take lithium carbonate as prescribed, usually in 2 to 4 doses daily due to a short half-life. Taking lithium carbonate with food will help decrease GI distress.

- Encourage clients to adhere to laboratory appointments needed to monitor lithium carbonate effectiveness and adverse effects. Emphasize the high risk of toxicity due to the narrow therapeutic range.

- Provide nutritional counseling. Stress the importance of adequate fluid and sodium intake.

- Instruct clients to monitor for signs of toxicity and when to contact the provider. Clients should stop taking medication and seek medical attention if experiencing diarrhea, vomiting, or excessive sweating.

MEDICATION CLASSIFICATION: MOOD-STABILIZING ANTIEPILEPTIC DRUGS (AEDS)

- Select Prototype Medications:
    - Carbamazepine (Tegretol)
    - Valproic acid (Depakote)
    - Lamotrigine (Lamictal)

Purpose

- Expected Pharmacological Action
    - AEDs help treat and manage bipolar disorders by various mechanisms, which include:
        - Slowing the entrance of sodium and calcium back into the neuron and, thus extending the time it takes for the nerve to return to its active state
        - Potentiating the inhibitory effects of gamma butyric acid
        - Inhibiting glutamic acid (glutamate) which in turn suppresses CNS excitation
- Therapeutic Uses
    - Treatment of manic and depressive episodes, prevention of relapse of mania and depressive episodes. Especially useful for clients with mixed mania and rapid-cycling bipolar disorders.

Complications

SIDE/ADVERSE EFFECTS	NURSING INTERVENTIONS/CLIENT EDUCATION
Carbamazepine	
Cognitive function is minimally affected, but CNS effects may include nystagmus, double vision, vertigo, staggering gait, headache	• Administer low doses initially, then gradually increase dosage. • Advise clients that symptoms should subside within a few weeks. • Administer dose at bedtime.
Blood dyscrasias (leukopenia, anemia, thrombocytopenia)	• Obtain the client's baseline CBC and platelet count and perform ongoing monitoring. • Observe clients for signs of bruising and bleeding of gums.
Teratogenesis	• Advise clients to avoid use in pregnancy.
Hypo-osmolarity (promotes secretion of ADH, which inhibits water excretion by the kidneys and places clients with heart failure at risk for fluid overload)	• Monitor serum sodium. • Monitor clients for edema, decrease in urine output, and hypertension.
Skin disorders (dermatitis, rash, Stevens-Johnson syndrome)	• Treat mild reactions with anti-inflammatory or antihistamine medications. • Advise clients to wear sunscreen. • Instruct clients to notify the provider if rash occurs.

SIDE/ADVERSE EFFECTS	NURSING INTERVENTIONS/CLIENT EDUCATION
Valproic acid	
GI (nausea, vomiting, indigestion)	• Advise clients that symptoms are usually self-limiting. • Advise clients to take medication with food or to request an enteric-coated formulation.
Hepatotoxicity (anorexia, nausea, vomiting, fatigue, abdominal pain, jaundice)	• Monitor baseline liver function and monitor liver function regularly. • Advise clients to observe for signs and symptoms and to notify the provider if they occur. • Administer the lowest effective dose.
Pancreatitis (nausea, vomiting, and abdominal pain)	• Advise clients to observe for signs and symptoms and to notify the provider immediately if they occur. • Monitor amylase levels. • Recognize that the medication will be discontinued if pancreatitis develops.
Thrombocytopenia	• Advise clients to observe for signs and symptoms such as bruising, and to notify the provider if these occur. • Monitor the client's platelet counts.
Teratogenesis	• Advise clients to avoid use in pregnancy.
Lamotrigine	
Common effects include double or blurred vision, dizziness, headache, nausea, and vomiting.	• Caution clients about performing activities requiring concentration.
Serious skin rashes including Stevens-Johnson syndrome	• Instruct clients to discontinue the medication and to notify the provider if a rash occurs.

 Contraindications/Precautions

- These medications are in Pregnancy Risk Category D and can result in birth defects.

- Carbamazepine is contraindicated in clients with bone marrow suppression or with bleeding disorders.

- Valproic acid is contraindicated in clients who have liver disorders.

Interactions

MEDICATION/FOOD INTERACTIONS	NURSING INTERVENTIONS/CLIENT EDUCATION
Carbamazepine	
• Carbamazepine decreases the effects of oral contraceptives and warfarin (Coumadin) because of stimulation of hepatic drug-metabolizing enzymes.	• Advise clients to use an alternate form of birth control. • Monitor for therapeutic effects of warfarin. • Administer adjusted dosages as prescribed.
• Grapefruit juice inhibits metabolism, thus increasing carbamazepine levels.	• Advise clients to avoid intake of grapefruit juice.
• Phenytoin and phenobarbital decrease the effects of carbamazepine by stimulating metabolism.	• Monitor phenytoin and phenobarbital levels. • Adjust dosage of medications as prescribed.
MEDICATION/FOOD INTERACTIONS	NURSING INTERVENTIONS/CLIENT EDUCATION
Valproic acid	
• Phenytoin and phenobarbital: Concurrent use with valproic acid increases the levels of these medications. • Combining valproic acid with topiramate (Topamax) may cause hyperammonemia and severe CNS effects.	• Monitor phenytoin and phenobarbital levels. • Adjust dosage of medications as prescribed. • Monitor ammonia levels. • Advise clients to notify the provider of symptoms.
Lamotrigine	
• Concurrent use of carbamazepine, phenytoin, and phenobarbital promotes liver drug-metabolizing enzymes, thereby decreasing the effect of lamotrigine.	• Monitor for therapeutic effects. • Administer adjusted dosages of medications as prescribed.
• Valproic acid: concurrent use inhibits medication-metabolizing enzymes and thus increases the half-life of lamotrigine.	• Monitor for adverse effects. • Adjust dosage of medications as prescribed.

Nursing Evaluation of Medication Effectiveness

- Depending on therapeutic intent, effectiveness may be evidenced by:

    o Relief of acute manic symptoms (flight of ideas, obsessive talking, agitation) or depressive symptoms (fatigue, poor appetite, psychomotor retardation)

    o Verbalizing improvement in mood

    o Ability to perform ADLs

    o Improved sleeping and eating habits

    o Greater interaction with peers

APPLICATION EXERCISES

1. A client who has been taking lithium carbonate (Eskalith) for several months, and whose mania has been stabilized, has a serum lithium level of 1.4 mEq/L. Which of the following manifestations should the nurse expect to find?

    A. Coarse tremors

    B. Muscle weakness

    C. Extreme polyuria

    D. Seizures

2. A client who started taking lithium carbonate a month ago tells the nurse she has just begun taking multiple daily doses of ibuprofen (Motrin) for tension headaches. Should the client avoid ibuprofen? Why or why not? What, if any, is the appropriate action for the nurse to take?

3. A nurse is caring for a client who has been taking lithium carbonate for almost a year. The nurse knows that the client's lithium carbonate levels should be monitored

    A. every 2-3 days.

    B. every 1-2 weeks.

    C. every 1-3 months.

    D. every 6 months.

4. A client has a prescription for valproic acid (Depakote). Which of the following laboratory values should the nurse anticipate monitoring for a client taking this medication? (Select all that apply.)

    _____ Thrombocyte count

    _____ WBC count

    _____ Amylase level

    _____ Liver function tests

    _____ Serum potassium level

APPLICATION EXERCISES ANSWER KEY

1. A client who has been taking lithium carbonate (Eskalith) for several months, and whose mania has been stabilized, has a serum lithium level of 1.4 mEq/L. Which of the following manifestations should the nurse expect to find?

   A. Coarse tremors

   B. Muscle weakness

   C. Extreme polyuria

   D. Seizures

   The therapeutic range for lithium in a client who has been taking the medication for some time is 0.4-1.0 mEq/L. Muscle weakness may occur as an early sign of lithium carbonate toxicity when the serum level is above the expected reference range but less than 1.5 mEq/L. Coarse tremors may occur at a lithium carbonate level of 1.5-2.0 mEq/L. Extreme polyuria and seizures may occur at a level of 2.0-2.5 mEq/L.

 NCLEX® Connection: Pharmacological Therapies, Medication Administration

2. A client who started taking lithium carbonate a month ago tells the nurse she has just begun taking multiple daily doses of ibuprofen (Motrin) for tension headaches. Should the client avoid ibuprofen? Why or why not? What, if any, is the appropriate action for the nurse to take?

   NSAIDs such as ibuprofen increase the renal reabsorption of lithium carbonate, possibly leading to lithium carbonate toxicity. Therefore, this client should avoid NSAIDs. The nurse should notify the provider about the client's headaches and ibuprofen use.

 NCLEX® Connection: Pharmacological Therapies, Adverse Effects/Contraindications/Side Effects/Interactions

3. A nurse is caring for a client who has been taking lithium carbonate for almost a year. The nurse knows that the client's lithium carbonate levels should be monitored

   A. every 2-3 days.

   B. every 1-2 weeks.

   C. every 1-3 months.

   D. every 6 months.

   After the client has been stabilized on lithium carbonate therapy, it is important that a lithium carbonate level be checked every 1-3 months. At the beginning of lithium carbonate therapy, levels are checked every 2-3 days.

 NCLEX® Connection: Pharmacological Therapies, Expected Actions/Outcomes

4. A client has a prescription for valproic acid (Depakote). Which of the following laboratory values should the nurse anticipate monitoring for a client taking this medication? (Select all that apply.)

X	**Thrombocyte count**
	WBC count
X	**Amylase level**
X	**Liver function tests**
	Serum potassium level

    Valproic acid may lead to thrombocytopenia, pancreatitis, or liver disease. The nurse should plan to monitor the thrombocyte count, amylase level, and liver function tests. Monitoring the WBC count and serum potassium level would not give information regarding an adverse effect of this medication.

 NCLEX® Connection: Pharmacological Therapies, Adverse Effects/Contraindications/Side Effects/Interactions

UNIT 2	MEDICATIONS AFFECTING THE NERVOUS SYSTEM
Chapter 10	Psychoses

 Overview

- Schizophrenia is the primary reason for the administration of antipsychotic medications.

  - The clinical course of schizophrenia usually involves acute exacerbations with intervals of semiremission.

  - Use medications to treat:

    - Positive symptoms related to behavior, thought, and speech (agitation, delusions, hallucinations, tangential speech patterns)

    - Negative symptoms (social withdrawal, lack of emotion, lack of energy [anergia], flattened affect, decreased motivation, decreased pleasure in activities)

  - The goals of psychopharmacological treatment for schizophrenia include:

    - Suppressing acute episodes

    - Preventing acute recurrence

    - Maintaining the highest possible level of functioning

- Conventional antipsychotic medications mainly control the positive symptoms, such as hallucinations, delusions, and bizarre behavior of psychosis. Use these medications for clients who are:

  - Using them successfully and can tolerate the side effects

  - Violent or particularly aggressive

- Atypical antipsychotic agents are medications of choice for clients receiving initial treatment and for treating breakthrough episodes in clients on conventional medication therapy, because they are more effective with fewer adverse effects.

  - Advantages of atypical antipsychotic agents include:

    - Relief of both the positive and negative symptoms of the disease

    - Decrease in affective symptoms (depression, anxiety) and suicidal behaviors

    - Improvement of neurocognitive defects, such as poor memory

    - Fewer or no extrapyramidal symptoms (EPS), including tardive dyskinesia (TD), because of less dopamine blockade

- Fewer anticholinergic adverse effects because most atypical antipsychotics, with the exception of clozapine (Clozaril), cause little or no blockade of cholinergic receptors
- Less relapse

MEDICATION CLASSIFICATION: ANTIPSYCHOTICS – CONVENTIONAL

- Select Prototype Medication – Chlorpromazine (Thorazine) – low potency
- Other Medications:
  - Haloperidol (Haldol) – High potency
  - Fluphenazine (Prolixin) – High potency
  - Thiothixene (Navane) – High potency

Purpose

- Expected Pharmacological Action
  - The conventional antipsychotic medications block dopamine (D_2), acetylcholine, histamine, and norepinephrine (NE) receptors in the brain and periphery.
  - Inhibition of psychotic symptoms is believed to be a result of D_2 blockade in the brain.
- Therapeutic Uses
  - Treatment of acute and chronic psychosis
  - Schizophrenia
  - Bipolar disorders (primarily the manic phase)
  - Tourette's syndrome
  - Delusional and schizoaffective disorders
  - Dementia
  - Prevention of nausea/vomiting through blocking of dopamine in the chemoreceptor trigger zone of the medulla

Complications

SIDE/ADVERSE EFFECTS	NURSING INTERVENTIONS/CLIENT EDUCATION
Acute dystonia: • Severe spasms of tongue, neck, face, or back. This is a crisis situation which requires rapid treatment.	• Begin to monitor for side effects anywhere between 5 hr to 5 days after administration of the first dose. • Treat with anticholinergic agents, such as benztropine (Cogentin) or diphenhydramine (Benadryl).
Parkinsonism • Bradykinesia, rigidity, shuffling gait, drooling and tremors	• Observe for signs and symptoms within 1 month of initiation of therapy. • Treat with benztropine, diphenhydramine, or amantadine (Symmetrel).
Akathisia • Inability to sit or stand still; Continual pacing and agitation	• Observe for signs and symptoms within 2 months of the initiation of treatment. • Manage symptoms with a beta-adrenergic blocker, benzodiazepine, or anticholinergic medication.
Late EPS, TD • Involuntary movements of the tongue and face, such as lip-smacking, which cause speech and/or eating disturbances • TD may also include involuntary movements of arms, legs, or trunk.	• Recognize that manifestations may occur months to years after the start of therapy, and may improve following medication change or may be permanent. • Administer the lowest dosage possible to control symptoms. • Evaluate clients after 12 months of therapy and then every 3 months. If signs of TD appear, tell clients the provider will decrease the dosage or prescribe a different medication. • Use the Abnormal Involuntary Movement Scale (AIMS) to screen for the presence of EPS.
Neuroleptic malignant syndrome • Sudden high-grade fever, blood pressure fluctuations, dysrhythmias, muscle rigidity, and change in level of consciousness developing into coma	• Stop antipsychotic medication. • Assist with transfer to medical unit for cooling measures, administration of dantrolene (Dantrium) and bromocriptine (Parlodel), maintenance of hydration and treatment of dysrhythmias. • Administer atypical agent as prescribed.

Anticholinergic effects
• Dry mouth
• Blurred vision
• Photophobia
• Urinary hesitancy/retention
• Constipation
• Tachycardia
	• Suggest these strategies to decrease anticholinergic effects:
	  ○ Chewing sugarless gum
	  ○ Sipping water
	  ○ Avoiding hazardous activities
	  ○ Wearing sunglasses when outdoors
	  ○ Eating foods high in fiber
	  ○ Participating in regular exercise
	  ○ Maintaining fluid intake of 2 to 3 L of water each day from food and beverage sources
	  ○ Voiding just before taking medication

SIDE/ADVERSE EFFECTS	NURSING INTERVENTIONS/CLIENT EDUCATION
Orthostatic hypotension	• Inform clients that they should develop tolerance in 2 to 3 months. • In the hospital setting, monitor the client's blood pressure and heart rate for orthostatic changes. If a significant decrease in blood pressure and/or increase in heart rate are noted, do not administer the medication, and notify the provider. • Instruct clients about the signs of orthostatic hypotension (lightheadedness, dizziness). Instruct clients to change positions slowly and to sit or lie down if symptoms occur.
Sedation	• Inform clients that effects should diminish within a few weeks. • Instruct clients to take this medication at bedtime to avoid daytime sleepiness. • Advise clients not to drive until sedation has subsided.
Neuroendocrine effects • Gynecomastia (breast enlargement), galactorrhea, and menstrual irregularities	• Advise clients to observe for manifestations and to notify the provider if these occur.
Seizures • The greatest risk for developing seizures is in clients with existing seizure disorders.	• Advise clients to report seizure activity to the provider. • Inform clients with a seizure disorder that an increase in antiseizure medication may be necessary.
Sexual dysfunction (common in both males and females)	• Advise clients of possible side effects. • Encourage clients to report side effects to the provider. Tell clients the provider may decrease the dosage or prescribe a different medication.
Skin effects • Effects include photosensitivity resulting in severe sunburn, and contact dermatitis from handling medications.	• Advise clients to avoid excessive exposure to sunlight, to use sunscreen, and to wear protective clothing. • Advise clients to avoid direct contact with medication.
Agranulocytosis	• Advise clients to observe for signs of infection (fever, sore throat), and to notify the provider if these occur. • If signs of infection appear, obtain the client's baseline WBC. Expect the provider to discontinue the medication if infection is present.
Prolongation of Q-T interval leading to fatal dysrhythmias with chlorpromazine or haloperidol	• Obtain the client's baseline ECG and serum potassium and magnesium levels prior to treatment and periodically throughout the treatment period. • Assist with maintaining serum potassium and magnesium levels within expected reference range.

Contraindications/Precautions

- These medications are contraindicated for clients in a coma, and clients who have severe depression, Parkinson's disease, prolactin-dependent cancer of the breast, and severe hypotension.

- Use of conventional antipsychotic medications is contraindicated in older clients with dementia.

- Use cautiously in clients with glaucoma, paralytic ileus, prostate enlargement, heart disorders, liver or kidney disease, and seizure disorders.

Interactions

MEDICATION/FOOD INTERACTIONS	NURSING INTERVENTIONS/CLIENT EDUCATION
Concurrent use of anticholinergic agents with these medications will increase anticholinergic effects.	• Advise clients to avoid over-the-counter medications that contain anticholinergic agents, such as sleep aids.
Alcohol, opioids, and antihistamines have additive CNS depressant effects.	• Advise clients to avoid alcohol and other medications that cause CNS depression. • Advise clients to avoid hazardous activities such as driving.
By activating dopamine receptors, levodopa counteracts the effects of antipsychotic agents.	• Avoid concurrent use of levodopa and other direct dopamine receptor agonists.
Tricyclic antidepressants, amiodarone (Cordarone), erythromycin (Biaxin) prolong QT and can further prolong QT interval with chlorpromazine or haloperidol	• Avoid concurrent use with other medications that prolong QT interval.

Nursing Administration

- Monitor clients to differentiate between EPS and worsening of psychotic disorder.

- Administer anticholinergics, beta-adrenergic blockers, and benzodiazepines to control early EPS. If symptoms are intolerable, the provider may prescribe a low-potency or an atypical antipsychotic agent.

- Advise clients that antipsychotic medications do not cause addiction.

- Advise clients to take medication as prescribed and to take it on a regular schedule.

- Advise clients that some therapeutic effects may be noticeable within a few days, but significant improvement may take 2 to 4 weeks, and possibly several months for full effects.

- Consider depot preparations administered IM once every 2 to 4 weeks for clients with difficulty maintaining medication regimen. Inform clients that lower doses can be used with depot preparations, which will decrease the risk of adverse effects and the development of tardive dyskinesia.

- Start administration with BID dosing, then switch to daily dosing at bedtime to decrease daytime drowsiness and promote sleep.

MEDICATION CLASSIFICATION: ANTIPSYCHOTICS – ATYPICAL

- Select Prototype Medication – Risperidone (Risperdal)

- Other Medications:

  o Olanzapine (Zyprexa)

  o Quetiapine (Seroquel)

  o Aripiprazole (Abilify)

  o Ziprasidone (Geodon)

  o Clozapine (Clozaril)

Purpose

- Expected Pharmacological Action

  o These antipsychotic agents work mainly by blocking serotonin, and to a lesser degree, dopamine receptors. These medications also block receptors for norepinephrine, histamine, and acetylcholine.

- Therapeutic Uses

  o Schizophrenia (negative and positive symptoms)

  o Psychosis induced by levodopa therapy

  o Relief of psychotic symptoms in other disorders such as bipolar disorders

Complications

SIDE/ADVERSE EFFECTS	NURSING INTERVENTIONS/CLIENT EDUCATION
New onset of diabetes mellitus or loss of glucose control in clients who have diabetes	• Obtain the client's baseline fasting blood glucose level and monitor throughout treatment. • Instruct clients to report symptoms (increased thirst, urination, and appetite).
Weight gain	• Advise clients to follow a healthy, low-calorie diet, engage in regular exercise, and monitor weight.
Hypercholesterolemia with increased risk for hypertension and other cardiovascular disease	• Monitor cholesterol, triglycerides, and blood glucose level if weight gain is greater than 14 kg (30 lb).
Orthostatic hypotension	• Monitor the client's blood pressure and heart rate for orthostatic changes. Instruct clients to change positions slowly.
Anticholinergic effects such as urinary hesitancy or retention, dry mouth	• Monitor for these effects and report their occurrence to the provider. • Educate clients about measures to relieve dry mouth, such as sipping fluids.
Agitation, dizziness, sedation, and sleep disruption	• Monitor for these effects and report to the provider if they occur. • Administer alternative medication if prescribed.
May cause mild EPS, such as tremor	• Monitor for and teach clients to recognize EPS. • Use AIMS test to screen for EPS.

 Contraindications/Precautions

- Risperidone is Pregnancy Risk Category C.

- Use is contraindicated for clients with dementia. Use of all atypical antipsychotic medications may cause death related to cerebrovascular accident or infection.

- Clients should avoid the use of alcohol.

- Use cautiously in clients who have cardiovascular or cerebrovascular disease, seizures, or diabetes mellitus. Obtain a fasting blood glucose level for clients who have diabetes mellitus, and monitor blood glucose carefully.

- Other atypical antipsychotic agents

MEDICATION	FORMULATIONS	COMPLICATIONS
Olanzapine	• Tablets • Oral solution • Short-acting injectable	• Olanzapine has a low risk of EPS. • Olanzapine has a high risk for diabetes, weight gain, and dyslipidemia. • Other adverse effects include sedation, orthostatic hypotension, and anticholinergic effects.
Quetiapine	• Tablets	• Quetiapine has a low risk of EPS. • Quetiapine has a moderate risk for diabetes, weight gain, and dyslipidemia. • Other effects include cataracts, sedation, orthostatic hypotension, and anticholinergic effects. • Clients should have screening eye exam and then every 6 months.
Aripiprazole	• Tablets • Oral solution	• Aripiprazole has low or no risk of EPS, diabetes, weight gain, dyslipidemia, hypotension, and anticholinergic effects. • Other adverse effects include headache, anxiety, insomnia, sedation, and gastrointestinal upset.
Ziprasidone • Affects both dopamine and serotonin; use for clients with concurrent depression	• Capsules • Short-acting injectable	• Ziprasidone has a low risk of EPS, diabetes, weight gain, and dyslipidemia. • Other effects include sedation, orthostatic hypotension, anticholinergic effects, and rash. • ECG changes and QT prolongation, which may lead to torsades de pointes.
Clozapine • The first atypical antipsychotic developed; no longer considered a first-line medication for schizophrenia because of its adverse effects	• Tablets	• Clozapine has a low risk of EPS. • High risk of weight gain, diabetes, and dyslipidemia. • Agranulocytosis may occur. Obtain the client's baseline WBC and then monitor weekly. • Monitor clients for signs of infection (fever, sore throat, lesions in mouth), and notify the provider if symptoms occur. • Other adverse effects include sedation, orthostatic hypotension, and anticholinergic effects.

Interactions

MEDICATION/FOOD INTERACTIONS	NURSING INTERVENTIONS/CLIENT EDUCATION
Immunosuppressive medications, such as anticancer medications, can further suppress immune function in clients taking clozapine.	• Avoid use in clients taking clozapine.
Alcohol, opioids, and antihistamines have additive CNS depressant effects.	• Advise clients to avoid alcohol and other medications that cause CNS depression. • Advise clients to avoid hazardous activities, such as driving.
By activating dopamine receptors, levodopa counteracts the effects of antipsychotic agents.	• Avoid concurrent use of levodopa and other direct dopamine receptor agonists.
Tricyclic antidepressants, amiodarone (Cordarone), and clarithromycin (Biaxin) prolong QT interval and thus increase the risk of cardiac dysrhythmias in clients taking ziprasidone.	• Use is contraindicated with ziprasidone
Barbiturates and phenytoin (Dilantin) stimulate hepatic medication-metabolizing enzymes and thereby decrease drug levels of aripiprazole, quetiapine, and ziprasidone.	• Monitor medication effectiveness.
Fluconazole (Diflucan) inhibits hepatic medication-metabolizing enzymes and thereby increases levels of aripiprazole, quetiapine, and ziprasidone	• Monitor medication effectiveness.

Nursing Administration

- Administer by oral or IM route. Risperidone is also available as a depot injection administered IM once every 2 weeks. Use for clients with difficulty adhering to medication regimen. Therapeutic effect occurs 4 to 6 weeks after the first depot injection.

- Advise clients that low doses of medication are given initially and are then gradually increased.

- Use oral disintegrating tablets for clients who may attempt to "cheek" (or pocket) tablets or have difficulty swallowing them.

Nursing Evaluation of Medication Effectiveness

- Depending on therapeutic intent, effectiveness may be evidenced by:

    o Improvement of symptoms (prevention of acute psychotic symptoms, absence of hallucinations, delusions, anxiety, and hostility)

    o Improvement in ability to perform ADLs

    o Improvement in ability to interact socially with peers

    o Improvement of sleeping and eating habits

APPLICATION EXERCISES

1. A nurse is caring for a client who takes chlorpromazine (Thorazine) for schizophrenia. For which of the following symptoms should the nurse expect to see improvement? (Choose all that apply)

   _____ Poverty of speech

   _____ Bizarre behavior

   _____ Impaired social interactions

   _____ Hallucinations

   _____ Decreased motivation

2. A nurse is reinforcing teaching for a client who has a new prescription for olanzapine (Zyprexa). Which of the following practices should the client be taught about in order to prevent a common adverse effect of olanzapine?

   A. Increasing daily exercise

   B. Preventing exposure to sunlight

   C. Avoiding a low-sodium diet

   D. Taking afternoon naps

3. A client has been taking chlorpromazine (Thorazine) for several years for paranoid schizophrenia. Which of the following recent manifestations should lead the nurse to suspect that the client is developing tardive dyskinesia?

   A. Hand tremors

   B. Shuffling gait

   C. Painful neck spasms

   D. Lip-smacking

4. A nurse is caring for a client who has a new prescription for clozapine (Clozaril). The nurse will be monitoring the client's WBC count results every two weeks. For what reason is the WBC monitored in this client?

APPLICATION EXERCISES ANSWER KEY

1. A nurse is caring for a client who takes chlorpromazine (Thorazine) for schizophrenia. For which of the following symptoms should the nurse expect to see improvement? (Choose all that apply)

    _X_ **Poverty of speech**

    _X_ **Bizarre behavior**

    _____ Impaired social interactions

    _X_ **Hallucinations**

    _____ Decreased motivation

    A client taking a conventional antipsychotic medication, such as chlorpromazine, should see improvement in positive symptoms such as poverty of speech, bizarre behavior and hallucinations. Chlorpromazine is not very effective for negative symptoms such as impaired social interactions and decreased motivation.

     NCLEX® Connection: Pharmacological Therapies, Expected Actions/Outcomes

2. A nurse is reinforcing teaching for a client who has a new prescription for olanzapine (Zyprexa). Which of the following practices should the client be taught about in order to prevent a common adverse effect of olanzapine?

    A. Increasing daily exercise

    B. Preventing exposure to sunlight

    C. Avoiding a low-sodium diet

    D. Taking afternoon naps

    Increasing daily exercise is a strategy important for a client who takes olanzapine because weight gain, diabetes, and hypercholesterolemia are common adverse effects of this medication. Preventing exposure to sunlight, avoiding a low-sodium diet, and taking afternoon naps will not help prevent adverse effects of this medication.

     NCLEX® Connection: Pharmacological Therapies, Adverse Effects/Contraindications/Side Effects/Interactions

3. A client has been taking chlorpromazine (Thorazine) for several years for paranoid schizophrenia. Which of the following recent manifestations should lead the nurse to suspect that the client is developing tardive dyskinesia?

   A. Hand tremors

   B. Shuffling gait

   C. Painful neck spasms

   D. Lip-smacking

   Involuntary twisting or writhing movements of the face or tongue, including lip-smacking, are early manifestations of tardive dyskinesia, which usually occurs months or years after beginning therapy with a traditional antipsychotic medication. Hand tremors and shuffling gait are manifestations of Parkinsonism, which can occur early in therapy with a traditional antipsychotic medication. Painful neck spasms are manifestations of dystonia, which usually occurs within hours or days following initiation of therapy with a traditional antipsychotic medication.

    NCLEX® Connection: Pharmacological Therapies, Adverse Effects/Contraindications/Side Effects/Interactions

4. A nurse is caring for a client who has a new prescription for clozapine (Clozaril). The nurse will be monitoring the client's WBC count results every two weeks. For what reason is the WBC monitored in this client?

   Clozapine may cause the rare, but very serious adverse effect of agranulocytosis during the first six months of therapy. The nurse should monitor lab results for a decrease in the normal white blood count.

    NCLEX® Connection: Pharmacological Therapies, Adverse Effects/Contraindications/Side Effects/Interactions

UNIT 2	MEDICATIONS AFFECTING THE NERVOUS SYSTEM
Chapter 11	Behavioral Disorders

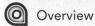 Overview

- Use various medications to manage behavioral disorders in children and adolescents. Reinforce to parents that pharmacological management should be accompanied by behavioral modification techniques.

- Medications include selective serotonin reuptake inhibitors, tricyclic antidepressants, antipsychotics, nonbarbiturate anxiolytics, CNS stimulants, and norepinephrine selective reuptake inhibitors.

MEDICATION CLASSIFICATION: SELECTIVE SEROTONIN REUPTAKE INHIBITORS (SSRIS)

- Select Prototype Medication – Fluoxetine (Prozac)

- Other Medications:

  o Citalopram (Celexa)

  o Escitalopram (Lexapro)

  o Paroxetine (Paxil)

  o Sertraline (Zoloft)

Purpose

- Expected Pharmacological Action

  o SSRIs selectively block reuptake of the monoamine neurotransmitter serotonin in the synaptic space, thereby intensifying the effects that can be produced.

- Therapeutic Uses

  o Major depression

  o Bulimia nervosa

  o Panic, school phobia, separation anxiety disorder

  o Posttraumatic stress disorder (PTSD)

  o Obsessive compulsive disorder (OCD)

  o Attention-deficit hyperactivity disorder (ADHD) in children (and adults)

Complications

SIDE/ADVERSE EFFECTS	NURSING INTERVENTIONS/CLIENT EDUCATION
CNS stimulation (inability to sleep, agitation, anxiety)	• Advise clients and families to notify provider as dose may need to be lowered. • Advise clients to take dose in the morning. • Advise clients to avoid chocolate and caffeinated beverages. • Suggest relaxation exercises to promote sleep.
Weight loss early in therapy, may be followed by weight gain with long-term treatment	• Monitor the client's weight. • Encourage clients to participate in regular exercise and to follow a healthy, well-balanced diet. • Assist clients with maintaining appropriate weight.
Serotonin syndrome may begin 2 to 72 hr after starting treatment and it can be lethal. Symptoms include: • Mental confusion, difficulty concentrating • Agitation • Anxiety • Hallucinations • Incoordination, hyperreflexia • Tremors • Fever • Diaphoresis	• Advise clients and families to observe for symptoms and to notify the provider immediately and stop the medication if symptoms occur.
Withdrawal syndrome (headache, nausea, visual disturbances, anxiety)	• Reinforce to clients and families how to slowly taper the medication dosage after a long period of use to avoid withdrawal symptoms.
Rash	• Advise clients and families to treat a rash with an antihistamine and to notify the provider.
Sleepiness, faintness, lightheadedness	• Advise clients that these side effects are not common, but can occur.
Gastrointestinal (GI) bleeding	• Use caution with clients with history of GI bleeding and ulcers, and with clients taking other medications that affect blood coagulation.

Bruxism	• Advise clients to report to the provider, who may:
	  ○ Switch clients to another class of medication
	  ○ Treat bruxism with low-dose buspirone
	• Advise clients to use mouthguard during sleep.

Contraindications/Precautions

- Contraindicated in clients taking MAOIs and tricyclic antidepressants (TCAs).

- Use cautiously in clients with liver and renal dysfunction, cardiac disease, seizure disorders, diabetes, ulcers, and a history of GI bleeding.

Interactions

MEDICATION/FOOD INTERACTIONS	NURSING INTERVENTIONS/CLIENT EDUCATION
MAOIs and TCAs - concurrent use increases the risk of serotonin syndrome.	• Avoid concurrent use.
Fluoxetine can displace warfarin (Coumadin) from bound protein and result in increased warfarin levels.	• Monitor the client's prothrombin time (PT) and INR levels. • Check clients for signs of bleeding and administer new dosage as prescribed.
Fluoxetine can increase the levels of TCAs and lithium.	• Avoid concurrent use.
Fluoxetine suppresses platelet aggregation and thus increases the risk of bleeding when used concurrently with NSAIDs and anticoagulants.	• Advise clients and families to monitor for signs of bleeding (bruising, hematuria) and to notify the provider if they occur.

Nursing Administration

- Check use of alcohol and other CNS depressants, especially with adolescents.

- Instruct clients to take medication with food to decrease GI distress.

- Encourage clients and families to administer the medication in the morning to minimize sleep disturbances.

- Instruct clients and families to administer the medication on a daily basis to establish therapeutic plasma levels.

- Suggest weekly dosing for clients with difficulty adhering to the medication regimen.

- Assist clients with adherence by informing them that therapeutic effects may not be experienced for 1 to 3 weeks.

- Instruct clients and families to continue therapy after improvement in symptoms. Sudden discontinuation of medication can result in relapse.

Nursing Evaluation of Medication Effectiveness

- Depending on therapeutic intent, effectiveness may be evidenced by the following:

  o For depression:

    ▪ Verbalizing improvement in mood

    ▪ Improved sleeping and eating habits

    ▪ Increased interaction with peers

  o For ADHD:

    ▪ Decreased hyperactivity

    ▪ Increased level of concentration

MEDICATION CLASSIFICATION: TRICYCLIC ANTIDEPRESSANTS (TCAS)

- Select Prototype Medication – Amitriptyline (Elavil)

- Other Medications:

  o Imipramine (Tofranil)

  o Clomipramine (Anafranil)

  o Nortriptyline (Aventyl)

Purpose

- Expected Pharmacological Action

  o These medications block reuptake of the monoamine neurotransmitters norepinephrine and serotonin in the synaptic space, thereby intensifying the effects that these neurotransmitters produce.

- Therapeutic Uses

  o Depression

  o Depressive episodes of bipolar disorders

  o Autistic disorder

  o ADHD

  o Panic, school phobia, separation anxiety disorder

  o PTSD

  o OCD

Complications

SIDE/ADVERSE EFFECTS	NURSING INTERVENTIONS/CLIENT EDUCATION
Orthostatic hypotension	o Monitor blood pressure with first dose. Instruct clients to change positions slowly.
Anticholinergic effects • Dry mouth • Blurred vision • Photophobia • Urinary hesitancy or retention • Constipation • Tachycardia	• Instruct clients and families about ways to minimize anticholinergic effects. These include: o Chewing sugarless gum o Sipping on water o Avoiding hazardous activities o Wearing sunglasses when outdoors o Eating foods high in fiber o Participating in regular exercise o Increasing fluid intake to at least 2 to 3 L/day from beverages or food sources o Voiding just before taking medication • Advise clients and families to notify the provider if symptoms are intolerable.
Weight gain	• Monitor the client's weight. • Encourage clients to participate in regular exercise and to follow a healthy, low-caloric diet.
Sedation	• Advise clients that this side effect usually diminishes over time. • Advise clients to avoid hazardous activities such as driving if sedation is excessive. • Advise clients and families to administer the medication at bedtime to minimize daytime sleepiness and to promote sleep.
Toxicity resulting in cholinergic blockade and cardiac toxicity evidenced by dysrhythmias, mental confusion, and agitation, followed by seizures and coma	• Give clients who are acutely ill a 1-week supply of medication. • Obtain the client's baseline ECG. • Monitor vital signs frequently. • Monitor clients for signs of toxicity and notify the provider if signs of toxicity occur.
Decreased seizure threshold	• Monitor clients who have seizure disorders.
Excessive sweating	• Inform clients of this side effect.

 Contraindications/Precautions

- Use cautiously in clients who have seizure disorders; diabetes; liver, kidney and respiratory disorders; and hyperthyroidism.

Interactions

MEDICATION/FOOD INTERACTIONS	NURSING INTERVENTIONS/CLIENT EDUCATION
Concurrent use of monoamine oxidase inhibitors (MAOIs) may cause hypertension.	Avoid concurrent use with TCAs.
Antihistamines and other anticholinergic agents have additive anticholinergic effects.	Avoid concurrent use with TCAs.
Alcohol, benzodiazepines, opioids, and antihistamines cause additive CNS depression when used concurrently.	Advise clients to avoid other CNS depressants.

Nursing Administration

- Instruct clients and families to administer the medication as prescribed on a daily basis to establish therapeutic serum levels.

- Assist with the client's medication regimen adherence by informing the client that therapeutic effects may not be experienced for 1 to 3 weeks. Full therapeutic effects may take 2 to 3 months.

- Instruct clients and families to continue therapy after improvement in symptoms. Sudden discontinuation of the medication can result in relapse.

Nursing Evaluation of Medication Effectiveness

- Depending on therapeutic intent, effectiveness may be evidenced by the following:

  o For depression:

    - Verbalizing improvement in mood

    - Improved sleeping and eating habits

    - Increased interaction with peers

  o For autistic disorder – Decreased anger and compulsive behavior

  o For ADHD – Decreased hyperactivity, increased level of concentration

MEDICATION CLASSIFICATION: ATYPICAL ANXIOLYTIC: NONBARBITURATE ANXIOLYTIC

- Select Prototype Medication – Buspirone (BuSpar)

Purpose

- Expected Pharmacological Action

  o The exact anti-anxiety mechanism of this medication is unknown. Buspirone binds to serotonin and dopamine receptors. There is no potential for abuse, and use of buspirone does not result in sedation or potentiate the effects of other CNS depressants.

- Therapeutic Uses

  o Panic disorder, obsessive-compulsive disorder, social anxiety disorder, and post-traumatic stress disorder

Complications

SIDE/ADVERSE EFFECTS	NURSING INTERVENTIONS/CLIENT EDUCATION
CNS effects (dizziness, nausea, headache, light-headedness, agitation)	• Advise clients to take with food to decrease nausea. • Instruct clients that most side effects are self-limiting.

 Contraindications/Precautions

- Buspirone is contraindicated for concurrent use with MAOI antidepressants or for 14 days after MAOIs are discontinued. Hypertensive crisis may result.

Interactions

MEDICATION/FOOD INTERACTIONS	NURSING INTERVENTIONS/CLIENT EDUCATION
Erythromycin, ketoconazole, and grapefruit juice increase the effects of buspirone.	• Take complete medication history. • Advise clients to avoid drinking grapefruit juice.

Nursing Administration

- Advise clients to take the medication with meals to prevent gastric irritation.

- Advise clients and families that effects do not occur rapidly and may take a week to start, and several more weeks for the full benefit to be felt.

- Advise clients and families to administer the medication on a regular basis and not PRN.

Nursing Evaluation of Medication Effectiveness

- Depending on therapeutic intent, effectiveness may be evidenced by the following:

  o For depression:

   ▪ Verbalizing improvement in mood

   ▪ Improved sleeping and eating habits

   ▪ Increased interaction with peers

  o For anxiety disorders:

   ▪ Decrease in anxiety symptoms

   ▪ Improvement in functioning

MEDICATION CLASSIFICATION: CNS STIMULANTS

- Select Prototypes and Other Medications

MEDICATION	SHORT-ACTING	INTERMEDIATE-ACTING	LONG-ACTING
Methylphenidate	Ritalin, Methylin	Ritalin SR, Methylin ER	Ritalin LA, Concerta, Daytrana (transdermal)
Dexmethylphenidate	Focalin		
Dextroamphetamine	DextroStat		Dexedrine Spansule
Amphetamine mixture	Adderall		Adderall-XR

Purpose

- Expected Pharmacological Action

  o These medications raise the levels of norepinephrine, serotonin, and dopamine into the CNS.

- Therapeutic Uses

  o ADHD

  o Conduct disorder

Complications

SIDE/ADVERSE EFFECTS	NURSING INTERVENTIONS/CLIENT EDUCATION
CNS stimulation (insomnia, restlessness)	• Advise clients and families to observe for symptoms and notify the provider if they occur. • Administer the last dose of the day before 4 p.m.
Weight loss, possible growth suppression	• Monitor the client's height and weight and compare to baseline height and weight. • Administer medication immediately before, with, or right after meals. • Promote good nutrition. • Encourage children and adolescents to eat at regular meal times and avoid unhealthy foods for snacks.
Cardiovascular effects (dysrhythmias, chest pain, high blood pressure) • These medications may increase the risk of sudden death in clients with heart abnormalities.	• Monitor the client's vital signs and ECG. • Advise clients and families to observe for symptoms and to notify the provider if they occur.

SIDE/ADVERSE EFFECTS	NURSING INTERVENTIONS/CLIENT EDUCATION
Development of psychotic symptoms such as hallucinations, paranoia	• Instruct clients and families to report symptoms immediately and to discontinue the medication if they occur.
Withdrawal reaction	• Advise clients not to stop taking medication suddenly. Doing so may lead to depression and severe fatigue.
Hypersensitivity skin reaction to transdermal methylphenidate (hives, papules)	• Remove the patch and notify the provider.

 Contraindications/Precautions

- These medications are contraindicated in clients who have a history of drug abuse, cardiovascular disorders, severe anxiety, and psychosis.

Interactions

MEDICATION/FOOD INTERACTIONS	NURSING INTERVENTIONS/CLIENT EDUCATION
Concurrent use of MAOIs may cause hypertensive crisis.	• Avoid concurrent use.
Concurrent use of caffeine may increase CNS stimulant effects.	• Instruct clients to avoid foods that contain caffeine.
Methylphenidate inhibits metabolism of phenytoin (Dilantin), warfarin (Coumadin), and phenobarbital, leading to increased serum levels.	• Monitor clients for adverse effects (CNS depression, signs of bleeding). • Concurrent use of these medications should be used cautiously.
OTC cold and decongestant medications with sympathomimetic action can increase CNS stimulant effects.	• Instruct clients and families to avoid use of OTC medications.

Nursing Administration

- Advise clients to swallow sustained-release tablets whole and to not chew or crush the tablets.

- Reinforce to clients and families the importance of administering the medication on a regular schedule.

- Reinforce to clients who use transdermal medication (Daytrana) to place the patch on one hip daily in the morning and leave it in place no longer than 9 hr. Alternate hips daily.

- Instruct clients and families that ADHD is not cured by medication and that an overall treatment plan should include family therapy and cognitive therapy.

- Instruct families that these medications have special handling procedures controlled by federal law. Medication refills require handwritten prescriptions.

- Instruct families in safety and storage of medications.

- Advise clients and families that these medications have a high potential for abuse.

Nursing Evaluation of Medication Effectiveness

- Depending on therapeutic intent, effectiveness may be evidenced by:

    o Improvement of symptoms of ADHD, such as increased ability to focus and complete tasks, to interact with peers, and to manage impulsivity

    o Improved ability to stay awake

MEDICATION CLASSIFICATION: NOREPINEPHRINE SELECTIVE REUPTAKE INHIBITOR

- Select Prototype Medication – Atomoxetine (Strattera)

Purpose

- Expected Pharmacological Action

    o Blocks reuptake of norepinephrine at synapses in the CNS. Atomoxetine is not a stimulant medication.

- Therapeutic Uses

    o ADHD

Complications

- Atomoxetine is usually tolerated well with minimal side effects.

SIDE/ADVERSE EFFECTS	NURSING INTERVENTIONS/CLIENT EDUCATION
Appetite suppression, weight loss, growth suppression	<ul><li>Monitor the client's height and weight and compare to baseline height and weight.</li><li>Administer medication immediately before, with, or right after meals.</li><li>Encourage children and adolescents to eat at regular meal times and avoid unhealthy foods for snacks.</li></ul>
GI effects (nausea and vomiting)	<ul><li>Advise client to take with food if these occur.</li></ul>
Suicidal ideation (in children and adolescents)	<ul><li>Monitor clients for signs of depression.</li><li>Advise clients and families to report change in mood, excessive sleeping, agitation, and irritability.</li></ul>
Hepatotoxicity	<ul><li>Advise client to report signs of liver damage (flu-like symptoms, yellowing skin, abdominal pain).</li></ul>

Contraindications/Precautions

- Use cautiously in clients with cardiovascular disorders.

Medication/Food Interactions

MEDICATION/FOOD INTERACTIONS	NURSING INTERVENTIONS
• Concurrent use of MAOIs may cause hypertensive crisis.	• Avoid concurrent use within 2 weeks of each other.
• Paroxetine (Paxil), fluoxetine (Prozac), or quinidine gluconate (Quinaglute Dura-tabs) inhibit hepatic metabolizing enzymes, thereby increasing levels of atomoxetine.	• Instruct clients and families to watch for and report increased adverse reactions of atomoxetine. • Concurrent use may require a reduction in the dosage of atomoxetine.

Nursing Administration

- Note any changes in the child's behavior related to dosing and timing of medications.

- Administer the medication in a daily dose in the morning, or in two divided doses, morning and afternoon, with or without food.

- Instruct clients that effects may take at least 1 week to fully develop.

Nursing Evaluation of Medication Effectiveness

- Depending on therapeutic intent, effectiveness may be evidenced by:

  o Improvement of symptoms of ADHD, such as increase in ability to focus and complete tasks, interact with peers, and manage impulsivity.

MEDICATION CLASSIFICATION: ANTIPSYCHOTICS – ATYPICAL

- Select Prototype Medication – Risperidone (Risperdal)

- Other Medications:

  o Olanzapine (Zyprexa)

  o Quetiapine (Seroquel)

Purpose

- Expected Pharmacological Action

  o These antipsychotic agents work mainly by blocking serotonin, and to a lesser degree, dopamine receptors. These medications also block receptors for norepinephrine, histamine, and acetylcholine.

- Therapeutic Uses
  - Pervasive development disorders (PDD) including autistic disorder
  - Conduct disorder
  - Post-Traumatic Stress Disorder (PTSD)
  - Relief of psychotic symptoms

Complications

SIDE/ADVERSE EFFECTS	NURSING INTERVENTIONS/CLIENT EDUCATION
Onset of diabetes or loss of glucose control in clients with diabetes	• Obtain the client's baseline fasting blood glucose level and monitor periodically throughout treatment. • Instruct clients and families to report symptoms such as increased thirst, urination, and appetite.
Weight gain	• Advise clients to follow a healthy, low-caloric diet, engage in regular exercise, and monitor weight gain.
Hypercholesterolemia with increased risk for hypertension and other cardiovascular disease	• Monitor cholesterol, triglycerides, and blood glucose if weight gain is more than 14 kg (30.8 lb).
Orthostatic hypotension	• Monitor blood pressure with first dose. Instruct clients to change positions slowly.
Anticholinergic effects (urinary hesitancy or retention, dry mouth)	• Encourage client to use measures to relieve dry mouth such as sipping fluids throughout the day.
Agitation, dizziness, sedation, and sleep disruption	• Administer an alternative medication if prescribed.
May cause mild extrapyramidal side effects, such as tremor	• Monitor for and instruct clients and families to recognize extrapyramidal side effects. These are usually dose-related.

 Contraindications/Precautions

- Clients should avoid the use of alcohol.

- Use cautiously in clients with cardiovascular disease, seizures, or diabetes mellitus. Obtain a baseline fasting blood glucose level for clients with diabetes mellitus and monitor blood glucose level closely.

Interactions

MEDICATION/FOOD INTERACTIONS	NURSING INTERVENTIONS/CLIENT EDUCATION
• Alcohol, opioids, and antihistamines cause additive CNS depressant effects.	• Advise clients to avoid alcohol • Advise clients to avoid hazardous activities, such as driving.
• Barbiturates and phenytoin (Dilantin) promote hepatic drug-metabolizing enzymes, thereby decreasing drug levels of quetiapine.	• Monitor medication effectiveness.
• Medications that inhibit CYP3A4, such as fluconazole (Diflucan), inhibit hepatic drug-metabolizing enzymes, thereby increasing drug levels of aripiprazole, quetiapine, and ziprasidone.	• Monitor for adverse effects.

Nursing Administration

- Administer by oral or IM route (risperidone and olanzapine).

- Advise clients that low doses of medication are given initially and are then gradually increased.

Nursing Evaluation of Medication Effectiveness

- Depending on therapeutic intent, effectiveness may be evidenced by the following:

   o For PDD: Reduction of hyperactivity and improvement in mood

   o For conduct disorder: Decrease in aggressiveness

   o For PTSD:

      ▪ Decrease in aggressiveness and reduction of flashbacks

      ▪ Improvement of psychotic symptoms (prevention of acute psychotic symptoms and absence of hallucinations, delusions, anxiety, and hostility)

      ▪ Improvement in ability to perform ADLs

      ▪ Improvement in ability to interact socially with peers

      ▪ Improvement of sleeping and eating habits

APPLICATION EXERCISES

1. A nurse is caring for an adolescent in an inpatient facility who has been diagnosed with major depressive disorder. The client has just begun taking a new prescription for fluoxetine (Prozac). What changes in the client's weight should the nurse expect to see while he takes fluoxetine?

2. A nurse is caring for an adolescent client who is taking amitriptyline (Elavil) for depression. For which of the following should the nurse monitor this client while taking amitriptyline?

   A. Diarrhea

   B. Bradycardia

   C. Increased salivation

   D. Urinary hesitation

3. A nurse is caring for a school-age child who recently began a prescription for atomoxetine (Strattera). For which of the following should the nurse monitor the child?

   A. Pale-colored urine

   B. Upper abdominal tenderness

   C. Seizure activity

   D. Blurred vision

4. A nurse is reinforcing teaching for a school-age child and his parents regarding the proper use of methylphenidate (Daytrana) transdermal patch. Which of the following statements by the child demonstrates appropriate understanding of the teaching?

   A. "I will change to a new patch every other day right after breakfast."

   B. "I will take the old patch off every morning before breakfast and put on a new patch."

   C. "I will take the patch off no more than 9 hours after putting it on every day."

   D. "I will change the patch once every week."

5. A child experiencing psychotic symptoms is beginning a new prescription for risperidone (Risperdal). The nurse plans to monitor periodic results of which of the following laboratory values while the client takes the medication?

   A. WBC count

   B. Hgb and HCT

   C. Fasting blood glucose

   D. Serum sodium

APPLICATION EXERCISES ANSWER KEY

1. A nurse is caring for an adolescent in an inpatient facility who has been diagnosed with major depressive disorder. The client has just begun taking a new prescription for fluoxetine (Prozac). What changes in the client's weight should the nurse expect to see while he takes fluoxetine?

    Fluoxetine may cause an initial loss of weight, but over a long course of therapy with this medication, weight gain may occur. It is important for the nurse to monitor the client's weight throughout therapy and to encourage good nutritional habits.

 NCLEX® Connection: Pharmacological Therapies, Adverse Effects/Contraindications/Side Effects/Interactions

2. A nurse is caring for an adolescent client who is taking amitriptyline (Elavil) for depression. For which of the following should the nurse monitor this client while taking amitriptyline?

    A. Diarrhea

    B. Bradycardia

    C. Increased salivation

    D. Urinary hesitation

    Urinary hesitation or retention is an anticholinergic adverse effect which may occur in clients taking amitriptyline. Other possible anticholinergic effects include constipation (not diarrhea), tachycardia (not bradycardia), and dry month (not increased salivation).

 NCLEX® Connection: Pharmacological Therapies, Adverse Effects/Contraindications/Side Effects/Interactions

3. A nurse is caring for a school-age child who recently began a prescription for atomoxetine (Strattera). For which of the following should the nurse monitor the child?

    A. Pale-colored urine

    B. Upper abdominal tenderness

    C. Seizure activity

    D. Blurred vision

    Liver damage may occur while taking atomoxetine and the nurse should monitor for signs such as upper abdominal tenderness, jaundice, and elevated liver enzymes. Darkening of urine, rather than pale-colored urine, may occur from liver damage. Seizures and blurred vision are not adverse effects of atomoxetine.

 NCLEX® Connection: Pharmacological Therapies, Adverse Effects/Contraindications/Side Effects/Interactions

4. A nurse is reinforcing teaching for a school-age child and his parents regarding the proper use of methylphenidate (Daytrana) transdermal patch. Which of the following statements by the child demonstrates appropriate understanding of the teaching?

    A. "I will change to a new patch every other day right after breakfast."

    B. "I will take the old patch off every morning before breakfast and put on a new patch."

    C. "I will take the patch off no more than 9 hours after putting it on every day."

    D. "I will change the patch once every week."

To prevent interfering with sleep, instruct clients and families to remove the methylphenidate transdermal patch no longer than 9 hours after it is applied every day.

 NCLEX® Connection: Pharmacological Therapies, Medication Administration

5. A child experiencing psychotic symptoms is beginning a new prescription for risperidone (Risperdal). The nurse plans to monitor periodic results of which of the following laboratory values while the client takes the medication?

    A. WBC count

    B. Hgb and HCT

    C. Fasting blood glucose

    D. Serum sodium

Use of risperidone over time can cause elevated blood glucose and diabetes mellitus. The nurse should plan to monitor this laboratory value throughout treatment with risperidone. WBC count, Hgb and HCT, and serum sodium do not need to be monitored for a client taking risperidone.

 NCLEX® Connection: Pharmacological Therapies, Adverse Effects/Contraindications/Side Effects/Interactions

UNIT 2	MEDICATIONS AFFECTING THE NERVOUS SYSTEM

Chapter 12   Substance Abuse

 Overview

- Abstinence syndrome occurs when a client abruptly withdraws from a drug on which he is physically dependent.

- Symptoms of abstinence syndrome can be distressing and may lead to coma and death.

- Major Drugs of Abuse

SUBSTANCE	WITHDRAWAL SYMPTOMS
Alcohol	• Effects usually start within 4 to 12 hr of the last intake of alcohol, peak after 24 to 48 hr and then subside within 5 to 7 days unless alcohol withdrawal delirium occurs. • Symptoms include nausea; vomiting; tremors; restlessness and inability to sleep; depressed mood or irritability; increased heart rate, blood pressure, respiratory rate, and temperature; diaphoresis and tonic-clonic seizures. Illusions are also common. • Alcohol withdrawal delirium may occur 2 to 3 days after cessation of alcohol, may last 2 to 3 days, and is considered a medical emergency. Findings include severe disorientation, psychotic symptoms (hallucinations), severe hypertension, and cardiac dysrhythmias that may progress to death.
Opioids, including heroin and prescription medications	• Characteristic withdrawal syndrome occurs within 1 hr to several days of cessation of drug use. • Symptoms include agitation, insomnia, flu-like symptoms, rhinorrhea, yawning, sweating, and diarrhea. • Symptoms are non-life-threatening, although suicidal ideation may occur.
Nicotine	• Abstinence syndrome is evidenced by irritability, nervousness, restlessness, insomnia, and difficulty concentrating.

MEDICATIONS TO SUPPORT WITHDRAWAL/ABSTINENCE FROM ALCOHOL

Detoxification

INTENDED EFFECTS	NURSING INTERVENTIONS/CLIENT EDUCATION
Benzodiazepines: chlordiazepoxide (Librium), diazepam (Valium), lorazepam (Ativan)	
• Maintenance of the client's vital signs within expected reference range • Decrease in the risk of seizures and delirium tremens • Decrease in the intensity of symptoms	• Obtain the client's baseline vital signs. • Monitor the client's vital signs and neurological status on an ongoing basis. • Provide for seizure precautions (padded side rails and suction equipment at bedside).
Adjunct medications: carbamazepine (Tegretol), clonidine (Catapres), propranolol (Inderal)	
• Decrease in seizures 　○ Carbamazepine • Depression of autonomic response (decrease in blood pressure, heart rate, and diaphoresis) 　○ Clonidine and propranolol • Decrease in cravings 　○ Propranolol	• Provide for seizure precautions (padded side rails and suction equipment at bedside). • Obtain the client's baseline vital signs and continue to monitor on a regular basis.

Abstinence Maintenance (Following Detoxification)

INTENDED EFFECTS	NURSING INTERVENTIONS/CLIENT EDUCATION
Disulfiram (Antabuse)	
• Disulfiram is a daily oral medication that is a type of aversion (behavioral) therapy. • Using disulfiram concurrently with alcohol will cause acetaldehyde syndrome to occur. • Effects include nausea, vomiting, weakness, sweating, palpitations, and hypotension. • Acetaldehyde syndrome can progress to respiratory depression, cardiovascular suppression, seizures, and death.	• Inform clients of the potential dangers of drinking any alcohol. • Advise clients to avoid any products that contain alcohol (cough syrups, aftershave lotion). • Encourage clients to wear a medical alert bracelet. • Encourage clients to participate in a 12-step self-help program. • Advise clients that medication effects (potential for acetaldehyde syndrome with alcohol ingestion) persist for 2 weeks following discontinuation of disulfiram.

INTENDED EFFECTS	NURSING INTERVENTIONS/CLIENT EDUCATION
Naltrexone (ReVia)	
Naltrexone is a pure opioid antagonist that suppresses the craving and pleasurable effects of alcohol (also used for opioid withdrawal).	• Obtain an accurate history to determine if clients are also dependent on opioids. Use of naltrexone will initiate withdrawal syndrome. • Advise clients to take the medication with meals to decrease gastrointestinal distress. • Suggest monthly IM injections for clients with difficulty adhering to regimen.
Acamprosate (Campral)	
Acamprosate decreases unpleasant effects resulting from abstinence (anxiety, restlessness).	• Inform clients that diarrhea may result. • Advise clients to maintain adequate fluid intake and to receive adequate rest. • Advise clients to avoid use in pregnancy.

MEDICATIONS TO SUPPORT WITHDRAWAL/ABSTINENCE FROM OPIOIDS

INTENDED EFFECTS	NURSING INTERVENTIONS/CLIENT EDUCATION
Methadone (Dolophine)	
• Methadone is an oral opioid agonist that replaces the opioid to which clients are addicted. • This will prevent abstinence syndrome from occurring and remove the need for clients to obtain illegal drugs. • Use for withdrawal and long-term maintenance. • Dependence will be transferred from the illegal opioid to methadone.	• Inform clients that the methadone dose must be slowly tapered to produce detoxification. • Encourage clients to participate in a 12-step self-help program. • Inform clients that they must receive the medication from an approved treatment center.
Clonidine (Catapres)	
• Clonidine assists with withdrawal of symptoms related to autonomic hyperactivity (diarrhea, nausea, vomiting). • Clonidine therapy does not reduce the craving for opioids.	• Obtain baseline vital signs. • Advise clients to avoid activities that require mental alertness until drowsiness subsides. • Encourage clients to chew gum or suck on hard candy and to sip small amounts of water or suck on ice chips to treat dry mouth.
Buprenorphine (Subutex), buprenorphine combined with naloxone (Suboxone)	
• Use agonist-antagonist opioids for detoxification and maintenance. • These medications decrease feelings of craving and may be effective in maintaining adherence.	• Inform clients that medication must be administered from an approved treatment center. • Administer sublingually.

MEDICATIONS TO SUPPORT WITHDRAWAL/ABSTINENCE FROM NICOTINE

INTENDED EFFECTS	NURSING INTERVENTIONS/CLIENT EDUCATION
Bupropion (Wellbutrin Zyban)	
Bupropion decreases nicotine craving and symptoms of withdrawal.	• To treat dry mouth, encourage clients to chew gum or suck on hard candy and to sip small amounts of water or suck on ice chips. • Advise clients to avoid caffeine and other CNS stimulants to control insomnia.
Nicotine replacement therapy (nicotine gum [Nicorette] and nicotine patch [Nicotrol])	

These nicotine replacements are pharmaceutical product substitutes for the nicotine in cigarettes or chewing tobacco.	• Instruct clients to avoid using any nicotine products while pregnant or breastfeeding.
	• For use of nicotine gum advise clients:
	  ○ that use of chewing gum is not recommended for longer than 6 months.
	  ○ to chew gum slowly and intermittently over 30 min.
	  ○ to avoid eating or drinking 15 min prior to and while chewing the gum.
	• For use of a nicotine patch advise clients to:
	  ○ apply a nicotine patch to an area of clean, dry skin each day.
	  ○ avoid using any nicotine products while the patch is on.
	  ○ follow product directions for dosage times.
	  ○ stop using patches and to notify the provider if local skin reactions occur.
	  ○ remove the patch prior to MRI scan and replace when the scan is completed.

Nursing Evaluation of Medication Effectiveness

- Depending on therapeutic intent, effectiveness may be evidenced by:

    o   Absence of injury

    o   Abstinence from substance

    o   Regular attendance at self-help group

APPLICATION EXERCISES

1. A nurse is monitoring a client who is receiving doses of lorazepam (Ativan) during withdrawal from alcohol. The nurse notes that the client's blood pressure is becoming stabilized and closer to his expected range. What other manifestations should the nurse expect to see as withdrawal symptoms abate?

2. A nurse is reinforcing teaching to a client who has a new prescription for clonidine (Catapres) to assist with maintenance of abstinence from opioids. Which of the following statements by the client requires further instruction?

   A. "I can chew gum to help relieve a side effect of this medication."

   B. "This medication will help take away my craving for drugs."

   C. "I will probably be drowsy at first while taking this medication."

   D. "This medication should relieve the nausea that has been bothering me."

3. Match the treatment goal with the appropriate medication.

_____	Alcohol withdrawal	A. Methadone (Dolophine)
_____	Heroin withdrawal	B. Naloxone (Narcan)
_____	Nicotine withdrawal	C. Bupropion (Wellbutrin)
_____	Alcohol abstinence	D. Chlordiazepoxide (Librium)
_____	Opioid overdose	E. Disulfiram (Antabuse)

APPLICATION EXERCISES ANSWER KEY

1. A nurse is monitoring a client who is receiving doses of lorazepam (Ativan) during withdrawal from alcohol. The nurse notes that the client's blood pressure is becoming stabilized and closer to his expected range. What other manifestations should the nurse expect to see as withdrawal symptoms abate?

    The nurse should expect to see pulse, respirations, and temperature return to expected baseline. Nausea and vomiting should decrease, and appetite should return. Agitation, anxiety, and restlessness diminish, and the client should be able to sleep. Tremors decrease. Any illusions which were present should disappear.

 NCLEX® Connection: Pharmacological Therapies, Expected Actions/Outcomes

2. A nurse is reinforcing teaching to a client who has a new prescription for clonidine (Catapres) to assist with maintenance of abstinence from opioids. Which of the following statements by the client requires further instruction?

    A. "I can chew gum to help relieve a side effect of this medication."

    B. "This medication will help take away my craving for drugs."

    C. "I will probably be drowsy at first while taking this medication."

    D. "This medication should relieve the nausea that has been bothering me."

    Clonidine relieves symptoms of opioid withdrawal, but does not relieve craving for opioids. Instruct clients to relieve dry mouth by chewing gum, sipping water, and sucking hard candies. Clonidine may cause drowsiness at first, and the client should not operate hazardous machinery while drowsiness is present. The symptoms of opioid withdrawal that clonidine relieves includes nausea, vomiting, and diarrhea.

 NCLEX® Connection: Pharmacological Therapies, Expected Actions/Outcomes

3. Match the treatment goal with the appropriate medication.

D	Alcohol withdrawal	A. Methadone (Dolophine)
A	Heroin withdrawal	B. Naloxone (Narcan)
C	Nicotine withdrawal	C. Bupropion (Wellbutrin)
E	Alcohol abstinence	D. Chlordiazepoxide (Librium)
B	Opioid overdose	E. Disulfiram (Antabuse)

 NCLEX® Connection: Pharmacological Therapies, Expected Actions/Outcomes

UNIT 2	MEDICATIONS AFFECTING THE NERVOUS SYSTEM
Chapter 13	Chronic Neurological Disorders

 Overview

- Use medications for chronic neurologic disorders to manage symptoms and improve quality of life.

- Chronic neurologic disorders include myasthenia gravis, Parkinson's disease, and seizure disorder.

MEDICATION CLASSIFICATION: CHOLINESTERASE INHIBITORS

- Select Prototype Medication – Neostigmine (Prostigmin)

- Other Medications:

  ○ Ambenonium (Mytelase)

  ○ Pyridostigmine (Mestinon)

  ○ Edrophonium (Tensilon)

Purpose

- Expected Pharmacological Action

  ○ Cholinesterase inhibitors prevent the enzyme cholinesterase (ChE) from inactivating acetylcholine (ACh), thereby increasing the amount of ACh available at receptor sites. Transmission of nerve impulses is improved at all sites responding to ACh as a transmitter.

- Therapeutic Uses

	NEOSTIGMINE	AMBENOMIUM	PYRIDOSTIGMINE	EDROPHONIUM
Treatment of myasthenia gravis	X	X	X	
Diagnosis of myasthenia gravis				X
Reversal of nondepolarizing neuromuscular blocking agents	X		X	X

Complications

SIDE/ADVERSE EFFECTS	NURSING INTERVENTIONS/CLIENT EDUCATION
Excessive muscarinic stimulation as evidenced by increased gastrointestinal (GI) motility, increased GI secretions, bradycardia, and urinary urgency	• Advise clients of potential side effects. If effects become intolerable, instruct clients to notify the provider. • Treat side effects with atropine.
Cholinergic crisis (excessive muscarinic stimulation and respiratory depression from neuromuscular blockade)	• Monitor clients receiving atropine for muscarinic effects. • Assist with emergency respiratory care.

 Contraindications/Precautions

- Cholinesterase inhibitors are Pregnancy Risk Category C.

- These medications are contraindicated in clients with obstruction of GI and genitourinary (GU) system, peptic ulcer disease, asthma, and coronary insufficiency.

Interactions

MEDICATION/FOOD INTERACTIONS	NURSING INTERVENTIONS/CLIENT EDUCATION
Atropine counteracts the effects of neostigmine.	• Atropine is used to treat neostigmine toxicity.
Neostigmine reverses neuromuscular blockade caused by neuromuscular blocking agents after surgical procedures and overdose.	• Monitor clients for return of respiratory function. Support respiratory function as necessary. If used to treat overdose, provide mechanical ventilation until clients have regained full muscle function.
Succinylcholine increases neuromuscular blockade.	• Avoid concurrent use.

Nursing Administration

- Neostigmine may be given PO, IM, IV, or subcutaneously.

- Instruct clients to take medications as prescribed.

- Advise clients that dosage is very individualized, starts at very low doses, and is titrated until desired muscle function is achieved.

- Encourage clients to participate in self-dosage adjustments. Have clients:

  o Keep records of medication administration and effects.

  o Recognize signs of inadequate dosing, such as difficulty swallowing, and signs of overmedication, such as urinary urgency.

  o Modify dosage based on response.

- Advise clients to wear a medical alert bracelet.

Nursing Evaluation of Medication Effectiveness

- Depending on therapeutic intent, effectiveness may be evidenced by:

  o Fewer episodes of fatigue

  o Improvement in strength as demonstrated by improved ability to chew, swallow, and perform activities of daily living (ADLs) such as bathing, walking, eating, and dressing

MEDICATION CLASSIFICATION: ANTI-PARKINSON'S MEDICATIONS

- Select Prototype Medications:

  o Dopaminergics – Levodopa (Dopar, Larodopa) or levodopa plus carbidopa (Sinemet)

  o Dopamine agonists – Pramipexole (Mirapex)

  o Centrally acting anticholinergics – Benztropine (Cogentin)

  o Dopamine releaser (Antiviral) – Amantadine (Symmetrel)

- Other Medications:

  o Dopamine agonists – Ropinirole (Requip), bromocriptine (Parlodel)

  o Centrally acting anticholinergics – Trihexyphenidyl (Artane)

Purpose

- Expected Pharmacological Action

  o These medications do not halt the progression of Parkinson's disease (PD). However, they do offer symptomatic relief from dyskinesias (bradykinesia, resting tremors, and muscle rigidity) and an increase in the ability to perform ADLs by maintaining the balance between dopamine and ACh in the extrapyramidal nervous system.

CLASSIFICATIONS	EXPECTED PHARMACOLOGICAL ACTION
Dopaminergics	• Levodopa crosses the blood-brain barrier and is taken up by dopaminergic nerve terminals and converted to dopamine (DA). This newly synthesized DA is released into the synaptic space and causes stimulation of DA receptors. • Use carbidopa to augment levodopa by decreasing the amount of levodopa that is converted to DA in the intestine and periphery. This results in greater amounts of levodopa reaching the CNS.
Dopamine agonists	• These agents act directly on DA receptors.
Centrally acting anticholinergics	• These agents block ACh at muscarinic receptors, which assists in maintaining balance between dopamine and ACh in the brain.
Antiviral	• Antivirals stimulate DA release, prevent dopamine reuptake, and may block cholinergic and glutamate receptors.

- Therapeutic Uses

  o Use levodopa as a first-line medication for PD treatment.

  o Use pramipexole as monotherapy in early-stage PD and use in conjunction with levodopa in late-stage PD. It is used more often in younger clients who are better able to tolerate daytime drowsiness and orthostatic hypotension.

Complications

SIDE/ADVERSE EFFECTS	NURSING INTERVENTIONS/CLIENT EDUCATION
Dopaminergics: levodopa (Usually dose dependent)	
Nausea and vomiting, drowsiness	• Administer with food in small doses, and at the start of treatment.
Dyskinesias (head bobbing, tics, grimacing, tremors)	• Administer a decreased dosage. The decrease may result in resumption of PD symptoms.
Orthostatic hypotension	• Monitor the client's blood pressure. • Instruct clients about signs of orthostatic hypotension (lightheadedness, dizziness). Instruct clients to change positions slowly and to sit or lie down if symptoms occur.
Cardiovascular effects from beta, stimulation (tachycardia, palpitations, irregular heartbeat)	• Monitor the client's vital signs. • Monitor ECG. • Notify the provider if symptoms occur. • Use cautiously in clients who have cardiovascular disorders.
Psychosis (visual hallucinations, nightmares)	• Administer antipsychotic medications as prescribed.
Discoloration of sweat and urine	• Advise clients that this is a harmless side effect.
Activation of malignant melanoma	• Avoid use of medication in clients who have skin lesions that have not been diagnosed.
Dopamine agonists: pramipexole	
Sudden inability to stay awake	• Advise clients to notify the provider immediately if this occurs.
Daytime sleepiness	• Advise clients of the potential for drowsiness and to avoid hazardous activities. • Advise clients to avoid other CNS depressants such as alcohol.
Orthostatic hypotension	• Instruct clients about the signs of orthostatic hypotension (lightheadedness, dizziness). Instruct clients to change positions slowly and to sit or lie down if symptoms occur.
Psychosis (visual hallucinations, nightmares)	• Administer an atypical antipsychotic medication if symptoms occur.
Dyskinesias (head bobbing, tics, grimacing, tremors)	• Decrease dosage of medication.
Nausea	• Advise clients to take medication with food.

SIDE/ADVERSE EFFECTS	NURSING INTERVENTIONS/CLIENT EDUCATION
Centrally acting anticholinergics: benztropine	
Nausea, vomiting	• Advise clients to take medication with food but to avoid high-protein snacks.
Anticholinergic effects (dry mouth, blurred vision, mydriasis, urinary hesitancy or retention, constipation)	• Advise clients to observe for symptoms and notify the provider if they occur. • Monitor I&O and check clients for urinary retention. • Advise clients to chew sugarless gum, eat foods high in fiber, and increase fluid intake to 2 to 3 L/day from beverage and food sources.
Antihistamine effects (sedation, drowsiness)	• Advise clients to avoid hazardous activities while taking the medication.
Antiviral: amantadine	
CNS effects (confusion, dizziness, restlessness)	• Advise clients to avoid hazardous activities while taking the medication.
Anticholinergic effects (dry mouth, blurred vision, mydriasis, urinary hesitancy or retention, constipation)	• Advise clients to observe for symptoms and notify the provider. • Monitor I&O and check clients for hesitancy or urinary retention. • Advise clients to chew sugarless gum, eat high-fiber foods, and increase fluid intake to 2 to 3 L/day from beverage and food.
Discoloration of skin, also called livido reticularis	• Advise clients that discoloration of the skin will subside when the medication is discontinued.
Levodopa plus carbidopa	
Abnormal movements, psychiatric disorders	• Advise clients of potential side effects and to notify the provider if they occur.

 Contraindications/Precautions

- ○ Levodopa
    - ■ This medication is Pregnancy Risk Category C.
    - ■ Contraindicated in clients with malignant melanoma.
    - ■ Do not use within 2 weeks of MAOI use.

    - ■ Use cautiously in clients who have heart disease, clients who have psychiatric disorders, and older adult clients.
- ○ Pramipexole
    - ■ This medication is Pregnancy Risk Category C.
    - ■ Use cautiously in clients with liver and kidney impairment.

- o Benztropine
    - Contraindicated in clients with narrow-angle glaucoma, myasthenia gravis, and obstruction of the GI or GU system.

    - Use cautiously in older adults, debilitated clients, clients who have enlarged prostate glands, hypertension, and renal and liver disease.

Interactions

MEDICATION/FOOD INTERACTIONS	NURSING INTERVENTIONS/CLIENT EDUCATION
Dopaminergics: levodopa	
Proteins interfere with levodopa absorption and transport across the blood-brain barrier. High-protein meals decrease therapeutic effects.	• Proteins trigger an "off episode." • Advise clients to avoid high-protein meals and snacks.
Conventional-antipsychotic agents (chlorpromazine [Compazine], haloperidol [Haldol]) decrease therapeutic effects.	• Avoid concurrent use. • If clients experience levodopa-induced psychosis, administer an atypical antipsychotic agent.
Pyridoxine (vitamin B_6) decreases therapeutic effects.	• Advise clients to avoid vitamin preparations that contain pyridoxine.
Concurrent use of MAOIs may result in hypertensive crisis.	• Avoid concurrent use.
Carbidopa, dopamine agonists, anticholinergics, Catechol O-methyltransferase (COMT) inhibitors, and dopamine releasers increase therapeutic effects.	• Use these medications concurrently to increase the beneficial effects of levodopa, but this increases the risk of adverse effects such as psychosis.
Dopamine agonists: pramipexole	
Use with levodopa can decrease motor control fluctuations and allow for lower dosage of levodopa. Concurrent use can also increase the risk of orthostatic hypotension and dyskinesias.	• Monitor clients for these interactions.
Levodopa plus carbidopa	
Beneficial interactions include allowing for lower dosage of levodopa, reduced cardiovascular responses to dopamine in the periphery, and decreased nausea.	• Monitor clients for therapeutic effects.

Nursing Administration

- Instruct family members to assist clients with the medication at home.

- Instruct clients about the possible sudden loss of the effects of medication and to notify the provider if symptoms occur.

- Inform clients that effects may not be noticeable for several weeks to several months.

- Instruct clients that a medication "holiday" may be prescribed, but will take place in an inpatient setting.

- Advise clients to avoid high-protein meals and snacks.

Nursing Evaluation of Medication Effectiveness

- Depending on therapeutic intent, effectiveness may be evidenced by:

  o Improvement of symptoms as demonstrated by absence of tremors, and reduction of irritability and stiffness.

  o Increase in ability to perform ADLs.

MEDICATION CLASSIFICATION: ANTIEPILEPTICS (AEDs)

- Select Prototype Medications:

  o Barbiturates: *— Suppress central nervous system*

    - Phenobarbital (Luminal)

    - Primidone (Mysoline)

  o Phenytoin (Dilantin)

  o Carbamazepine (Tegretol)

  o Ethosuximide (Zarontin)

  o Valproic acid (Depakote) *— treat various types of seizure*

  o Gabapentin (Neurontin)

  o Benzodiazepines:

    - Diazepam (Valium)

    - Lorazepam (Ativan)

- Other Medications:

  o Lamotrigine (Lamictal)

  o Oxcarbazepine (Trileptal)

Purpose

- Expected Pharmacological Action

  o AEDs control seizure disorders by various mechanisms, which include:

    - Slowing the entrance of sodium and calcium back into the neuron and, thus extending the time it takes for the nerve to return to its active state.

    - Suppressing neuronal firing, which decreases seizure activity and prevents propagation of seizure activity into other areas of the brain.

    - Decreasing seizure activity by enhancing the inhibitory effects of gamma butyric acid (GABA).

- Therapeutic Uses

MEDICATION	THERAPEUTIC USES
Phenobarbital	• Use for partial seizures and generalized tonic-clonic seizures. • This medication is not effective against absence seizures.
Phenytoin	• Use for all major forms of epilepsy except absence seizures. • Use IV route for status epilepticus. • Use for dysrhythmias with QT prolongation.
Carbamazepine	• Use for the treatment of partial (simple and complex) seizures, tonic-clonic seizures, bipolar disorder, and trigeminal and glossopharyngeal neuralgias.
Ethosuximide	• Use only for absence seizures.
Valproic acid	• Use for partial, generalized, and absence seizures; bipolar disorder; and migraine headaches.
Gabapentin	• Use as a single agent for control of partial seizures. • This medication is also used for neuropathic pain and the prevention of migraine headaches.
Diazepam or lorazepam	• Use IV route for status epilepticus.

Complications

SIDE/ADVERSE EFFECTS	NURSING INTERVENTIONS/CLIENT EDUCATION
Barbiturates: phenobarbital	
CNS effects in adults manifest as drowsiness, sedation, confusion, and anxiety. In children, CNS effects manifest as irritability and hyperactivity.	• Advise clients to observe for symptoms and to notify the provider if they occur. • Advise clients to avoid hazardous activities, such as driving.
Toxicity (nystagmus, ataxia, respiratory depression, coma, pinpoint pupils, hypotension, death)	• Stop medication. Administer oxygen and assist with emergency care. • Monitor the client's vital signs.

SIDE/ADVERSE EFFECTS	NURSING INTERVENTIONS/CLIENT EDUCATION
Hydantoins: phenytoin	
CNS effects (nystagmus, sedation, ataxia, cognitive impairment, double vision)	• Monitor for symptoms and notify the provider if symptoms occur.
Gingival hyperplasia (softening and overgrowth of gum tissue, tenderness, and bleeding gums)	• Advise clients to maintain good oral hygiene (dental flossing, massaging gums).
Skin rash	• Instruct clients to stop the medication and notify the provider.
Teratogenic (cleft palate, heart defects)	• Avoid use in pregnancy.
Cardiovascular effects (dysrhythmias, hypotension)	• Monitor clients receiving IV therapy for adverse CV effects.
Endocrine and other effects (coarsening of facial features, hirsutism, and interference with vitamin D metabolism)	• Instruct clients to report changes. • Encourage clients to consume adequate amounts of calcium and vitamin D.
Carbamazepine	
Cognitive function is minimally affected, but CNS effects (nystagmus, double vision, vertigo, staggering gait, headache) can occur.	• Administer in low doses initially and then gradually increase dosage. • Instruct clients to administer the dose at bedtime.
Blood dyscrasias (leukopenia, anemia, thrombocytopenia)	• Obtain the client's baseline and perform ongoing monitoring of CBC and platelet count. • Observe clients for signs of bruising and bleeding of gums.
Hypo-osmolarity (Carbamazepine promotes secretion of ADH, which inhibits water excretion by the kidneys and places clients who have heart failure at risk for fluid overload.	• Monitor serum sodium periodically. • Monitor clients for edema, decrease in urine output, and hypertension.
Skin disorders (dermatitis, rash, Stevens-Johnson syndrome)	• Treat mild reactions with anti-inflammatory or antihistamine medications. • Instruct clients to notify the provider of severe reaction. The medication should be discontinued.
Ethosuximide	
GI effects (nausea, vomiting)	• Administer with food.
CNS effects (sleepiness, lightheadedness, fatigue)	• Administer low initial dosage. • Advise clients to avoid hazardous activities, such as driving.

SIDE/ADVERSE EFFECTS	NURSING INTERVENTIONS/CLIENT EDUCATION
Valproic acid	
GI effects (nausea, vomiting, indigestion)	• Advise clients to take medication with food. Enteric-coated formulation can decrease symptoms.
Hepatotoxicity (anorexia, abdominal pain, jaundice)	• Check baseline liver function and monitor liver function periodically. • Advise clients to observe for signs (anorexia, nausea, vomiting, abdominal pain, jaundice), and notify the provider if symptoms occur. • Administer in lowest effective dose.
Pancreatitis as evidenced by nausea, vomiting, and abdominal pain	• Advise clients to observe for symptoms and to notify the provider immediately if these symptoms occur. • Monitor amylase levels. • Medication should be discontinued if pancreatitis develops.
Thrombocytopenia	• Advise clients to observe for symptoms such as bruising, and to notify the provider if these occur. • Monitor the client's platelet counts.
Gabapentin	
CNS effects (drowsiness, nystagmus)	• Administer low initial dosage. • Advise clients to avoid hazardous activities, such as driving.
Diazepam	
Respiratory depression	• Monitor the client's vital signs. • Have resuscitation equipment ready. • Administer oxygen.
Anterograde amnesia	• Monitor clients for memory loss. • Notify the provider if symptoms occur.

 Contraindications/Precautions

- Phenobarbital, phenytoin, carbamazepine and valproic acid are Pregnancy Risk Category D.

- Barbiturates are contraindicated in clients with intermittent porphyria.

- Phenytoin is contraindicated in clients with sinus bradycardia, sinoatrial blocks, second- and third-degree AV block, or Stokes-Adams syndrome.

- Carbamazepine is contraindicated in clients with bone marrow suppression or bleeding disorders.

- Valproic acid is contraindicated in clients with liver disorders and children less than 3 yr of age.

Interactions

MEDICATION/FOOD INTERACTIONS	NURSING INTERVENTIONS/CLIENT EDUCATION
Phenytoin	
Phenytoin causes a decrease in the effects of oral contraceptives, warfarin (Coumadin), and glucocorticoids because of the stimulation of hepatic drug-metabolizing enzymes.	• Inform clients of interaction, and provider may need to adjust the dosage of oral contraceptives. Suggest use of an alternative form of birth control. • Monitor for therapeutic effects of warfarin with PT and INR. Provider may adjust dosage.
Alcohol, diazepam (Valium), cimetidine (Tagamet), and valproic acid decrease phenytoin levels.	• Advise clients to avoid alcohol use. • Monitor phenytoin serum levels.
Carbamazepine (Tegretol), phenobarbital, and chronic alcohol use increase phenytoin levels.	• Encourage clients to avoid use of alcohol.
Additive CNS depressant effects can occur with concurrent use of CNS depressants (barbiturates, alcohol).	• Advise clients to avoid concurrent use of alcohol and other CNS depressants.
Carbamazepine	
Carbamazepine causes a decrease in the effects of oral contraceptives and warfarin (Coumadin) because of the stimulation of hepatic drug-metabolizing enzymes.	• Inform clients of interaction and provider may need to adjust the dosage of oral contraceptives. Suggest use of an alternative form of birth control. • Monitor for therapeutic effects of warfarin with PT and INR. • Provider may adjust dosage.
Grapefruit juice inhibits metabolism, and thus increases carbamazepine levels.	• Advise clients to avoid intake of grapefruit juice.
Phenytoin and phenobarbital decrease the effects of carbamazepine.	• Avoid concurrent use.
Valproic acid	
Concurrent use with valproic acid increases the levels of phenytoin and phenobarbital.	• Monitor phenytoin and phenobarbital levels. • Adjust dosage of medications as prescribed.

Nursing Administration

- Monitor therapeutic serum levels. Be aware of therapeutic levels for medications prescribed. Notify the provider of results.

- Advise clients taking antiepileptic medications that treatment provides for control of seizures, not cure of disorder.

- Encourage clients to keep a seizure frequency diary to monitor effectiveness of therapy.

- Advise clients to take medications as prescribed and not to stop medications without consulting the provider. Sudden cessation of medication may trigger seizures.

- Advise clients to avoid hazardous activities (driving, operating heavy machinery) until seizures are fully controlled.

- Advise clients who are traveling to carry extra medication to avoid interruption of treatment in locations where their medication is not available.

- Advise clients of childbearing age to avoid pregnancy, because medications may cause birth defects and congenital abnormalities.

- Advise clients that phenytoin has a narrow therapeutic range, and strict adherence to the medication regimen is imperative to prevent toxicity or therapeutic failure.

Nursing Evaluation of Medication Effectiveness

- Depending on therapeutic intent, effectiveness may be evidenced by:

  o Absence or decreased occurrence of seizures

  o Ability to perform ADLs

  o Absence of injury

APPLICATION EXERCISES

1. Clients who take phenytoin must perform good oral hygiene. Why is oral hygiene important for these clients?

2. A client has been diagnosed with absence seizures. The nurse should recognize that which of the following medications are used to treat this type of seizure? (Select all that apply.)

   _____   Phenytoin (Dilantin) ❡

   _____   Ethosuximide (Zarontin) ✔

   _____   Gabapentin (Neurontin) ❡

   _____   Carbamazepine (Tegretol)

   _____   Valproic acid (Depakote) ✔

3. A nurse is caring for a client who is taking valproic acid (Depakote) to prevent seizures. What laboratory values should the nurse plan to monitor for this client?

4. A client who has Parkinson's disease is prescribed levodopa/carbidopa (Sinemet) and pramipexole (Mirapex). For which of the following should the nurse monitor this client?

   A. Urinary hesitancy

   B. Watery diarrhea

   C. Weight gain

   D. Orthostatic hypotension

5. A client with Parkinson's disease has a new prescription for levodopa (Dopar). Which of the following findings should the nurse watch for in this client? (Select all that apply.)

   _____   Hallucinations

   _____   Memory loss

   _____   Mania

   _____   Paranoid ideas

   _____   Nightmares

APPLICATION EXERCISES ANSWER KEY

1. Clients who take phenytoin must perform good oral hygiene. Why is oral hygiene important for these clients?

    Gingival hyperplasia, an overgrowth of gum tissue, may occur in clients who take phenytoin. Bleeding gums, and swelling and tenderness of tissue, may result. The client should brush well, floss between teeth, and perform gum massage to minimize this adverse reaction.

 NCLEX® Connection: Pharmacological Therapies, Adverse Effects/Contraindications/Side Effects/Interactions

2. A client has been diagnosed with absence seizures. The nurse should recognize that which of the following medications are used to treat this type of seizure? (Select all that apply.)

    _____ Phenytoin (Dilantin)

    __X__ **Ethosuximide (Zarontin)**

    _____ Gabapentin (Neurontin)

    _____ Carbamazepine (Tegretol)

    __X__ **Valproic acid (Depakote)**

    Use ethosuximide and valproic acid to treat absence seizures. Phenytoin is effective against all major forms of seizures except absence seizures. Use gabapentin as a single agent for control of partial seizures. Use carbamazepine for the treatment of partial (simple and complex) seizures, tonic-clonic seizures, bipolar disorder, and trigeminal and glossopharyngeal neuralgias.

 NCLEX® Connection: Pharmacological Therapies, Expected Actions/Outcomes

3. A nurse is caring for a client who is taking valproic acid (Depakote) to prevent seizures. What laboratory values should the nurse plan to monitor for this client?

    Severe hepatotoxicity and pancreatitis may occur in the client taking valproic acid. The nurse should plan to monitor periodic liver function tests and amylase values. The nurse should also reinforce teaching about manifestations of hepatotoxicity (nausea, anorexia, abdominal pain, and jaundice) and pancreatitis (abdominal pain, nausea, vomiting, and weight loss) for the client to report to the provider.

 NCLEX® Connection: Pharmacological Therapies, Adverse Effects/Contraindications/Side Effects/Interactions

4. A client who has Parkinson's disease is prescribed levodopa/carbidopa (Sinemet) and pramipexole (Mirapex). For which of the following should the nurse monitor this client?

    A. Urinary hesitancy

    B. Watery diarrhea

    C. Weight gain

    D. Orthostatic hypotension

    Orthostatic hypotension is an adverse effect of both levodopa/carbidopa and pramipexole. When both medications are prescribed, the incidence of orthostatic hypotension is very high. Memory loss, diarrhea, and weight gain are not adverse effects of either medication.

 NCLEX® Connection: Pharmacological Therapies, Adverse Effects/Contraindications/Side Effects/Interactions

5. A client with Parkinson's disease has a new prescription for levodopa (Dopar). Which of the following findings should the nurse watch for in this client? (Select all that apply.)

    __X__   **Hallucinations**

    _____   Memory loss

    _____   Mania

    __X__   **Paranoid ideas**

    __X__   **Nightmares**

    Psychotic behaviors which may occur in clients taking levodopa include visual hallucinations, paranoid ideas, and vivid dreams or nightmares. Memory loss and mania are not manifestations seen in clients taking this medication.

 NCLEX® Connection: Pharmacological Therapies, Adverse Effects/Contraindications/Side Effects/Interactions

UNIT 2	MEDICATIONS AFFECTING THE NERVOUS SYSTEM

Chapter 14   Eye and Ear Disorders

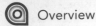 Overview

- Eye Disorders

    - Glaucoma is the leading cause of blindness in the United States. Damage to the optic nerve occurs when aqueous humor is not allowed to exit from the anterior chamber of the eye. This results in the buildup of aqueous humor, increased intraocular pressure (IOP), and loss of vision.

        - Types of glaucoma include:

            - Primary open-angle glaucoma (POAG)

                - POAG occurs in about 90% of people in the U.S. who have glaucoma.

                - Peripheral vision is lost gradually, with central visual field loss occurring if damage to the optic nerve continues.

                - Symptoms usually occur only with widespread damage. IOP greater than 21 mm Hg is the highest risk factor for POAG.

                - Treatment includes medication therapy to reduce IOP. Surgical intervention is indicated if IOP cannot be reduced by medications.

            - Angle-closure glaucoma

                - This is an acute disorder with a sudden onset, resulting in irreversible blindness within 1 to 2 days without emergency treatment.

                - Symptoms include acute onset of ocular pain, seeing halos around lights, blurred vision, and photophobia. The optic nerve is damaged when the aqueous humor builds up as a result of displacement of the iris.

        - Treat POAG with the following medications:

            - Beta-adrenergic blockers – Nonselective and beta$_1$ selective

            - Alpha$_2$-adrenergic agonists

            - Prostaglandin analogs

            - Cholinergic agonists

            - Carbonic anhydrase inhibitors

            - Nonselective adrenergic agonists

        - Use osmotic agents as first-line medications to control symptoms of angle-closure glaucoma until corrective surgery can be implemented.

- Ear Disorders

  o Acute otitis media

    ■ This condition occurs most often in young children.

    ■ A bacterial or a viral infection causes a buildup of fluid in the middle ear (middle ear effusion).

    ■ The major symptom is acute onset of pain. Objective findings include erythema, bulging of the tympanic membrane, and fever.

    ■ Treatment for bacterial infection, especially in infants and young children, is an antibiotic (oral penicillins and other antimicrobials). Treatment for viral infection is symptomatic.

      □ Because of the increase in antibiotic-resistant bacteria, the current trend is to observe children over age 2 and prescribe antibiotics only if symptoms do not resolve or worsen over several days.

    ■ Yearly influenza vaccinations and vaccinations with pneumococcal conjugate vaccine (PCV) can reduce the incidence of acute otitis media in infants and children.

  o Otitis externa

    ■ This condition, also known as "swimmer's ear," is caused by a bacterial infection of the external auditory canal.

    ■ Any object that abrades or leaves moisture in the canal facilitates colonization of bacteria and the onset of otitis externa.

    ■ Otitis externa is usually treated by topical antimicrobial/anti-inflammatory combination. Treatment usually resolves infection within 10 days.

    ■ Incidence of acute otitis media in infants and children can be reduced by yearly influenza vaccination and vaccination with pneumococcal conjugate vaccine (PCV).

MEDICATIONS FOR EYE DISORDERS

MEDICATION CLASSIFICATION: BETA-ADRENERGIC BLOCKERS

- Nonselective beta adrenergic blockers (which have both beta$_1$ and beta$_2$ properties):

  o Timolol (Timoptic, Betimol)

  o Carteolol (Ocupress)

  o Metipranolol (OptiPranolol)

  o Levobunolol (Betagan Liquifilm, AKBeta)

- Selective beta$_1$ adrenergic blockers – Betaxolol (Betoptic) and levobetaxolol (Betaxon)

Purpose

- Expected Pharmacological Action

  o Beta-adrenergic blockers decrease IOP by decreasing the amount of aqueous humor produced.

- Therapeutic Uses

  o Use topical beta-adrenergic blockers to treat POAG. They may also be prescribed in combination with other topical medications to lower IOP.

  o May use to treat angle-closure glaucoma on an emergency basis.

Complications

SIDE/ADVERSE EFFECTS	NURSING INTERVENTIONS/CLIENT EDUCATION
Reports of temporary stinging discomfort in the eye immediately after drop is instilled	• Educate clients that this effect is transient.
Occasional conjunctivitis, blurred vision, photophobia, dry eyes	• Instruct clients to report symptoms to the provider.
Systemic effects of beta blockade on heart and lungs may occur.	• Warn clients that overdose could cause or increase the chance of systemic effects. • When taking beta$_1$ blockers, clients should monitor pulse rate for bradycardia. • Use beta$_1$ blockers for clients who have chronic respiratory disease.

 Contraindications/Precautions

- Betaxolol and levobetaxolol are contraindicated for clients who have bradycardia and AV heart block, and use cautiously in clients who have heart failure.

Interactions

MEDICATION/FOOD INTERACTIONS	NURSING INTERVENTIONS/CLIENT EDUCATION
Oral beta-adrenergic blockers or calcium channel blockers can increase cardiovascular and respiratory effects.	• Instruct clients to inform the provider if they are taking any of these medications.
Beta-adrenergic blockers can interfere with some effects of insulin.	• Advise clients who have diabetes to monitor their blood glucose levels.

Nursing Administration

- Instill one drop in the affected eye once or twice daily as prescribed.

- Review the proper method of instilling eye drops and provide instruction to a family member if indicated.

- Use sterile technique when handling the applicator portion of the container. Avoid touching any part of the applicator and keep the lid in place when not in use.

- Hold gentle pressure on the nasolacrimal duct for 30 to 60 seconds immediately after instilling the drop(s) to prevent or minimize any expected systemic effect.

- Monitor pulse rate/rhythm as indicated for beta-adrenergic blocker.

 View Media Supplement: Administration of Eye Medications (Video)

MEDICATION CLASSIFICATION: ALPHA$_2$ ADRENERGIC AGONISTS

- Select Prototype Medication – Brimonidine (Alphagan)

- Other Medication– Apraclonidine (Iopidine)

Purpose

- Expected Pharmacological Action

  o Brimonidine decreases production and may also decrease the outflow of aqueous humor to lower IOP.

- Therapeutic Uses

  o Use brimonidine as a first-line medication for long-term topical treatment of POAG.

  o Use apraclonidine only as a short-term therapy for POAG; also use preoperatively for laser eye surgeries.

Complications

SIDE/ADVERSE EFFECTS	NURSING INTERVENTIONS/CLIENT EDUCATION
Localized stinging discomfort and pruritus of conjunctiva; sensation that a foreign body is in the eye.	• Advise clients not to rub their eyes.
Blurred vision, headache, dry mouth	• Instruct clients to report symptoms.
Reddened sclera caused by blood-vessel engorgement	• Inform clients of the possibility of this effect.
Hypotension, drowsiness (brimonidine crosses the blood-brain barrier)	• Advise clients to use caution with driving and other tasks, and to inform the provider if dizziness and/or weakness occur.

 ### Contraindications/Precautions

- Advise clients who wear soft contact lenses to administer brimonidine with lenses removed. Delay insertion of the contact lens at least 15 minutes after administration to prevent absorption of medication into the lens.

Interactions

MEDICATION/FOOD INTERACTIONS	NURSING INTERVENTIONS/CLIENT EDUCATION
Antihypertensive medications may intensify hypotension caused by brimonidine.	Instruct clients to inform the provider if they are taking any antihypertensive medications.

Nursing Administration

- Review proper method of administering eye drops and minimizing systemic effects.

- Monitor blood pressure for hypotension as needed.

MEDICATION CLASSIFICATION: PROSTAGLANDIN ANALOGS

- Select Prototype Medication – Latanoprost (Xalatan)

- Other Medications:

   o Travoprost (Travatan)

   o Bimatoprost (Lumigan)

Purpose

- Expected Pharmacological Action

   o Latanoprost increases aqueous humor outflow through relaxation of ciliary muscle.

- Therapeutic Uses

   o Topical first-line medications for clients with POAG and ocular hypertension

Complications

SIDE/ADVERSE EFFECTS	NURSING INTERVENTIONS/CLIENT EDUCATION
Permanent increased brown pigmentation, usually occurring in individuals with brown-colored iris (May also cause pigmentation of lids, lashes)	• Inform clients about the possibility of this effect.
Stinging, burning, reddened conjunctiva	• Instruct clients not to rub their eyes.
Blurred vision	• Instruct clients to report to the provider.
Migraine (rare adverse effect)	• Instruct clients to report to the provider.

Second-line Topical Medications for Glaucoma

CLASSIFICATION	PROTOTYPE	PURPOSE	SIDE/ADVERSE EFFECTS
Direct-acting cholinergic agonist	Pilocarpine (Isopto Carpine, Pilocar)	• Second-line treatment for POAG; lowers IOP indirectly through ciliary contraction • Use to treat angle-closure glaucoma	• Retinal detachment • System effects, such as bradycardia • Decreased visual acuity
Carbonic anhydrase inhibitor	Dorzolamide (Trusopt) Also available in combination with Timolol (called Cosopt)	• Second-line treatment for POAG, which decreases aqueous humor production • Timolol/dorzolamide combination produces increased effect of both medications	• Localized allergic reactions in up to 15% of clients • Blurred vision, dryness, photophobia
Nonselective adrenergic agonist	Dipivefrin (Propine)	• Converted to epinephrine after administration • Increases outflow of aqueous humor in POAG	• Local eye irritation, headache • Contraindicated for clients with angle-closure glaucoma

MEDICATION CLASSIFICATION: OSMOTIC AGENTS

- Select Prototype Medication – Mannitol (Osmitrol) IV

- Other Medications:

  o Urea (Ureaphil) IV

  o Glycerin (Osmoglyn) PO

  o Isosorbide (Ismotic) PO

Purpose

- Expected Pharmacological Action

  o Osmotic agents decrease intraocular pressure rapidly by drawing fluid rapidly from the anterior chamber of the eye.

- Therapeutic Uses

  o Treat rapid progression of angle-closure glaucoma to prevent blindness.

MEDICATION CLASSIFICATION: CARBONIC ANHYDRASE INHIBITOR (SYSTEMIC)

- Select Prototype Medication – Acetazolamide (Diamox)

- Other Medications – Methazolamide (GlaucTabs, Neptazane)

Purpose

- Expected Pharmacological Action

  ○ Reduces production of aqueous humor by causing diuresis through renal effects

- Therapeutic Uses

  ○ Use to quickly lower IOP in clients for whom other medications have been ineffective.

  ○ Use as an emergency medication prior to surgery for acute angle-closure glaucoma and as a second-line medication for treatment of POAG.

  ○ Glaucoma, acute mountain sickness, seizures, and heart failure (as a diuretic)

Complications

SIDE/ADVERSE EFFECTS	NURSING INTERVENTIONS/CLIENT EDUCATION
• Severe allergic reactions (anaphylaxis) • Possible cross-sensitivity with sulfonamides	• Reinforce to clients about signs/symptoms to report. • Ask about sulfonamide allergy.
• Rare serious blood disorders, such as bone marrow depression	• Reinforce to clients to recognize and immediately report symptoms.
• Gastrointestinal (GI) side effects (nausea and diarrhea)	• Report GI symptoms and weight loss to provider.
• Electrolyte depletion (sodium and potassium), altered liver function	• Prepare clients for the need to obtain regular laboratory testing.
• Generalized flu-like symptoms (headache, fever, body aches)	• Instruct clients about possible reactions.
• Central nervous system disturbances (paresthesias of extremities, fatigue, sleepiness, rarely seizures)	• Educate clients about possible reactions. • Tell clients the provider may discontinue the medication.
• Glucose disturbances in clients with diabetes mellitus	• Reinforce to clients who have diabetes to closely monitor blood glucose levels and watch for signs of hypo- or hyperglycemia.

 ## Contraindications/Precautions:

- Acetazolamide is Pregnancy Risk Category C

- Use during lactation only after evaluation by the provider.

Interactions

MEDICATION/FOOD INTERACTIONS	NURSING INTERVENTIONS/CLIENT EDUCATION
Serious effects, such as metabolic acidosis, can occur in clients using high-dose aspirin.	• Question clients about aspirin use and notify the provider.
Acetazolamide may increase the risk of toxic effects of quinidine.	• Instruct clients to notify the provider of concurrent use and to watch for signs of toxicity such as decreased heart rate.
Acetazolamide may decrease blood levels of lithium.	• Reinforce to clients taking lithium to watch for increased symptoms of mania. Monitor levels regularly.
Acetazolamide may increase osteomalacia, an adverse effect of phenytoin.	• Reinforce to clients taking phenytoin to watch for bone pain or weakness and report symptoms to the provider.
Sodium bicarbonate increases the risk of kidney stones.	• Question clients about the use of sodium bicarbonate and other over-the-counter antacids.

Nursing Administration

- Administer acetazolamide orally as a tablet or a capsule. It is also available for parenteral administration.

Nursing Evaluation of Medication Effectiveness

- Depending on therapeutic intent, effectiveness may be evidenced by:

  o Reduced IOP

  o Safe self-administration of medication

  o Prevention or minimization of systemic effects

MEDICATIONS FOR EAR DISORDERS

MEDICATION CLASSIFICATION: ANTIMICROBIALS

- Select Prototype Medication – Amoxicillin (Amoxil)

- Other Medication – Amoxicillin/clavulanate (Augmentin) PO

- Use the following antibiotics to treat acute otitis media in clients who have a penicillin allergy or penicillin-resistant otitis media.

  o Ceftriaxone (Rocephin) IM, IV (severe illness)

  o Cefdinir (Omnicef) PO

  o Cefuroxime (Ceftin) PO, IM, IV

      ○   Cefpodoxime (Vantin) PO

      ○   Azithromycin (Zithromax) PO, IV

      ○   Clindamycin (Cleocin), PO, IM, IV (a macrolide antibiotic)

Purpose

- Expected Pharmacological Action

  ○ Eradication of infection

- Therapeutic Uses

  ○ Otitis media and various other bacterial infections throughout the body

Complications

SIDE/ADVERSE EFFECTS	NURSING INTERVENTIONS/CLIENT EDUCATION
Possible allergic reaction is the most common risk when taking penicillin.	• Question clients and their families regarding the presence of penicillin or other antibiotic allergy. • Administer an alternative medication if prescribed. • Perform a skin test for sensitivity.
GI upset (usually less with amoxicillin than with ampicillin)	• Educate families to inform the provider of severe diarrhea, especially in an infant or young child.
Suprainfection with other microbes, such as oral candidiasis	• Instruct clients and their families to report symptoms of new infection to the provider.

 Contraindications/Precautions

- Amoxicillin is contraindicated for clients with severe allergy to penicillin, cephalosporins

- Use cautiously in infants less than 3 months of age because of immature renal system and increased risk for toxicity.

Nursing Administration

- Advise clients that amoxicillin is usually prescribed 3 times daily, PO.

- Advise clients that amoxicillin may be taken with meals.

- As with all antibiotics, instruct clients to take full course of medication.

Nursing Evaluation of Medication Effectiveness

- Depending on therapeutic intent, effectiveness may be evidenced by:

  ○ No presence of infection

  ○ No reoccurrence of infection

MEDICATION CLASSIFICATION: FLUOROQUINOLONE ANTIBIOTIC PLUS STEROID MEDICATION

- Select Prototype Medication – Ciprofloxacin plus dexamethasone (Cipro HC) otic drops
- Other Medications:
    - Acetic acid 2% solution otic drops (Vasolate)
    - Ciprofloxacin plus dexamethasone otic drops (Ciprodex)
    - Ofloxacin otic drops (Floxin)

Purpose

- Expected Pharmacological Action
    - The bactericidal effect of the ciprofloxacin and anti-inflammatory effect of the dexamethasone should decrease pain, edema, and erythema in the ear canal.
- Therapeutic Uses
    - Otitis externa

Complications

SIDE/ADVERSE EFFECTS	NURSING INTERVENTIONS/CLIENT EDUCATION
CNS effects (dizziness, lightheadedness, tremors, restlessness, convulsions)	• Instruct clients to inform the provider if any of these occur.
Rash	• Question clients and their families about allergies to fluoroquinolone antibiotics or to steroids such as dexamethasone or cortisone.

Nursing Administration

- Review the method for instilling otic drops.
- Inform clients that movement of the tragus or pinna may be very painful when instilling otic drops.
- Instruct clients to warm the medication by gently rolling the container between hands before instilling drops. Cold drops may cause dizziness.
- Instruct clients to maintain a side-lying position for 30 to 60 seconds with the affected ear up after instilling drops.
- Instruct clients to prevent otic medications from being placed in the eye or ingested orally.

 View Media Supplement: Administration of Ear Medications (Video)

- Reinforce to clients and their families to prevent otitis externa by:

  o Keeping foreign bodies, such as cotton swabs, out of the ear canal, and avoiding the use of manual measures to remove cerumen.

  o Drying the ear canal after bathing or swimming, using a towel and tilting the head to promote drainage.

  o Avoiding the use of earplugs except for swimming.

Nursing Evaluation of Medication Effectiveness

- Depending on therapeutic intent, effectiveness may be evidenced by:

  o Subsiding of symptoms

  o Use of measures to prevent reinfection

APPLICATION EXERCISES

1. After instilling an eye drop that has a systemic effect, the nurse should press on which of the following to prevent absorption into the circulation?

    A. The bony orbit

    B. The nasolacrimal duct

    C. The conjunctival sac

    D. The outer canthus of the eye

2. A client has a new prescription for brimonidine (Alphagan) ophthalmic, 1 drop daily in his right eye. He tells the nurse that he wears soft contact lenses and wants to know if he can put the drop in his eye with the lens in place. What should the nurse tell this client?

3. A nurse is caring for a client who has just been diagnosed with primary open-angle glaucoma (POAG) during a screening examination. Which of the following data collection findings should the nurse expect?

    A. Sudden loss of central vision

    B. Intraocular pressure 19 mm Hg

    C. No reports of pain

    D. Intact peripheral vision

4. A nurse is preparing to administer timolol (Timoptic) ophthalmic drops into the eye of a client who has glaucoma. For which of the following adverse effects should this client be monitored?

    A. Hypertension

    B. Bradycardia

    C. Seizures

    D. Jaundice

5. A nurse is caring for a preschooler who has been diagnosed with bilateral otitis externa. She has a new prescription for ciprofloxacin plus dexamethasone (Cipro HC) otic drops. The child's mother asks the nurse what type of medication is in the drops. What should the nurse reply?

APPLICATION EXERCISES ANSWER KEY

1. After instilling an eye drop that has a systemic effect, the nurse should press on which of the following to prevent absorption into the circulation?

   A. The bony orbit

   B. The nasolacrimal duct

   C. The conjunctival sac

   D. The outer canthus of the eye

   The nurse should gently press the nasolacrimal duct with a gloved hand and a clean tissue for 30 to 60 seconds. This prevents movement of the medication into the circulation and thus minimizes or prevents systemic effects from taking place. Pressing any of the other structures will not prevent medication from reaching circulation.

 NCLEX® Connection: Pharmacological Therapies, Medication Administration

2. A client has a new prescription for brimonidine (Alphagan) ophthalmic, 1 drop daily in his right eye. He tells the nurse that he wears soft contact lenses and wants to know if he can put the drop in his eye with the lens in place. What should the nurse tell this client?

   The nurse should tell the client to remove the contact lens, instill the ophthalmic drop and then wait at least 15 min before putting the contact lens back in place.

 NCLEX® Connection: Pharmacological Therapies, Medication Administration

3. A nurse is caring for a client who has just been diagnosed with primary open-angle glaucoma (POAG) during a screening examination. Which of the following data collection findings should the nurse expect?

   A. Sudden loss of central vision

   B. Intraocular pressure 19 mm Hg

   C. No reports of pain

   D. Intact peripheral vision

   The client diagnosed with POAG during a screening exam is likely to have no pain or visual disturbances. The client with POAG has a loss of peripheral vision, but central vision remains intact unless there is damage to the optic nerve caused by progressive disease. An intraocular pressure of 21 mm Hg or greater characterizes POAG.

 NCLEX® Connection: Physiological Adaptations, Basic Pathophysiology

4. A nurse is preparing to administer timolol (Timoptic) ophthalmic drops into the eye of a client who has glaucoma. For which of the following adverse effects should this client be monitored?

   A. Hypertension

   B. Bradycardia

   C. Seizures

   D. Jaundice

   Since timolol is a nonselective beta-adrenergic blocking agent, a possible adverse effect includes that of beta blockade on the heart and respiratory systems. The nurse should monitor the pulse for bradycardia. Hypertension, seizures, and jaundice are not adverse effects of timolol.

 NCLEX® Connection: Pharmacological Therapies, Adverse Effects/Contraindications/Side Effects/Interactions

5. A nurse is caring for a preschooler who has been diagnosed with bilateral otitis externa. She has a new prescription for ciprofloxacin plus dexamethasone (Cipro HC) otic drops. The child's mother asks the nurse what type of medication is in the drops. What should the nurse reply?

   Ciprofloxacin is an antibiotic to treat the infection, and dexamethasone is an anti-inflammatory agent which will decrease swelling in the ear canal.

 NCLEX® Connection: Pharmacological Therapies, Expected Effects/Outcomes

UNIT 2	MEDICATIONS AFFECTING THE NERVOUS SYSTEM
Chapter 15	Miscellaneous Central Nervous System Medications

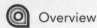 Overview

- Muscle relaxants and antispasmodic agents can affect both the central and peripheral nervous systems.

  - Use diazepam (Valium), baclofen (Lioresal), and dantrolene (Dantrium) for spasticity related to muscle injury, cerebral palsy, spinal cord injury, and multiple sclerosis.

  - Use bethanechol (Urecholine), a muscarinic agonist, for urinary retention.

  - Use oxybutynin (Ditropan), a muscarinic antagonist, for neurogenic bladder.

MEDICATION CLASSIFICATION: MUSCLE RELAXANTS AND ANTISPASMODICS

- Select Prototype Medication:

  - Centrally acting muscle relaxants – Diazepam (Valium)

  - Peripherally acting muscle relaxants – Dantrolene (Dantrium)

- Other Medications:

  - Centrally acting muscle relaxants:

    - Baclofen (Lioresal)

    - Cyclobenzaprine (Flexeril)

    - Metaxalone (Skelaxin)

    - Tizanidine (Zanaflex)

Purpose

EXPECTED PHARMACOLOGICAL ACTION	THERAPEUTIC USES
Diazepam	
Diazepam acts in the CNS to enhance GABA and produce sedative effects and depress spasticity of muscles.	• Relief of: ○ Muscle spasm related to muscle injury and spasticity ○ Anxiety and panic disorders ○ Insomnia ○ Status epilepticus ○ Alcohol withdrawal ○ Anesthesia induction
Cyclobenzaprine, metaxalone, tizanidine	
These medications act in the CNS to enhance GABA and produce sedative effects and depress spasticity of muscles.	Relief of muscle spasm related to muscle injury
Baclofen	
Baclofen acts in the CNS to enhance GABA, produce sedative effects, and depress spasticity of muscles.	Relief of spasticity related to cerebral palsy, spinal cord injury, and multiple sclerosis
Dantrolene	
Dantrolene is a peripherally acting muscle relaxant that acts directly on spastic muscles and inhibits muscle contraction by preventing release of calcium in skeletal muscles.	• Relief of spasticity related to cerebral palsy, spinal cord injury and multiple sclerosis • Treatment of malignant hyperthermia

Complications

SIDE/ADVERSE EFFECTS	NURSING INTERVENTIONS/CLIENT EDUCATION
All muscle relaxants and antispasmodics	
CNS depression (sleepiness, lightheadedness, fatigue)	• Start at low doses. • Inform clients of potential side effects. • Advise clients to avoid hazardous activities, such as driving, and concurrent use of other CNS depressants, such as alcohol.
Centrally acting agents: Diazepam, cyclobenzaprine, metaxalone, tizanidine	
Hepatic toxicity with metaxalone, tizanidine, (anorexia, nausea, vomiting, abdominal pain, jaundice)	• Obtain the client's baseline liver function and perform periodic follow-up liver function tests. • Observe clients for signs of toxicity, and notify the provider if they occur. • Start at low dose.
Physical dependence from chronic long-term use	• Advise clients not to discontinue medication abruptly.

SIDE/ADVERSE EFFECTS	NURSING INTERVENTIONS/CLIENT EDUCATION
Baclofen	
Nausea, constipation, and urinary retention	• Advise clients of side effects and notify the provider if symptoms occur. • Monitor the client's I&O. • Advise clients to increase intake of high-fiber foods.
Peripherally acting agent: Dantrolene	
Hepatic toxicity (anorexia, nausea, vomiting, abdominal pain, jaundice)	• Obtain the client's baseline liver function studies and perform periodic follow-up liver function tests. • Observe clients for signs of toxicity and notify the provider if symptoms occur. • Start at low doses.
Muscle weakness	• Monitor effectiveness of medication.

 Contraindications/Precautions

- Baclofen and dantrolene

  o Pregnancy Risk Category C

- Diazepam

  o Pregnancy Risk Category D

- Use these medications cautiously in clients with impaired liver and renal function.

Interactions

MEDICATION/FOOD INTERACTIONS	NURSING INTERVENTIONS/CLIENT EDUCATION
CNS depressants (alcohol, opioids, antihistamines) have additive CNS depressant effects.	• Advise clients to avoid concurrent use.

Nursing Administration

- Instruct clients to take medications as prescribed.

- Reinforce to clients how to taper dose when discontinuing medication to avoid withdrawal reaction after long-term use.

- Advise clients to avoid CNS depressants while using these medications.

- Provide assistance as needed in self-administration of medication and performance of ADLs.

Nursing Evaluation of Medication Effectiveness

- Depending on therapeutic intent, effectiveness may be evidenced by:

  o Absence of muscle rigidity and spasms, good range of motion

  o Absence of pain

  o Increased ability to perform ADLs

MEDICATION CLASSIFICATION: MUSCARINIC AGONISTS

- Select Prototype Medication – Bethanechol (Urecholine)

Purpose

- Expected Pharmacological Action

  o Stimulation of muscarinic receptors of the genitourinary (GU) tract, thereby causing relaxation of the trigone and sphincter muscles and contraction of the detrusor muscle

- Therapeutic Uses

  o Nonobstructive urinary retention, usually postoperatively or postpartum

Complications

SIDE/ADVERSE EFFECTS	NURSING INTERVENTIONS/CLIENT EDUCATION
Extreme muscarinic stimulation may result in sweating, tearing, urinary urgency, bradycardia and hypotension.	Instruct clients to report symptoms if they occur.

 Contraindications/Precautions

- Contraindicated in clients with urinary or gastrointestinal (GI) obstruction, peptic ulcer disease, coronary insufficiency, asthma and hyperthyroidism

Nursing Administration

- Administer by oral route, 1 hr before or 2 hr after meals to prevent nausea/vomiting.

- Monitor I & O.

Nursing Evaluation of Medication Effectiveness

- Depending on therapeutic intent, effectiveness may be evidenced by:

  o Relief of urinary retention

MEDICATION CLASSIFICATION: MUSCARINIC ANTAGONISTS

- Select Prototype Medication:

  o Selective M3-muscarinic receptor – Oxybutynin (Ditropan), oxybutynin transdermal system (Oxytrol)

- Other Medications:

  o Selective M3-muscarinic receptor – Darifenacin (Enablex)

  o Nonselective – Tolterodine (Detrol)

Purpose

- Expected Pharmacological Action

  o Inhibiting muscarinic receptors of the detrusor muscle of the bladder, which prevents contractions of the bladder and the urge to void

- Therapeutic Uses

  o Overactive bladder

Complications

SIDE/ADVERSE EFFECTS	NURSING INTERVENTIONS/CLIENT EDUCATION
Anticholinergic effects (constipation, dry mouth, blurred vision, photophobia, dry eyes)	Instruct clients to increase dietary fiber, consume 2 to 3 L/day of fluid from beverage and food sources, sip fluids, and avoid hazardous activities if vision is impaired.
CNS effects (hallucinations, confusion, insomnia, nervousness)	Instruct clients to report symptoms to the provider. Tell clients the provider may discontinue the medication.

Contraindications/Precautions

- These medications are contraindicated in clients who have glaucoma, myasthenia gravis, paralytic ileus, GI or GU obstruction, or urinary retention.

- Use cautiously in children and older adults.

- Use cautiously in clients who have gastroesophageal reflux disease (GERD), heart failure, or kidney or liver impairment.

Interactions

MEDICATION/FOOD INTERACTIONS	NURSING INTERVENTIONS/CLIENT EDUCATION
Antihistamines, tricyclic antidepressants, or phenothiazines used concurrently can result in extreme muscarinic blockage.	Avoid concurrent use.

Nursing Administration

- Oral oxybutynin – Use extended-release formulations to minimize anticholinergic effects.

- Advise clients to swallow extended-release tablets and to avoid chewing or crushing the tablets.

- Instruct clients that the shell of extended-release tablets will be eliminated whole in the stool.

- Instruct clients to apply the transdermal patch two times a week. Instruct clients to apply to dry skin of hip, abdomen, or buttock and to rotate sites.

Nursing Evaluation of Medication Effectiveness

- Depending on therapeutic intent, effectiveness may be evidenced by:

  o Decrease of urinary urgency and frequency, nocturia, and urge incontinence

APPLICATION EXERCISES

1. A nurse is caring for a client who has a prescription for tizanidine (Zanaflex) for relief of muscle spasm following a back injury. Which of the following lab values should the nurse expect to monitor while the client is taking this medication?

    A. Serum creatinine

    B. Liver enzymes

    C. WBC count

    D. RBC count

2. A nurse is caring for a client who has been taking oral baclofen (Lioresal) three times daily for the past 8 months. The client says to the nurse, "I've been having problems with constipation, so I'm just going to stop taking this medication." What should be the nurse's response? Why?

3. A nurse is caring for a client who has been prescribed oxybutynin (Ditropan). What therapeutic outcomes should the nurse expect to see if this medication is helping the client?

APPLICATION EXERCISES ANSWER KEY

1. A nurse is caring for a client who has a prescription for tizanidine (Zanaflex) for relief of muscle spasm following a back injury. Which of the following lab values should the nurse expect to monitor while the client is taking this medication?

   A. Serum creatinine

   B. Liver enzymes

   C. WBC count

   D. RBC count

   An adverse effect of tizanidine, as well as metaxalone (Skelaxin) and the peripherally-acting, antispasmodic dantrolene (Dantrium), is liver damage. Monitor liver enzymes while the client is taking these medications. The nurse should notify the provider for manifestations of liver damage, such as abdominal pain, jaundice, anorexia, or nausea.

    NCLEX® Connection: Pharmacological Therapies, Adverse Effects/Contraindications/Side Effects/Interactions

2. A nurse is caring for a client who has been taking oral baclofen (Lioresal) three times daily for the past 8 months. The client says to the nurse, "I've been having problems with constipation, so I'm just going to stop taking this medication." What should be the nurse's response? Why?

   The nurse should advise the client to talk to his provider before stopping baclofen. The nurse should realize that abrupt withdrawal from baclofen following chronic use may cause severe reactions, such as seizures. If the client and his provider decide to stop the medication, withdrawal should be done gradually over 7-14 days. To prevent constipation, an adverse effect of the medication, advise the client to increase the amount of liquids and fiber in the diet, as well as taking stool softeners.

    NCLEX® Connection: Pharmacological Therapies, Adverse Effects/Contraindications/Side Effects/Interactions

3. A nurse is caring for a client who has been prescribed oxybutynin (Ditropan). What therapeutic outcomes should the nurse expect to see if this medication is helping the client?

   Oxybutynin is prescribed to decrease the urge to void by inhibiting muscarinic receptors of the detrusor muscle, which contracts the bladder. Expected outcomes might include a decrease of nocturia, voiding fewer times during the day, and/or decreasing incontinence.

    NCLEX® Connection: Pharmacological Therapies, Expected Actions/Outcomes

UNIT 2	MEDICATIONS AFFECTING THE NERVOUS SYSTEM
Chapter 16	Sedative-Hypnotics

 Overview

- Sedatives are CNS depressants that induce a sense of calm and decrease anxiety. Hypnotics are CNS depressants that induce sleep.

- IV anesthetics are usually administered during induction of general anesthesia. Most have a quick onset of action and short duration. These medications may be nonopioids such as thiopental (Pentothal), midazolam (Versed), diazepam (Valium) propofol (Diprivan), Ketamine (Ketalar) or opioids such as fentanyl (Sublimaze).

MEDICATION CLASSIFICATION: BENZODIAZEPINES

- Select Prototype Medication – Diazepam (Valium)

- Other Medications:

  o Alprazolam (Xanax)

  o Lorazepam (Ativan)

  o Chlordiazepoxide (Librium)

  o Temazepam (Restoril)

Purpose

- Expected Pharmacological Action

  o These medications enhance the action of gamma-amino butyric acid (GABA) in the CNS.

- Therapeutic Uses

  o Anxiety disorders

  o Seizure disorders

  o Insomnia

  o Muscle spasm

  o Alcohol withdrawal

  o Panic disorder

  o Induction of anesthesia

Complications

SIDE/ADVERSE EFFECTS	NURSING INTERVENTIONS/CLIENT EDUCATION
CNS depression (lightheadedness, drowsiness, incoordination)	• Advise clients to observe for symptoms and notify the provider if they occur. • Advise clients to avoid hazardous activities such as driving or operating heavy equipment/machinery.
Anterograde amnesia	• Advise clients to observe for symptoms and notify the provider if they occur.
Paradoxical response such as insomnia, excitation, euphoria, anxiety, rage	• Advise clients to observe for symptoms. If symptoms occur, instruct the client to notify the provider and stop the medication.
Respiratory depression, especially with IV administration	• Monitor the client's vital signs. • Have resuscitation equipment available.
Physical dependence • Withdrawal following short-term therapy manifests as anxiety, insomnia, tremors and dizziness. • Withdrawal following long-term therapy manifests as delirium, paranoia, panic, hypertension and seizures.	• Reinforce to clients how to slowly taper dose over weeks to months.
Acute toxicity; oral toxicity (drowsiness, lethargy, confusion); IV toxicity (respiratory depression)	• For oral toxicity, use gastric lavage followed by the administration of activated charcoal or saline cathartics. • Assist with clients with IV toxicity who are receiving flumazenil (Romazicon) to counteract sedation and reverse side effects. • Monitor the client's vital signs, maintain patent airway, and provide fluids to maintain blood pressure. • Have resuscitation equipment available.

 Contraindications/Precautions

- These medications are Pregnancy Risk Category D.

- These medications are contraindicated in clients who have sleep apnea, respiratory depression, organic brain disease, or during lactation.

- Use cautiously in clients who have a history of substance abuse, liver dysfunction, and renal failure.

Interactions

MEDICATION/FOOD INTERACTIONS	NURSING INTERVENTIONS/CLIENT EDUCATION
CNS depressants such as alcohol, barbiturates, and opioids cause additive CNS depressant effects.	• Take complete medication history to identify concurrent use of other CNS depressants. • Advise clients to avoid alcohol and other CNS depressants.

Nursing Administration

- Ensure proper route of administration.

    o Administer all agents by oral route.

    o Administer diazepam and lorazepam by IM and IV route.

- Advise clients to take the medication as prescribed and to avoid abrupt discontinuation of treatment to prevent withdrawal symptoms. Instruct clients that dose should be tapered over several weeks.

- Administer medication with meals. Advise clients to swallow sustained-release tablets and to avoid chewing or crushing the tablet.

- Inform clients about possible development of dependency during and after treatment, and to notify the provider if symptoms occur.

Nursing Evaluation of Medication Effectiveness

- Depending on therapeutic intent, effectiveness may be evidenced by:

    o Improvement of symptoms as evidenced by absence of panic attacks, decrease or absence of anxiety, normal sleep pattern, absence of seizures, absence of withdrawal symptoms from alcohol, and relaxation of muscles.

MEDICATION CLASSIFICATION: NONBENZODIAZEPINES

- Select Prototype Medication – Zolpidem (Ambien)

- Other Medications:

    o Zaleplon (Sonata)

    o Eszopiclone (Lunesta)

    o Trazodone (formerly known as Desyrel)

Purpose

- Expected Pharmacological Action

    o These medications enhance the action of gamma-amino butyric acid (GABA) in the CNS. This results in prolonged sleep duration and decreased awakenings. These medications do not function as antianxiety, muscle relaxant, or antiepileptic agents. There is a low risk of tolerance, abuse, and dependence.

- Therapeutic Uses

    o Management of insomnia

Complications

SIDE/ADVERSE EFFECTS	NURSING INTERVENTIONS/CLIENT EDUCATION
Daytime sleepiness and lightheadedness	• Advise clients to take medication at bedtime. • Advise clients to allow for at least 8 hr of sleep when taking medication.

 ## Contraindications/Precautions

- Pregnancy Risk Category B

- Contraindicated in clients who are breastfeeding

- Use cautiously in older adult clients and in clients with impaired kidney, liver, and/or respiratory function.

Interactions

MEDICATION/FOOD INTERACTIONS	NURSING INTERVENTIONS/CLIENT EDUCATION
CNS depressants such as alcohol, barbiturates, and opioids cause additive CNS depression.	• Advise clients to avoid alcohol and other CNS depressants.

Nursing Administration

- Advise clients to take the medication just before bedtime.

- Administer all agents by oral route.

Nursing Evaluation of Medication Effectiveness

- Depending on therapeutic intent, effectiveness may be evidenced by:

    o Effective sleep pattern

MEDICATION CLASSIFICATION: MELATONIN AGONIST

- Select Prototype Medication – Ramelteon (Rozerem)

Purpose

- Expected Pharmacological Action
  - Activation of melatonin receptors
- Therapeutic Uses
  - Management of insomnia

Complications

SIDE/ADVERSE EFFECTS	NURSING INTERVENTIONS/CLIENT EDUCATION
Sleepiness, dizziness, fatigue	• Ramelteon is generally well tolerated. Instruct clients to notify the provider if symptoms occur. • Advise clients to avoid activities such as driving if symptoms occur.
Hormonal effects (amenorrhea, decreased libido, difficulty with fertility, galactorrhea)	• Instruct clients to notify the provider if symptoms occur. Tell clients the provider may discontinue medication.

 Contraindications/Precautions

- Pregnancy Category C
- Use cautiously in clients with liver disease.

Interactions

MEDICATION/FOOD INTERACTIONS	NURSING INTERVENTIONS/CLIENT EDUCATION
High-fat foods decrease absorption.	Instruct clients to take medication on an empty stomach.
Concurrent use of fluvoxamine (Luvox) can increase levels of ramelteon.	Avoid concurrent use.
CNS depressants such as opioids and alcohol can cause additive CNS depression.	Avoid concurrent use.

Nursing Administration

- Administer by oral route.
- Instruct clients to take medication 30 min prior to bedtime.
- Instruct clients to take medication on an empty stomach.

Nursing Evaluation of Medication Effectiveness

- Depending on therapeutic intent, effectiveness may be evidenced by:

    o   Improvement in sleep patterns

APPLICATION EXERCISES

1. A nurse is preparing to care for a client in the surgical unit who will be receiving lorazepam (Ativan) IV. For what adverse effect should the nurse monitor this client?

2. A nurse is caring for a client who received moderate sedation with diazepam (Valium) IV and is now in the surgical unit. The client's respiration decreases to 10/min. Which of the following medications should the nurse anticipate being prescribed for this client?

   A. Ketamine (Ketalar)

   B. Naltrexone (ReVia)

   C. Flumazenil (Romazicon)

   D. Fluvoxamine (Luvox)

3. A nurse is reinforcing teaching for a client who has a new prescription for ramelteon (Rozerem). For which of the following adverse effects should the client be taught to notify the provider? (Select all that apply.)

   _____ Blurred vision

   _____ Amenorrhea

   _____ Productive cough

   _____ Discharge from the nipples

   _____ Decreased libido

4. A nurse is caring for several clients who have prescriptions for sedative-hypnotic medications. Which of the following medications should the nurse realize has the lowest risk for causing physical dependence?

   A. Alprazolam (Xanax)

   B. Chlordiazepoxide (Librium)

   C. Temazepam (Restoril)

   D. Zolpidem (Ambien)

APPLICATION EXERCISES ANSWER KEY

1. A nurse is preparing to care for a client in the surgical unit who will be receiving lorazepam (Ativan) IV. For what adverse effect should the nurse monitor this client?

    The nurse should monitor the client for respiratory depression, which is most likely to occur with IV administration of a benzodiazepine, such as lorazepam. Respiratory depression may also occur with oral benzodiazepines, especially if the medication is taken concurrently with another CNS depressant or alcohol.

     NCLEX® Connection: Pharmacological Therapies, Adverse Effects/ Contraindications/Side Effects/Interactions

2. A nurse is caring for a client who received moderate sedation with diazepam (Valium) IV and is now in the surgical unit. The client's respiration decreases to 10/min. Which of the following medications should the nurse anticipate being prescribed for this client?

    A. Ketamine (Ketalar)

    B. Naltrexone (ReVia)

    C. Flumazenil (Romazicon)

    D. Fluvoxamine (Luvox)

    Flumazenil (Romazicon) reverses toxicity to benzodiazepines, such as diazepam. Ketamine is an anesthetic agent, which will potentiate the effects of diazepam. Use naltrexone, an opioid antagonist, to suppress the craving and pleasurable effects of alcohol, and to assist with opioid withdrawal. Use fluvoxamine, an SSRI antidepressant, to manage depression.

     NCLEX® Connection: Pharmacological Therapies, Expected Actions/Outcomes

3. A nurse is reinforcing teaching for a client who has a new prescription for ramelteon (Rozerem). For which of the following adverse effects should the client be taught to notify the provider? (Select all that apply.)

_____	Blurred vision
X	**Amenorrhea**
_____	Productive cough
X	**Discharge from the nipples**
X	**Decreased libido**

    Amenorrhea, galactorrhea (discharge from the nipples), and decreased libido are adverse effects of ramelteon for which the client should be taught to notify the provider. Blurred vision and productive cough are not adverse effects of this medication.

     NCLEX® Connection: Pharmacological Therapies, Adverse Effects/Contraindications/Side Effects/Interactions

4. A nurse is caring for several clients who have prescriptions for sedative-hypnotic medications. Which of the following medications should the nurse realize has the lowest risk for causing physical dependence?

    A. Alprazolam (Xanax)

    B. Chlordiazepoxide (Librium)

    C. Temazepam (Restoril)

    D. Zolpidem (Ambien)

Use zolpidem (Ambien), a nonbenzodiazepine medication, to treat insomnia. It has a very low risk for dependence, tolerance, and abuse. Alprazolam, chlordiazepoxide, and temazepam are all benzodiazepines and may cause physical dependence in clients.

 NCLEX® Connection: Pharmacological Therapies, Adverse Effects/ Contraindications/Side Effects/Interactions

UNIT 3: MEDICATIONS AFFECTING THE RESPIRATORY SYSTEM

- Airflow Disorders
- Upper Respiratory Disorders

NCLEX® CONNECTIONS

When reviewing the chapters in this section, keep in mind the relevant sections of the NCLEX® outline, in particular:

CLIENT NEEDS: PHARMACOLOGICAL THERAPIES

Relevant topics/tasks include:
- Adverse Effects/Contraindications/Side Effects/Interactions
  - Identify symptoms of an allergic reaction.
- Expected Actions/Outcomes
  - Use resources to check on purposes and actions of pharmacological agents.
- Medication Administration
  - Reinforce client teaching on client self administration of medications.

UNIT 3   MEDICATIONS AFFECTING THE RESPIRATORY SYSTEM

Chapter 17   Airflow Disorders

 Overview

- Asthma is a chronic inflammatory disorder of the airways. It is an intermittent and reversible airflow obstruction that affects the bronchioles. The obstruction occurs either by inflammation or airway hyper-responsiveness leading to bronchoconstriction.

- Medication management usually addresses both inflammation and bronchoconstriction. These same medications may be used in symptomatic treatment of chronic obstructive pulmonary disease (COPD).

- Medications include:

- Bronchodilator agents such as beta-adrenergic agonists, methylxanthines, inhaled anticholinergics, and anti-inflammatory agents such as glucocorticoids, mast cell stabilizers, and leukotriene modifiers.

 View Media Supplement: Bronchoconstriction (Animation)

MEDICATION CLASSIFICATION: BETA$_2$-ADRENERGIC AGONISTS

- Select Prototype Medication – Albuterol (Proventil, Ventolin)

- Other Medications:

    o   Formoterol (Foradil Aerolizer)

    o   Salmeterol (Serevent)

    o   Terbutaline (Brethine)

    o   Levalbuterol (Xopenex)

Purpose

- Expected Pharmacological Action

    o   Beta-adrenergic agonists act by selectively activating the beta$_2$ receptors in the bronchial smooth muscle, resulting in bronchodilation and symptomatic relief. This results in:

        ▪   Relief of bronchospasm

        ▪   Inhibition of histamine release

        ▪   Increased ciliary motility

- Therapeutic Uses

MEDICATION	ROUTE	THERAPEUTIC USES
Albuterol (Proventil, Ventolin)	• Inhaled, short-acting • Oral, long-acting	• Prevention of asthma attack (exercise-induced) • PRN treatment for ongoing asthma attack • Long-term control of asthma
Formoterol (Foradil Aerolizer) Salmeterol (Serevent)	• Inhaled, long-acting	• Adjunct treatment for long-term control of asthma
Terbutaline (Brethine)	• Oral, long-acting	• Adjunct treatment for long-term control of asthma

Complications

SIDE/ADVERSE EFFECTS	NURSING INTERVENTIONS/CLIENT EDUCATION
Inhaled agents (short- and long-acting) have minimal adverse effects.	• Use as directed.
Oral agents can cause tachycardia and angina because of activation of alpha$_1$ receptors in the heart.	• Advise clients to observe for signs and symptoms (chest, jaw, or arm pain or palpitations) and to notify the provider if they occur. • Instruct clients on how to check pulse and to report an increase of greater than 20 to 30 beats/min. • Advise clients to avoid caffeine. • Tell clients the provider may decrease dosage.
Tremors caused by activation of beta$_2$ receptors in skeletal muscle	• Tell clients that tremors usually resolve with continued medication use. • Tell clients the provider may decrease dosage.

 Contraindications/Precautions

- Beta-adrenergic agonists are Pregnancy Risk Category C.

- These agents are contraindicated in clients with tachydysrhythmias.

- Use cautiously in clients who have diabetes, hyperthyroidism, hypertension, and angina.

Interactions

MEDICATION/FOOD INTERACTIONS	NURSING INTERVENTIONS/CLIENT EDUCATION
Use of beta-adrenergic blockers (propranolol) can negate effects of both medications.	• Avoid concurrent use.
MAOIs and tricyclic antidepressants can increase the risk of tachycardia and angina.	• Instruct clients to report changes in heart rate and chest pain.

Nursing Administration

- Instruct clients to follow manufacturer's instructions for use of device – Metered-dose inhaler (MDI), dry-powder inhaler (DPI), and nebulizer.

 View Media Supplement: Metered-Dose Inhaler (Image)

- When clients are prescribed an inhaled beta-adrenergic agonist and an inhaled glucocorticoid, advise clients to inhale the beta-adrenergic agonist before inhaling the glucocorticoid. The beta-adrenergic agonist promotes bronchodilation and enhances absorption of the glucocorticoid.

- Advise clients not to exceed prescribed dosages.

- Ensure that clients know the appropriate dosage schedule (if the medication is to be taken on a fixed or a when-necessary schedule).

- Formoterol and salmeterol are both long-acting beta-adrenergic agonist inhalers. Instruct clients to use these agents every 12 hr for long-term control and not to abort an asthma attack. Instruct clients to use a short-acting beta-adrenergic agonist, such as albuterol, to treat an acute attack.

- Advise clients to observe for signs of an impending asthma attack and to keep a log of the frequency and intensity of attacks.

- Instruct clients to notify the provider if there is an increase in the frequency and intensity of asthma attacks.

Nursing Evaluation of Medication Effectiveness

- Depending on therapeutic intent, effectiveness may be evidenced by:

  ○ Long-term control of asthma attacks.

  ○ Prevention of exercise-induced asthma attack.

  ○ Resolution of asthma attack as evidenced by absence of shortness of breath, clear breath sounds, absence of wheezing, return of respiratory rate to baseline.

MEDICATION CLASSIFICATION: METHYLXANTHINES

- Select Prototype Medication – Theophylline (Theolair, Theo-24)

Purpose

- Expected Pharmacological Action

  ○ Theophylline causes relaxation of bronchial smooth muscle, resulting in bronchodilation.

- Therapeutic Uses

  ○ Long-term control of chronic asthma (oral)

  ○ Route of administration – Oral or IV (emergency use only)

Complications

SIDE/ADVERSE EFFECTS	NURSING INTERVENTIONS/CLIENT EDUCATION
• Mild toxicity reaction may include gastrointestinal (GI) distress and restlessness. • More severe reactions can occur with higher therapeutic levels and can include dysrhythmias and seizures.	• Monitor theophylline serum levels to keep within therapeutic range (5 to 15 mcg/mL). Side effects are unlikely to occur at levels less than 20 mcg/mL. • Instruct clients that periodic blood levels will be needed. Advise clients to report any symptoms of nausea, diarrhea, or restlessness that may indicate toxicity.

 Contraindications/Precautions

- Pregnancy Risk Category C

- Use cautiously in clients who have heart disease, hypertension, liver and renal dysfunction, and diabetes.

- Use cautiously in children and older adults.

Interactions

MEDICATION/FOOD INTERACTIONS	NURSING INTERVENTIONS/CLIENT EDUCATION
• Caffeine increases CNS and cardiac adverse effects of theophylline. • Caffeine can also increase theophylline levels.	• Advise clients to avoid consuming caffeinated beverages (coffee, caffeinated colas).
• Phenobarbital and phenytoin decrease theophylline levels.	• Concurrent use with these medications requires an increased theophylline dosage.
• Cimetidine (Tagamet), ciprofloxacin (Cipro), and other fluoroquinolone antibiotics increase theophylline levels.	• Concurrent use with these medications requires a decreased theophylline dosage.

Nursing Administration

- Advise clients to take the medication as prescribed. If a dose is missed, instruct clients not to double dose.

- Instruct clients not to chew or crush sustained-release preparations, but to swallow whole.

Nursing Evaluation of Medication Effectiveness

- Depending on therapeutic intent, effectiveness may be evidenced by:

  o Long-term control of asthma attacks.

MEDICATION CLASSIFICATION: INHALED ANTICHOLINERGICS

- Select Prototype Medication – Ipratropium (Atrovent)

- Other Medications – Tiotropium (Spiriva)

Purpose

- Expected Pharmacological Action

  o These medications block muscarinic receptors of the bronchi, resulting in bronchodilation.

- Therapeutic Uses

  o Relief of bronchospasm associated with chronic obstructive pulmonary disease

  o Allergen-induced and exercise-induced asthma

  o Route of administration – Inhalation

Complications

SIDE/ADVERSE EFFECTS	NURSING INTERVENTIONS/CLIENT EDUCATION
Local anticholinergic effects (dry mouth, hoarseness)	Advise clients to sip fluids and suck on hard candies to control dry mouth.

 ### Contraindications/Precautions

- Inhaled anticholinergics are Pregnancy Risk Category B.

- These agents are contraindicated in clients who have an allergy to peanuts because the medication preparations may contain soy lecithin.

- Use cautiously in clients who have narrow-angle glaucoma and benign prostatic hypertrophy (due to anticholinergic effects).

Nursing Administration

- Advise clients to rinse the mouth after inhalation to decrease unpleasant taste.

- Usual adult dosage is two puffs. Instruct clients to wait the length of time directed between puffs.

- If clients are prescribed two inhaled medications, instruct clients to wait at least 5 min between medications.

Nursing Evaluation of Medication Effectiveness

- Depending on therapeutic intent, effectiveness may be evidenced by:

  o Control of bronchospasm in clients with chronic obstructive pulmonary disease.

  o Prevention of allergen-induced and exercise-induced asthma attack.

MEDICATION CLASSIFICATION: GLUCOCORTICOIDS

- Select Prototype Medication:
  - ○ Inhalation – Beclomethasone (QVAR)
  - ○ Oral – Prednisone (Deltasone)
- Other Medications:
  - ○ Inhalation:
    - Budesonide (Pulmicort Flexhaler)
    - Fluticasone (Advair, Flovent)
    - Triamcinolone acetonide (Azmacort)
  - ○ Oral – Prednisolone (Prelone)
  - ○ IV:
    - Hydrocortisone sodium succinate (Solu-Cortef)
    - Methylprednisolone sodium succinate (Solu-Medrol)

Purpose

- Expected Pharmacological Action
  - ○ These medications prevent inflammation, suppress airway mucus production, and promote responsiveness of beta$_2$ receptors in the bronchial tree.
  - ○ The use of glucocorticoids does not provide immediate effects, but rather promotes decreased frequency and severity of exacerbations and acute attacks.
- Therapeutic Uses
  - ○ Use short-term IV agents as adjuncts for status asthmaticus and anaphylaxis.
  - ○ Use inhaled agents for long-term prophylaxis of asthma.
  - ○ Use short-term oral therapy to treat symptoms following an acute asthma attack.
  - ○ Use long-term oral therapy to treat chronic asthma.
  - ○ Use replacement therapy for primary adrenocortical insufficiency.
  - ○ Promote lung maturity and decrease respiratory distress in fetuses at risk for preterm birth.

Complications

SIDE/ADVERSE EFFECTS	NURSING INTERVENTIONS/CLIENT EDUCATION
Inhaled glucocorticoids	
Difficulty speaking, hoarseness, and candidiasis	• Advise clients to use a spacer with MDI except with beclomethasone inhaler. • Advise clients to rinse mouth or gargle with water or salt water after use. • Advise clients to monitor for redness, sores, or white patches and to report to the provider if they occur. Treat candidiasis with nystatin oral suspension.
Prednisone when used for 10 days or more can result in:	
Suppression of adrenal gland function, such as a decrease in the ability of the adrenal cortex to produce glucocorticoids, can occur with inhaled agents and oral agents.	• Administer oral glucocorticoid on an alternate-day dosing schedule. • Monitor the client's blood glucose levels. • Taper the client's dose.
Bone loss (can occur with inhaled agents and oral agents)	• Advise clients to perform weight-bearing exercises. • Advise clients to consume a diet with sufficient calcium and vitamin D intake. • Use the lowest dose possible to control symptoms. • Administer oral glucocorticoid on an alternate-day dosing schedule.
Hyperglycemia and glucosuria	• Monitor blood glucose levels of clients who have diabetes. • Administer an increased insulin dosage if indicated.
Myopathy as evidenced by muscle weakness	• Instruct clients to report signs of muscle weakness. • Tell clients the provider should decrease dosage.
Peptic ulcer disease	• Advise clients to avoid NSAIDs. • Advise clients to report black, tarry stools. Check stool for occult blood periodically. • Advise clients to take with food or meals.
Infection	• Advise clients to notify the provider if early signs of infection occur (sore throat, weakness, malaise).
Disturbances of fluid and electrolytes (fluid retention)	• Instruct clients to observe weight gain, edema, and muscle weakness.

Contraindications/Precautions

- Pregnancy risk category C

- Contraindicated in clients who have received a live virus vaccine

- Contraindicated in clients with systemic fungal infections

- Use cautiously in children, and in clients who have diabetes, hypertension, peptic ulcer disease, and/or renal dysfunction.

- Use cautiously in clients taking NSAIDs.

Interactions

MEDICATION/FOOD INTERACTIONS	NURSING INTERVENTIONS/CLIENT EDUCATION
Prednisone	
Concurrent use of potassium-depleting diuretics increases the risk of hypokalemia.	• Monitor potassium level and administer supplements as needed.
Concurrent use of NSAIDs increases the risk of GI ulceration.	• Advise clients to avoid use of NSAIDs. If GI distress occurs, instruct clients to notify the provider.
Concurrent use of glucocorticoids and hypoglycemic agents (oral and insulin) will counteract the effects.	• Instruct clients with diabetes to notify the provider if hyperglycemia occurs. The client may need increased dosage of hypoglycemic agents.

Nursing Administration

- Instruct clients to use glucocorticoid inhalers on a regular, fixed schedule for long-term therapy of asthma. Instruct clients not to use glucocorticoids to treat an acute attack.

- Administer using an MDI device, DPI, or nebulizer.

- Instruct clients to use a spacer with all preparations except beclomethasone.

- When a client is prescribed an inhaled beta-adrenergic agonist and an inhaled glucocorticoid, advise the client to inhale the beta-adrenergic agonist before inhaling the glucocorticoid. The beta-adrenergic agonist promotes bronchodilation and enhances absorption of the glucocorticoid.

- Instruct clients to use oral glucocorticoids short-term, 3 to 10 days following an acute asthma attack.

- If client is on long-term oral therapy, additional dosages of oral glucocorticoids are required in times of stress (infection, trauma).

- Clients who discontinue oral glucocorticoid medications or switch from oral to inhaled agents require additional doses of glucocorticoids during periods of stress.

Nursing Evaluation of Medication Effectiveness

- Depending on therapeutic intent, effectiveness may be evidenced by:

  o Long-term control of asthma attacks

  o Resolution of acute attack as demonstrated by absence of shortness of breath, clear breath sounds, absence of wheezing, and return of respiratory rate to baseline

MEDICATION CLASSIFICATION: MAST CELL STABILIZERS (ANTI-INFLAMMATORIES)

- Select Prototype Medication – Cromolyn sodium (Intal)

Purpose

- Expected Pharmacological Action

  o Anti-inflammatory action

    ▪ These medications stabilize mast cells, which inhibits the release of histamine and other inflammatory mediators.

    ▪ These medications suppress inflammatory cells (eosinophils, macrophages).

- Therapeutic Uses

  o Management of chronic asthma

  o Prophylaxis of exercise-induced asthma

  o Prevention of allergen-induced attack

  o Allergic rhinitis by intranasal route

  o Route of administration – Inhalation

Complications

- Safest of all asthma medications

- Safe to use for children

 ## Contraindications/Precautions

- These agents are Pregnancy Risk Category B.

- Fluorocarbons in aerosols make this medication contraindicated for clients who have coronary artery disease, dysrhythmias, and status asthmaticus.

- Use cautiously in clients with liver and kidney impairment.

Nursing Administration

- Advise clients to take medication 15 min before exercise or exposure to allergen.

- Advise clients that long-term prophylaxis may take several weeks for full therapeutic effects to be established.

- Advise clients that this is not a bronchodilator and is not intended for aborting an asthmatic attack.

- Instruct clients in the proper use of administration devices (nebulizer, MDI).

Nursing Evaluation of Medication Effectiveness

- Depending on therapeutic intent, effectiveness may be evidenced by:

  o Prevention of exercise- or allergen-induced bronchospasm

  o Decreased episodes of allergic rhinitis

  o Long-term control of asthma

MEDICATION CLASSIFICATION: LEUKOTRIENE MODIFIERS

- Select Prototype Medication – Montelukast (Singulair)
- Other Medication – Zileuton (Zyflo), zafirlukast (Accolate)

Purpose

- Expected Pharmacological Action

  o Leukotriene modifiers prevent the effects of leukotrienes, thereby suppressing inflammation, bronchoconstriction, airway edema, and mucus production.

- Therapeutic Uses

  o Long-term therapy of asthma in adults and children 15 years and older and to prevent exercise-induced bronchospasm.

  o Route of administration – Oral

Complications

SIDE/ADVERSE EFFECTS	NURSING INTERVENTIONS/CLIENT EDUCATION
Liver injury with use of zileuton (Zyflo) and zafirlukast (Accolate)	• Obtain baseline liver function tests and monitor periodically. • Advise clients to monitor for signs of liver damage (nausea, anorexia, abdominal pain). • Instruct clients to notify the provider if symptoms occur.

 Contraindications/Precautions

- Use cautiously in clients with liver dysfunction.

Interactions

MEDICATION/FOOD INTERACTIONS	NURSING INTERVENTIONS/CLIENT EDUCATION
Zileuton and zafirlukast inhibit metabolism of warfarin (Coumadin), leading to increased warfarin levels.	• Advise clients to observe for signs of bleeding and to notify the provider. • Monitor PT and INR levels.
Zileuton and Zafirlukast inhibit metabolism of theophylline, leading to increased theophylline levels.	• Monitor theophylline levels. • Advise clients to observe for signs of theophylline toxicity (nausea, vomiting, seizures), and to notify the provider.

Nursing Administration

- Advise clients to take zileuton as prescribed. Zileuton can be given with or without food.

- Advise clients not to take zafirlukast with food, and to administer it 1 hr before or 2 hr after meals.

- Advise clients to take montelukast once daily at bedtime.

Nursing Evaluation of Medication Effectiveness

- Depending on therapeutic intent, effectiveness may be evidenced by:

  o Prevention of exercise- or allergen-induced bronchospasm.

  o Decreased episodes of allergic rhinitis.

  o Long-term control of asthma.

APPLICATION EXERCISES

1. A nurse is reinforcing teaching to a client with asthma about how to use cromolyn (Intal). Which of the following should the nurse include in the teaching? (Select all that apply.)

    _____ Take the medication 15 min before exercising.

    _____ Follow a fixed-dosage schedule for long-term control of asthma.

    _____ Expect to lose weight while taking the medication.

    _____ Observe for adverse effects such as tremors, restlessness, and palpitations.

    _____ Do not crush or chew tablets.

2. A nurse is reinforcing teaching for a client with a prescription for a beclomethasone (QVAR) inhaler to be used for the long-term management of asthma. Which of the following dietary supplements should the client be sure to consume in sufficient amounts to prevent a deficiency while taking the QVAR inhaler?

    A. Iron and protein

    B. Calcium and vitamin D

    C. Vitamin B_{12} and folic acid

    D. Vitamins E and K

3. A nurse is to administer prescribed puffs of a beclomethasone (QVAR) inhaler and an albuterol (Proventil) inhaler to a hospitalized client newly diagnosed with asthma. Which of the following inhalers should the nurse administer to the client first? How long should the nurse wait before administering the second inhaled medication? Why?

4. A nurse is caring for a client who is prescribed oral prednisone (Deltasone) for the treatment of chronic asthma. The nurse should plan to monitor the client for which of the following findings?

    A. Weight loss

    B. Infection

    C. Hypoglycemia

    D. Angina pain

5. A nurse is reinforcing teaching for a client who has a new prescription for oral montelukast (Singular) as a maintenance therapy to prevent exacerbation of asthma. When should the client be taught to take this medication?

APPLICATION EXERCISES ANSWER KEY

1. A nurse is reinforcing teaching to a client with asthma about how to use cromolyn (Intal). Which of the following should the nurse include in the teaching? (Select all that apply.)

     X   **Take the medication 15 min before exercising.**

     X   **Follow a fixed-dosage schedule for long-term control of asthma.**

          Expect to lose weight while taking the medication.

          Observe for adverse effects such as tremors, restlessness, and palpitations.

          Do not crush or chew tablets.

   Use cromolyn for prophylactic treatment of asthma. Do not use to abort an asthma attack, but use to prevent exercise-induced bronchospasm. For long-term control, the client should take cromolyn on a fixed-dose schedule. Cromolyn does not promote weight loss, has no significant side effects, and is only given by inhalation.

 NCLEX® Connection: Pharmacological Therapies, Medication Administration

2. A nurse is reinforcing teaching for a client with a prescription for a beclomethasone (QVAR) inhaler to be used for the long-term management of asthma. Which of the following dietary supplements should the client be sure to consume in sufficient amounts to prevent a deficiency while taking the QVAR inhaler?

   A. Iron and protein

   B. Calcium and vitamin D

   C. Vitamin B_{12} and folic acid

   D. Vitamins E and K

   Since inhaled glucocorticoids may cause bone loss, it is important for the client to consume sufficient amounts of calcium and vitamin D during treatment with the QVAR inhaler. While adequate amounts of iron, protein, Vitamin B_{12}, folic acid, and vitamins E and K are important, the client should not require extra supplementation while taking the glucocorticoid inhaler.

 NCLEX® Connection: Pharmacological Therapies, Adverse Effects/Contraindications/Side Effects/Interactions

3. A nurse is to administer prescribed puffs of a beclomethasone (QVAR) inhaler and an albuterol (Proventil) inhaler to a hospitalized client newly diagnosed with asthma. Which of the following inhalers should the nurse administer to the client first? How long should the nurse wait before administering the second inhaled medication? Why?

When a client is prescribed an inhaled beta-adrenergic agonist, such as albuterol, and an inhaled glucocorticoid, such as beclomethasone, the beta-adrenergic agonist should be administered first; then the nurse should wait 5 min before administering the beclomethasone inhaler. The beta-adrenergic agonist promotes bronchodilation and enhances absorption of the glucocorticoid.

 NCLEX® Connection: Pharmacological Therapies, Medication Administration

4. A nurse is caring for a client who is prescribed oral prednisone (Deltasone) for the treatment of chronic asthma. The nurse should plan to monitor the client for which of the following findings?

A. Weight loss

B. Infection

C. Hypoglycemia

D. Angina pain

The client who takes prednisone (Deltasone) on a long-term basis is at risk for infection because the medication decreases the body's inflammatory response. The client is also at risk for weight gain and hyperglycemia. The client is not at risk for angina pain due to prednisone.

 NCLEX® Connection: Pharmacological Therapies, Adverse Effects/Contraindications/Side Effects/Interactions

5. A nurse is reinforcing teaching for a client who has a new prescription for oral montelukast (Singular) as a maintenance therapy to prevent exacerbation of asthma. When should the client be taught to take this medication?

For maintenance therapy to prevent exacerbation of asthma, the client should take montelukast once a day before bed. It can prevent symptoms of asthma during the night and improve the client's lung function the next morning.

 NCLEX® Connection: Pharmacological Therapies, Expected Actions/Outcomes

UNIT 3	MEDICATIONS AFFECTING THE RESPIRATORY SYSTEM
Chapter 18	Upper Respiratory Disorders

 Overview

- The medications in this section affect the CNS, nasal passages, or other parts of the respiratory system to treat the effects of allergic rhinitis or coughs from the common cold, influenza, and other disorders.

  o Use antihistamines to treat nausea, motion sickness, allergic reactions, and insomnia.

  o Use acetylcysteine, a mucolytic, as an antidote for acetaminophen toxicity.

- This section includes opioid and nonopioid antitussives, expectorants, mucolytics, decongestants, and antihistamine medications.

- Medications in this section are frequently combined for increased effectiveness. For example, an antitussive may be combined with an expectorant to better control a cough.

MEDICATION CLASSIFICATION: ANTITUSSIVES — OPIOIDS

- Select Prototype Medication – Codeine

- Other Medication – Hydrocodone

Purpose

- Expected Pharmacological Action

  o Codeine suppresses cough through its action on the central nervous system.

- Therapeutic Uses

  o Chronic nonproductive cough

Complications

SIDE/ADVERSE EFFECTS	NURSING INTERVENTIONS/CLIENT EDUCATION
CNS effects (dizziness, lightheadedness, drowsiness, respiratory depression)	• Obtain the client's baseline vital signs. • Monitor clients when ambulating. • Advise clients to lie down if feeling lightheaded. • Observe for signs of respiratory depression such as respiratory rate less than 12/min. Stimulate clients to breathe if respiratory depression occurs. It may be necessary to stop the medication and naloxone (Narcan) may need to be administered. • Advise clients to avoid driving while taking codeine.
GI distress (nausea, vomiting, constipation)	• Instruct clients to take oral codeine with food. • Advise clients to increase fluids and dietary fiber.
Potential for abuse	• Advise clients of the potential for abuse. • Use for short duration.

 Contraindications/Precautions

- Codeine is Pregnancy Category Risk C.

- This medication is contraindicated in clients who have acute asthma, head trauma, liver and renal dysfunction, and acute alcoholism.

 • Use cautiously in children, older adults, and clients with a history of substance abuse.

Nursing Administration

- Advise clients to avoid hazardous activities, such as driving while taking codeine.

- Advise clients to change positions slowly and to lie down if feeling dizzy.

- Advise clients to avoid alcohol and other CNS depressants while taking codeine.

MEDICATION CLASSIFICATION: ANTITUSSIVES — NON-OPIOIDS

- Select Prototype Medication – Dextromethorphan (found in many different products for cough, such as Robitussin and others)

- Other Medications – Benzonatate (Tessalon), diphenhydramine (Benadryl)

Purpose

- Expected Pharmacological Action

  o Dextromethorphan suppresses cough through its action on the CNS. Although not an opioid, it is derived from opioids.

- Therapeutic Uses

    o Cough suppression

Complications

- This medication has few adverse effects.

- Some mild nausea, dizziness, and sedation may occur.

- There is some potential for abuse.

 ## Contraindications/Precautions

- Pregnancy Category Risk C

Interactions

- May cause high fever when used within 2 weeks of MAOI antidepressants

Nursing Administration

- Instruct clients that some formulations may contain alcohol and/or sucrose.

- Available forms include capsules, lozenges (for clients older than 12 years), liquids, and syrups.

Nursing Evaluation of Medication Effectiveness

- Depending on therapeutic intent, effectiveness may be evidenced by:

    o Absence or decreased episodes of coughing.

MEDICATION CLASSIFICATION: EXPECTORANTS

- Select Prototype Medication– Guaifenesin (Mucinex)

Purpose

- Expected Pharmacological Action

    o Guaifenesin promotes increased cough production through increasing mucous secretion (stimulates flow of respiratory tract secretions). These actions increase the ability to cough and thus decrease chest congestion.

- Therapeutic Uses

    o Although guaifenesin is available as an expectorant alone (Mucinex), it is most often combined with antitussives (either opioid or nonopioid), or a decongestant for treating symptoms of colds, allergic rhinitis, or for cough caused by lower respiratory disorders.

Complications

SIDE/ADVERSE EFFECTS	NURSING INTERVENTIONS/CLIENT EDUCATION
Gastrointestinal (GI) upset	• Advise clients to take with food if gastrointestinal upset occurs.
Drowsiness, dizziness	• Advise clients to avoid hazardous activities (driving) if these reactions occur.
Allergic reaction (rash)	• Advise clients to stop taking guaifenesin and obtain medical care if rash or other symptoms of allergy occur.

 Contraindications/Precautions

- Guaifenesin is Pregnancy Risk Category C.

- Advise clients who are breastfeeding to talk to the provider before taking medications containing guaifenesin.

- Depending on the formulation and medication combinations, preparations containing guaifenesin may not be recommended for children.

Nursing Administration

- Advise clients to increase fluid intake when taking guaifenesin, in order to promote liquefying secretions.

- Instruct clients not to crush tablets and that capsules may be opened to sprinkle on foods.

- Advise clients to read over-the-counter labels carefully to discover what medications have been combined in the preparation used. Guaifenesin is frequently combined with other medications (antitussives, decongestants) as a liquid or syrup (for example, Mucinex D combines guaifenesin with the sympathomimetic decongestant, pseudoephedrine).

Nursing Evaluation of Medication Effectiveness

- Depending on therapeutic intent, effectiveness may be evidenced by the following:

  o Cough is more productive and mucous is easier to expectorate

  o Chest congestion is decreased

MEDICATION CLASSIFICATION: MUCOLYTICS

- Select Prototype Medication – Acetylcysteine (Mucomyst, Acetadote)

- Other Medication – Hypertonic saline

Purpose

- Expected Pharmacological Action

    o   Mucolytics enhance the flow of secretions in the respiratory passages.

- Therapeutic uses

    o   Acute and chronic pulmonary disorders exacerbated by large amounts of secretions

    o   Cystic fibrosis

    o   Acetylcysteine is the antidote for acetaminophen poisoning.

Complications

SIDE/ADVERSE EFFECTS	NURSING INTERVENTIONS/CLIENT EDUCATION
Aspiration and bronchospasm when administered orally	• Monitor clients for signs of aspiration and bronchospasm. Stop medication immediately and notify the provider.

 ## Contraindications/Precautions

- Acetylcysteine is Pregnancy Risk Category B.

- Contraindicated for clients at risk for GI hemorrhage.

- Use cautiously in clients who have peptic ulcer disease, esophageal varices, and severe liver disease.

Nursing Administration

    o   Advise clients that acetylcysteine has an odor that smells like rotten eggs.

    o   Administer acetylcysteine by inhalation to liquefy nasal and bronchial secretions and facilitate coughing.

    o   Manage acetaminophen overdose with oral doses. Mix oral doses with fruit juice, cola drinks, or water. Administer doses every 4 hr for 72 hr. Be prepared to suction clients if aspiration occurs with oral administration

    o   Monitor clients receiving IV doses. Clients will receive three doses starting with loading dose, followed by the next dose to be infused over 4 hr, followed by the last dose infused over 16 hr.

Nursing Evaluation of Medication Effectiveness

- Depending on therapeutic intent, effectiveness may be evidenced by:

    o   Improvement of symptoms as demonstrated by regular respiratory rate, clear lung sounds, and increased ease of expectoration.

MEDICATION CLASSIFICATION: DECONGESTANTS

- Select Prototype Medication – Phenylephrine
- Other Medications:
  - Ephedrine
  - Naphazoline
  - Phenylpropanolamine

Purpose

- Expected Pharmacological Action
  - Sympathomimetic decongestants stimulate alpha$_1$-adrenergic receptors causing reduction in the inflammation of the nasal membranes.
- Therapeutic Uses
  - This medication can be used to treat allergic rhinitis by relieving nasal stuffiness.
  - This medication acts as a decongestant for clients with sinusitis and the common cold.

Complications

SIDE/ADVERSE EFFECTS	NURSING INTERVENTIONS/CLIENT EDUCATION
Rebound congestion secondary to prolonged use of topical agents	• Advise clients to use for short-term therapy, no more than 3 to 5 days. • Reinforce to clients how to taper use and discontinue medication using one nostril at a time.
CNS stimulation (agitation, nervousness, uneasiness)	• CNS stimulation is rare with the use of topical agents • Advise clients to observe for signs of CNS stimulation, and to notify the provider if symptoms occur. • Stop medication.
Vasoconstriction	• Advise clients who have hypertension and coronary artery disease to avoid using these medications.

Ⓢ Contraindications/Precautions

- These medications are contraindicated in clients who have chronic rhinitis.
- Use cautiously in clients who have coronary artery disease and hypertension.

Nursing Administration

- When administering nasal drops, instruct clients to be in the lateral, head-low position to increase the desired effect and to prevent swallowing the medication.

- Use drops for children to facilitate precise dosage and prevent toxicity.

- Educate clients in the differences between topical and oral agents.

  o Topical agents are usually more effective and work faster.

  o Topical agents have a shorter duration.

  o Vasoconstriction and CNS stimulation are uncommon with topical agents, but are a concern with oral agents.

  o Oral agents do not lead to rebound congestion.

- Advise clients to use topical decongestions for no longer than 3 to 5 days to avoid rebound congestion.

- Instruct clients not to exceed recommended doses.

Nursing Evaluation of Medication Effectiveness

- Depending on therapeutic intent, effectiveness may be evidenced by:

  o Improvement of symptoms (relief of congestion, increased ease of breathing, ability to sleep comfortably)

MEDICATION CLASSIFICATION: ANTIHISTAMINES

- Select Prototype Medications:

  o 1st generation H_1 antagonists:

    - Diphenhydramine (Benadryl)

    - Promethazine (Phenergan)

    - Dimenhydrinate (Dramamine)

- Other Medications:

  o 2nd generation H_1 antagonists:

    - Loratadine (Claritin)

    - Cetirizine (Zyrtec)

    - Fexofenadine (Allegra)

    - Desloratadine (Clarinex)

Purpose

- Expected Pharmacological Action

    o Antihistamine action is on the H_1 receptors, which results in the blocking of histamine release in the small blood vessels, capillaries, and nerves during allergic reactions. When used for upper respiratory infections, antihistamines relieve symptoms by suppressing mucous secretion because of their anticholinergic effect.

- Therapeutic Uses

    o 1st generation H_1 antagonists are used for:

        ■ Mild allergic reactions (seasonal allergic rhinitis, urticaria, mild transfusion reaction)

        ■ Anaphylaxis (hypotension, acute laryngeal edema, bronchospasm)

        ■ Motion sickness

        ■ Insomnia

Complications

SIDE/ADVERSE EFFECTS	NURSING INTERVENTIONS/CLIENT EDUCATION
1st generation H_1 antagonists	
Sedation	• Advise clients to take the medication at night to minimize daytime sedative effect. • Instruct clients to avoid hazardous activities (driving), consumption of alcohol, and other CNS depressant medications (barbiturates, benzodiazepines, opioids).
Anticholinergic effects (dry mouth, constipation)	• Advise clients to take sips of water, suck on sugarless candies, and maintain 2 to 3 L of water each day from food and beverage sources.
GI discomfort (nausea, vomiting, constipation)	• Advise clients to take antihistamine with meals.
Acute toxicity (flushed face, high fever, tachycardia, dry mouth, urinary retention, pupil dilation) – Children have symptoms of excitation, hallucinations, incoordination and seizures	• Advise clients to notify the provider if symptoms occur. • Administer activated charcoal and cathartic to decrease absorption of antihistamine. • Administer acetaminophen for fever. • Apply ice packs or sponge baths.

Contraindications/Precautions

- Antihistamines are contraindicated during the third trimester of pregnancy, for mothers who are breastfeeding, and for newborns. Newborns are sensitive to the adverse effects, such as sedation, of these medications.

- Use cautiously in children and older adults (impact of adverse effects).

- Use cautiously in clients who have asthma, urinary retention, open angle glaucoma, hypertension, and prostate hypertrophy (impact of anticholinergic medications).

Interactions

MEDICATION/FOOD INTERACTIONS	NURSING INTERVENTIONS/CLIENT EDUCATION
CNS depressants/alcohol cause additive CNS depression.	• Advise clients to avoid alcohol and medications causing CNS depression (opioids, barbiturates, and benzodiazepines).

Nursing Administration

- Advise clients taking first-generation medications to be aware of sedating effects.

Nursing Evaluation of Medication Effectiveness

- Depending on therapeutic intent, effectiveness may be evidenced by:

  o Improvement of allergic reaction (absence of rhinitis, urticaria)

  o Relief of symptoms of motion sickness (decreased nausea and vomiting)

APPLICATION EXERCISES

1. A nurse is caring for a client who states she has been taking phenylephrine (Neo-Synephrine) nasal drops for the past 10 days for her upper respiratory symptoms. The nurse should plan to monitor the client for which of the following findings?

    A. Sedation

    B. Nasal congestion

    C. Productive cough

    D. Constipation

2. A nurse is reinforcing teaching to a client regarding the self-administration of nasal drops for allergic rhinitis symptoms. The nurse should instruct the client to lie in which position to obtain the best effect of the medication?

3. Match the following medications to their therapeutic action:

    _____ Phenylephrine   A. Mucolytic

    _____ Acetylcysteine (Mucomyst)   B. Antitussive

    _____ Guaifenesin (Mucinex)   C. Expectorant

    _____ Dextromethorphan (Robitussin)   D. Decongestant

4. A nurse is caring for a preschool-age child who may have taken an overdose of diphenhydramine (Benadryl). To identify antihistamine toxicity, the nurse should plan to monitor the child for which of the following?

    A. Hallucinations

    B. Bradycardia

    C. Pinpoint pupils

    D. Pallor

5. A nurse is caring for a client who is taking 20 mg of liquid codeine six times daily as an antitussive medication. What potentially serious adverse effect should the nurse monitor the client for?

APPLICATION EXERCISES ANSWER KEY

1. A nurse is caring for a client who states she has been taking phenylephrine (Neo-Synephrine) nasal drops for the past 10 days for her upper respiratory symptoms. The nurse should plan to monitor the client for which of the following findings?

    A. Sedation

    B. Nasal congestion

    C. Productive cough

    D. Constipation

    When used for over 5 days, rebound nasal congestion may occur when taking topical sympathomimetic medications, such as phenylephrine. Insomnia, rather than sedation, is a possible adverse effect of the medication. Productive cough is not an expected adverse effect. Constipation, an anticholinergic adverse effect, is not caused by sympathomimetic medications, such as phenylephrine.

 NCLEX® Connection: Pharmacological Therapies, Adverse Effects/Contraindications/Side Effects/Interactions

2. A nurse is reinforcing teaching to a client regarding the self-administration of nasal drops for allergic rhinitis symptoms. The nurse should instruct the client to lie in which position to obtain the best effect of the medication?

    The client should lay in a lateral position with the head in a low position. This helps spread the nasal drops and allows the medication to be more effective. It also prevents swallowing the medication.

 NCLEX® Connection: Pharmacological Therapies, Medication Administration

3. Match the following medications to their therapeutic action:

D	Phenylephrine	A. Mucolytic
A	Acetylcysteine (Mucomyst)	B. Antitussive
C	Guaifenesin (Mucinex)	C. Expectorant
B	Dextromethorphan (Robitussin)	D. Decongestant

 NCLEX® Connection: Pharmacological Therapies, Expected Actions/Outcomes

4. A nurse is caring for a preschool-age child who may have taken an overdose of diphenhydramine (Benadryl). To identify antihistamine toxicity, the nurse should plan to monitor the child for which of the following?

    A. Hallucinations

    B. Bradycardia

    C. Pinpoint pupils

    D. Pallor

    In children, antihistamine toxicity may be manifested by hallucinations, ataxia, excitation, and seizures. Other findings in antihistamine toxicity may include tachycardia, dilated pupils, and flushed face.

 NCLEX® Connection: Pharmacological Therapies, Adverse Effects/Contraindications/Side Effects/Interactions

5. A nurse is caring for a client who is taking 20 mg of liquid codeine six times daily as an antitussive medication. What potentially serious adverse effect should the nurse monitor the client for?

    The nurse should monitor the client for respiratory depression, which is a potential problem for a client who is taking an opioid medication.

 NCLEX® Connection: Pharmacological Therapies, Adverse Effects/Contraindications/Side Effects/Interactions

UNIT 4: MEDICATIONS AFFECTING THE CARDIOVASCULAR SYSTEM

- Medications Affecting Urinary Output

- Medications Affecting Blood Pressure

- Cardiac Glycosides and Heart Failure

- Angina

- Antilipemic Agents

NCLEX® CONNECTIONS

When reviewing the chapters in this section, keep in mind the relevant sections of the NCLEX® outline, in particular:

CLIENT NEEDS: PHARMACOLOGICAL THERAPIES

Relevant topics/tasks include:
- Adverse Effects/Contraindications/Side Effects/Interactions
  - Implement procedures to counteract adverse effects of medications.
- Expected Actions/Outcomes
  - Apply knowledge of pathophysiology when addressing client pharmacological agents.
- Medication Administration
  - Regulate client intravenous (IV) rate.

UNIT 4	MEDICATIONS AFFECTING THE CARDIOVASCULAR SYSTEM
Chapter 19	Medications Affecting Urinary Output

 Overview

- Indications for medications that affect urinary output include management of blood pressure, excretion of edematous fluid related to heart failure, kidney and liver disease, and prevention of renal failure.

- Medications include high-ceiling loop diuretics, thiazide diuretics, and potassium-sparing diuretics.

MEDICATION CLASSIFICATION: HIGH CEILING LOOP DIURETICS

- Select Prototype Medication – Furosemide (Lasix)

- Other Medications:

    o Ethacrynic acid (Edecrin)

    o Bumetanide (Bumex)

    o Torsemide (Demadex)

Purpose

- Expected Pharmacological Action

    o High ceiling loop diuretics work in the ascending limb of loop of Henle to:

       ■ Block reabsorption of sodium and chloride and to prevent reabsorption of water

       ■ Cause extensive diuresis even with severe renal impairment

- Therapeutic Uses

    o Emergent need for rapid mobilization of fluid such as:

       ■ Pulmonary edema caused by heart failure

       ■ Conditions not responsive to other diuretics such as edema caused by liver, cardiac, or kidney disease; hypertension

    o Hypercalcemia related to kidney stone formation

- Route of administration – Oral, IV, IM

Complications

SIDE/ADVERSE EFFECTS	NURSING INTERVENTIONS/CLIENT EDUCATION
Dehydration, hyponatremia, hypochloremia	• Monitor clients for signs of dehydration – Dry mouth, increased thirst, minimal urine output, and weight loss. • Monitor electrolytes. • Report urine output less than 30 mL/hr. Stop medication and notify the provider. • If signs of headache and/or chest, calf, or pelvic pain occur, notify the provider. This may be an indication of thrombosis or embolism. • Start clients on low doses and monitor daily weights to minimize the risk for dehydration.
Hypotension	• Monitor the client's blood pressure. • Instruct clients about signs of orthostatic hypotension (lightheadedness, dizziness). Instruct clients to change positions slowly and to sit or lie down if symptoms occur.
Ototoxicity (transient with furosemide and irreversible with ethacrynic acid)	• Advise clients to notify the provider of tinnitus, which may indicate ototoxicity. • Avoid use with other ototoxic medications, such as gentamicin.
Hypokalemia (K+ less than 3.5 mEq/L)	• Monitor the client's cardiac status and potassium levels. • Report a decrease in potassium level (K+ less than 3.5 mEq/L). • Instruct clients to consume high-potassium foods such as bananas and potatoes. • Instruct clients regarding signs of hypokalemia such as nausea/vomiting and general weakness.
Other adverse effects (hyperglycemia, hyperuricemia, and decrease in calcium and magnesium levels)	• Monitor the client's blood glucose, uric acid, and calcium and magnesium levels. • Report elevated levels.

 Contraindications/Precautions

- Pregnancy Risk Category C

- Avoid using these medications during pregnancy unless absolutely required.

- Use cautiously in clients who have diabetes and/or gout.

Interactions

MEDICATION/FOOD INTERACTIONS	NURSING INTERVENTIONS/CLIENT EDUCATION
Digoxin (Lanoxin) toxicity can occur in the presence of hypokalemia.	• Monitor the client's cardiac status and potassium and digoxin levels. • Use potassium-sparing diuretics in conjunction with loop diuretics to reduce the risk of hypokalemia.
Concurrent use of antihypertensives can have additive hypotensive effect.	• Monitor the client's blood pressure.
Hyponatremia can lead to decrease in lithium carbonate (Eskalith) excretion, which may lead to toxicity.	• Monitor the client's lithium levels. Tell clients the provider may adjust the dosage.
NSAIDs reduce diuretic effect.	• Watch for a decrease in the effectiveness of the diuretic, such as a decrease in urine output.

(handwritten: 0·5-13)

Nursing Administration

- Obtain the client's baseline data to include orthostatic blood pressure, weight, electrolytes, and location and extent of edema.

- Weigh clients at the same time each day; usually upon awakening.

- Monitor the client's blood pressure and I&O.

- Avoid administering the medication late in the day to prevent nocturia. Usual dosing time is 0800 and 1400.

- Administer furosemide orally. Monitor clients receiving IV bolus dose.

- Notify the provider if the client's potassium level drops below 3.5 mEq/L. Prepare to administer a potassium supplement and apply a cardiac monitor to observe for dysrhythmias. *(handwritten: irregular heart beat)*

- Show clients who have hypertension how to self-monitor blood pressure and weight by keeping a log.

- Advise clients to get up slowly to minimize orthostatic hypotension. If faintness or dizziness occurs, instruct clients to sit or lie down.

- Instruct clients to report significant weight loss, hearing loss, lightheadedness, dizziness, gastrointestinal (GI) distress, and/or general weakness to the provider.

- Encourage clients to consume foods high in potassium, such as avocados and strawberries.

- Instruct clients with diabetes to monitor for elevated blood glucose levels.

- Instruct clients to observe for signs of low magnesium levels such as muscle twitching and tremors.

Nursing Evaluation of Medication Effectiveness

- Depending on therapeutic intent, effectiveness may be evidenced by:

  o Decrease in pulmonary or peripheral edema

  o Weight loss

  o Decrease in blood pressure

  o Increase in urine output

MEDICATION CLASSIFICATION: THIAZIDE DIURETICS

- Select Prototype Medication – Hydrochlorothiazide (HydroDIURIL)

- Other Medications:

  o Chlorothiazide (Diuril)

  o Methyclothiazide (Enduron)

  o Thiazide-type diuretics:

    ▪ Indapamide (Lozide, Lozol)

    ▪ Chlorthalidone (Hygroton)

    ▪ Metolazone (Zaroxolyn)

Purpose

- Expected Pharmacological Action

  o Thiazide diuretics work in the early distal convoluted tubule to:

    ▪ Block the reabsorption of sodium and chloride, and prevent the reabsorption of water at this site

    ▪ Promote diuresis when renal function is not impaired

- Therapeutic Uses

  o Essential hypertension

  o Management of edema of mild-to-moderate heart failure and liver and kidney disease

Complications

SIDE/ADVERSE EFFECTS	NURSING INTERVENTIONS/CLIENT EDUCATION
Dehydration	• Monitor clients for signs of dehydration (dry mouth, increased thirst, minimal urine output, weight loss). • Monitor electrolytes and daily weight. • Report urine output less than 30 mL/hr. Stop medication and notify the provider.

SIDE/ADVERSE EFFECTS	NURSING INTERVENTIONS/CLIENT EDUCATION
Hypokalemia (K+ less than 3.5 mEq/L)	• Monitor the client's cardiac status and K+ levels. • Report a decrease in K+ level (less than 3.5 mEq/L). • Instruct clients to consume foods high in potassium, such as spinach and tomatoes. • Instruct clients to recognize signs and symptoms of hypokalemia (nausea/vomiting, general weakness).
Hyperglycemia	• Monitor clients for an increase in blood glucose levels.

 Contraindications/Precautions

- Thiazide diuretics are Pregnancy Risk Category B. Avoid use during pregnancy and lactation. If a thiazide diuretic is indicated, advise clients not to breastfeed.

Interactions

MEDICATION/FOOD INTERACTIONS	NURSING INTERVENTIONS/CLIENT EDUCATION
Digoxin (Lanoxin) toxicity can occur in the presence of hypokalemia.	• Monitor the client's cardiac status and potassium and digoxin levels. • Use a potassium-sparing diuretic in conjunction with thiazide diuretics to reduce the risk of hypokalemia.
Antihypertensives have additive hypotensive effects.	• Monitor the client's blood pressure.
Hyponatremia can lead to decrease in lithium carbonate (Eskalith) excretion, which may lead to toxicity.	• Monitor the client's lithium levels. Tell clients the provider may adjust the dosage.
NSAIDs reduce diuretic effect.	• Watch for a decrease in the effectiveness of the diuretic, such as reduced urine output.

Nursing Administration

- Administer medications by oral route.

- Obtain the client's baseline data to include orthostatic blood pressure, weight, electrolytes, and location and extent of edema.

- Monitor the client's potassium levels.

- Instruct clients to take the medication first thing in the morning. For twice-a-day dosing, instruct clients to take the second dose by 1400 to prevent nocturia.

- Encourage clients to consume foods high in potassium and maintain adequate fluid intake (2 to 3 L per day, unless contraindicated).

- If GI upset occurs, advise clients to take the medication with or after meals.

- Instruct clients that the provider may prescribe alternate-day dosing to decrease electrolyte imbalances.

Nursing Evaluation of Medication Effectiveness

- Depending on therapeutic intent, effectiveness may be evidenced by:

  o Decrease in blood pressure

  o Decrease in edema

  o Increase in urine output

MEDICATION CLASSIFICATION: POTASSIUM-SPARING DIURETICS

- Select Prototype Medication – Spironolactone (Aldactone)

- Other Medications – Triamterene (Dyrenium), amiloride (Midamor)

Purpose

- Expected Pharmacological Action

  o Potassium-sparing diuretics work in the distal nephron to:

    ▪ Block the action of aldosterone (sodium and water retention), which results in potassium retention and the secretion of sodium and water.

- Therapeutic Uses

  o Heart failure

  o In primary hyperaldosteronism, potassium-sparing diuretics block actions of aldosterone.

- Route of administration – Oral

Complications

SIDE/ADVERSE EFFECTS	NURSING INTERVENTIONS/CLIENT EDUCATION
Hyperkalemia (K+ greater than 5.0 mEq/L)	• Monitor potassium level. Initiate cardiac monitoring for serum potassium greater than 5 mEq/L. • Treat hyperkalemia by discontinuing medication, restricting potassium in the diet, and insulin injections to drive potassium back into the cell.
Endocrine effects (impotence in male clients; irregularities of menstrual cycle in female clients)	• Advise clients to observe for side effects. • Advise clients to notify the provider if these responses occur.

Contraindications/Precautions

- Do not administer to clients who have hyperkalemia.

- Potassium-sparing diuretics are contraindicated in clients who have severe renal failure and anuria.

Interactions

MEDICATION/FOOD INTERACTIONS	NURSING INTERVENTIONS/CLIENT EDUCATION
Concurrent use of ACE inhibitors and angiotensin II receptor blockers increase the risk of hyperkalemia.	• Monitor the client's K+ levels. Notify the provider if K+ is greater than 5.0 mEq/L.
Concurrent use of potassium supplements increases the risk of hyperkalemia.	• Avoid concurrent use.

Nursing Administration

- Instruct clients that the onset of action for spironolactone is one to two days.

- Obtain the client's baseline data.

- Monitor the client's potassium levels regularly.

- Remind clients to avoid salt substitutes that contain potassium.

- Show clients how to self-monitor blood pressure.

- Instruct clients to keep a log of blood pressure and weight.

- Warn clients that triamterene may turn urine a pale, bluish color.

Nursing Evaluation of Medication Effectiveness

- Depending on therapeutic intent, effectiveness may be evidenced by:

  ○ Maintenance of normal potassium levels – Between 3.5 mEq/L and 5.0 mEq/L

  ○ Weight loss

  ○ Decrease in blood pressure and edema.

APPLICATION EXERCISES

1. A nurse is reinforcing teaching for a client who has hypertension and is prescribed hydrochlorothiazide (HydroDIURIL) twice daily. Which of the following instructions should the nurse include in the client's teaching?

    A. "You should avoid foods high in potassium."

    B. "Take the second dose of the day by early afternoon."

    C. "Watch for ankle swelling that may appear late in the evening.

    D. "Limit your daily fluid intake to 1½ L."

2. The nurse should monitor the client for the adverse effect of tinnitus and hearing loss when administering which of the following diuretics?

    A. Ethacrynic acid (Edecrin)

    B. Chlorothiazide (Diuril)

    C. Triamterene (Dyrenium)

    D. Metolazone (Zaroxolyn)

3. A client has a new prescription for spironolactone (Aldactone). Which of the following laboratory values should the nurse recognize as a reason to withhold the morning dose of the medication and notify the provider?

    A. Serum sodium 138 mEq/L

    B. Serum potassium 5.2 mEq/L

    C. Serum creatinine 1.2 mg/dL

    D. Serum chloride 106 mEq/L

4. A nurse is caring for a client who is prescribed daily doses of both digoxin (Lanoxin) and furosemide (Lasix). The client's potassium level is 3.2 mEq/L. For which of the following medication interactions is the client at risk?

    A. Toxic levels of furosemide

    B. Toxic levels of digoxin

    C. Sub-therapeutic levels of furosemide

    D. Sub-therapeutic levels of digoxin

APPLICATION EXERCISES ANSWER KEY

1. A nurse is reinforcing teaching for a client who has hypertension and is prescribed hydrochlorothiazide (HydroDIURIL) twice daily. Which of the following instructions should the nurse include in the client's teaching?

    A. "You should avoid foods high in potassium."

    B. "Take the second dose of the day by early afternoon."

    C. "Watch for ankle swelling that may appear late in the evening.

    D. "Limit your daily fluid intake to 1½ L."

    The second daily dose is usually taken by 1400 daily in order to allow for diuresis before bedtime. Encourage the client to eat foods high in potassium while taking hydrochlorothiazide to prevent hypokalemia. An expected effect of the thiazide diuretic is to decrease ankle swelling; it is not a potential adverse effect. Instruct clients taking hydrochlorothiazide to consume between 2 to 3 L of fluid daily in order to promote urine output.

 NCLEX® Connection: Pharmacological Therapies, Medication Administration

2. The nurse should monitor the client for the adverse effect of tinnitus and hearing loss when administering which of the following diuretics?

    A. Ethacrynic acid (Edecrin)

    B. Chlorothiazide (Diuril)

    C. Triamterene (Dyrenium)

    D. Metolazone (Zaroxolyn)

    The high-loop diuretic ethacrynic acid may cause irreversible hearing loss. The nurse should monitor the client for hearing loss and report to the provider if it occurs. Chlorothiazide (a thiazide diuretic), triamterene (a potassium-sparing diuretic), and metolazone (a thiazide-type diuretic) do not cause hearing loss.

 NCLEX® Connection: Pharmacological Therapies, Adverse Effects/Contraindications/Side Effects/Interactions

3. A client has a new prescription for spironolactone (Aldactone). Which of the following laboratory values should the nurse recognize as a reason to withhold the morning dose of the medication and notify the provider?

    A. Serum sodium 138 mEq/L

    B. Serum potassium 5.2 mEq/L

    C. Serum creatinine 1.2 mg/dL

    D. Serum chloride 106 mEq/L

    The nurse should not administer spironolactone, a potassium-sparing diuretic, if the serum potassium is higher than 5.0 mEq/L. The serum sodium, creatinine, and chloride levels are all within the expected reference range.

  NCLEX® Connection: Pharmacological Therapies, Adverse Effects/Contraindications/Side Effects/Interactions

4. A nurse is caring for a client who is prescribed daily doses of both digoxin (Lanoxin) and furosemide (Lasix). The client's potassium level is 3.2 mEq/L. For which of the following medication interactions is the client at risk?

    A. Toxic levels of furosemide

    B. Toxic levels of digoxin

    C. Sub-therapeutic levels of furosemide

    D. Sub-therapeutic levels of digoxin

    If potassium levels are decreased in the client who takes both a loop diuretic and digoxin, there is an increased risk for digoxin toxicity. The other choices are not potential interactions between the two medications when potassium levels are low.

  NCLEX® Connection: Pharmacological Therapies, Adverse Effects/Contraindications/Side Effects/Interactions

UNIT 4	MEDICATIONS AFFECTING THE CARDIOVASCULAR SYSTEM
Chapter 20	Medications Affecting Blood Pressure

Overview

- Guidelines for pharmacological management of hypertension can be found in The Seventh Report of the Joint National Committee on Prevention, Detection, Evaluation, and Treatment of High Blood Pressure (JNC 7) prepared by the US Department of Health and Human Services. Pharmacological management involves treatment with a single agent or a combination of medications.

- Classifications include:

  [handwritten: Treat Hypertension / Edema — Reduce the risk of death, stroke, heart attack heart failure, due to Hypertension.]

  o Thiazide diuretics

  o Angiotensin-converting enzyme (ACE) inhibitors

  o Angiotensin II receptor blockers (ARBS)

  [handwritten: Treat Heart failure, Controlling high blood pressure preventing Kidney failure in people.]

  o Calcium channel blockers (CCB)

  o Alpha-adrenergic blockers

  o Centrally acting alpha₂ agonists

  o Beta-adrenergic blockers

MEDICATION CLASSIFICATION: ANGIOTENSIN-CONVERTING ENZYME (ACE) INHIBITORS

- Select Prototype Medication – Captopril (Capoten) *[handwritten: — treat]*

- Other Medications:

  [handwritten: (1) Hypertension (2) Heart failure (3) To improve survival after a heart attack (4)]

  o Enalapril (Vasotec)

  o Enalaprilat (Vasotec IV)

  o Fosinopril (Monopril)

  o Lisinopril (Prinivil)

  o Ramipril (Altace)

Purpose

- Expected Pharmacological Action

  o ACE inhibitors produce their effects by blocking the production of angiotensin II, leading to:

    ■ Vasodilation (mostly arteriole).

    ■ Excretion of sodium and water, and retention of potassium by actions in the kidneys.

    ■ Reduction in pathological changes in the blood vessels and heart that result from the presence of angiotensin II and aldosterone.

- Therapeutic Uses

  o Hypertension

  o Heart failure

  o Myocardial infarction (to decrease mortality and to decrease risk of heart failure and left ventricular dysfunction)

  o Diabetic and nondiabetic nephropathy

  o For clients at high risk for a cardiovascular event, use ramipril to prevent MI, stroke, or death.

Complications

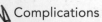

SIDE/ADVERSE EFFECTS	NURSING INTERVENTIONS/CLIENT EDUCATION
First-dose orthostatic hypotension	• If clients are already taking a diuretic, instruct them to withhold the medication temporarily for 2 to 3 days prior to the start of an ACE inhibitor. • Give first dose at bedtime. • Start treatment with a low dosage of the medication. • Monitor the client's blood pressure for 2 hr after initiation of treatment, if given during the day. • Instruct clients to change positions slowly and to lie down if feeling dizzy, lightheaded, or faint.
Cough related to inhibition of kinase II (alternative name for ACE) which results in increase in bradykinin	• Inform clients to withhold the medication and notify the provider if they experience a cough. The provider will then discontinue the medication.
Hyperkalemia	• Monitor potassium levels to maintain a level within the expected reference range of 3.5 to 5 mEq/L. • Advise clients to avoid the use of salt substitutes containing potassium.
Rash and dysgeusia (altered taste), primarily with captopril	• Instruct clients to inform the provider if these effects occur. • Instruct clients that symptoms will stop with discontinuation of the medication.

SIDE/ADVERSE EFFECTS	NURSING INTERVENTIONS/CLIENT EDUCATION
Angioedema (swelling of the tongue and oral pharynx)	• Treat severe effects with subcutaneous injection of epinephrine. • Tell clients the provider will discontinue the medication.
Neutropenia (rare but serious complication of captopril)	• Monitor the client's WBC counts every 2 weeks for 3 months, then periodically. • Inform clients to notify the provider at the first signs of infection. (fever, sore throat). The provider will discontinue the medication.

 Contraindications/Precautions

- These medications are Pregnancy Risk Category D during the second and third trimester, related to fetal injury.

- ACE inhibitors are contraindicated in clients with renal stenosis when present bilaterally or in a single remaining kidney.

- These medications are contraindicated in clients with a history of angioedema following use of an ACE inhibitor.

- Use cautiously in clients with renal impairment and collagen vascular disease because they are at greater risk for developing neutropenia. Closely monitor these clients for signs of infection.

Interactions

MEDICATION/FOOD INTERACTIONS	NURSING INTERVENTIONS/CLIENT EDUCATION
Diuretics can contribute to first-dose hypotension.	• Advise clients to temporarily stop taking diuretics 2 to 3 days before the start of therapy with an ACE inhibitor.
Antihypertensive medications may have an additive hypotensive effect.	• Advise clients that dosage of medication may need to be adjusted if ACE inhibitors are added to the treatment regimen.
Potassium supplements and potassium-sparing diuretics increase the risk of hyperkalemia.	• Advise clients to only take potassium supplements if prescribed by the provider. Clients should avoid salt substitutes that contain potassium.
ACE inhibitors can increase levels of lithium carbonate (Eskalith).	• Monitor the client's lithium levels to avoid toxicity.
Use of NSAIDs may decrease the antihypertensive effect of ACE inhibitors.	• Avoid concurrent use.
Concurrent use of ACE inhibitors and NSAIDs increases the risk of acute renal failure.	• Avoid concurrent use. May continue therapy with low-dose aspirin if indicated.

Nursing Administration

- Administer ACE inhibitors orally. Enalaprilat is the only ACE inhibitor for IV use.

- Advise clients that the medication may be prescribed as a single formulation or in combination with hydrochlorothiazide.

- Advise clients that blood pressure will be monitored after the first dose for at least 2 hr to detect hypotension.

- Instruct clients to take captopril at least 1 hr before meals. All other ACE inhibitors can be taken with or without food.

- Advise clients to notify the provider if cough, rash, dysgeusia (lack of taste), and/or signs of infection occur.

MEDICATION CLASSIFICATION: ANGIOTENSIN II RECEPTOR BLOCKERS (ARBS)

- Select Prototype Medication – Losartan (Cozaar)

- Other Medications:

    - Valsartan (Diovan)

    - Irbesartan (Avapro)

    - Candesartan (Atacand)

    - Olmesartan (Benicar)

Purpose

- Expected Pharmacological Action

    - These medications block the action of angiotensin II in the body. This results in:

        - Vasodilation (mostly arteriole)

        - Excretion of sodium and water, and retention of potassium (through effects on the kidney)

- Therapeutic Uses

    - Hypertension

    - Heart failure and prevention of mortality following MI

    - Stroke prevention

    - Delay progression of diabetic nephropathy

Complications

- The major difference between ARBs and ACE inhibitors is that cough and hyperkalemia are not side effects of ARBs.

SIDE/ADVERSE EFFECTS	NURSING INTERVENTIONS/CLIENT EDUCATION
Angioedema	• Advise clients to observe for signs and symptoms (skin wheals, swelling of tongue) and to notify the provider. • Treat severe effects with subcutaneous injection of epinephrine. • Medication should be discontinued.

 Contraindications/Precautions

- ARBs are contraindicated in second and third trimester related to fetal injury (Pregnancy Risk Category D).

- These medications are contraindicated in clients with renal stenosis when present bilaterally or in a single remaining kidney

- Use cautiously in clients who experienced angioedema with ACE inhibitor (not an absolute contraindication).

Interactions

MEDICATION/FOOD INTERACTIONS	NURSING INTERVENTIONS/CLIENT EDUCATION
Concurrent use with antihypertensive medications may have an additive effect.	• Advise clients that dosage of medication may need to be adjusted if ACE inhibitors are added to the treatment regimen.
Concurrent use of ARBs and NSAIDs increases the risk of acute renal failure.	• Avoid concurrent use. May continue therapy with low-dose aspirin if indicated.

Nursing Administration

- Administer medications by oral route.

- Advise clients that medication may be prescribed as a single formulation or in combination with hydrochlorothiazide.

- Advise clients that ARBs can be taken with or without food.

MEDICATION CLASSIFICATION: CALCIUM CHANNEL BLOCKERS

- Select Prototype Medications:

  o Nifedipine (Adalat, Procardia)

  o Verapamil (Calan)

  o Diltiazem (Cardizem)

- Other Medications:

  o Amlodipine (Norvasc)

  o Felodipine (Plendil)

  o Nicardipine (Cardene, Cleviprex)

Purpose

- Expected Pharmacological Action

MEDICATION	EXPECTED PHARMACOLOGICAL ACTION	SITE OF ACTION AT THERAPEUTIC DOSES
Nifedipine *Treat high Blood pressure, & prevent Angina (chest pain)*	• Blocking of calcium channels in blood vessels leads to vasodilation of peripheral arterioles and arteries/arterioles of the heart.	• Nifedipine acts primarily on arterioles. • Veins are not significantly affected.
Verapamil, diltiazem	• Blocking of calcium channels in blood vessels leads to vasodilation of peripheral arterioles and arteries/arterioles of the heart. • Blocking of calcium channels in the myocardium, the SA node, and the AV node leads to a decreased force of contraction, a decreased heart rate, and slowing of the rate of conduction through the AV node.	• These medications act on arterioles and the heart at therapeutic doses. • Veins are not significantly affected.

- Therapeutic Uses

Chest pain or stable Angina, pressure

MEDICATION	ANGINA PECTORIS	HYPERTENSION	CARDIAC DYSRHYTHMIAS (ATRIAL FIBRILLATION, ATRIAL FLUTTER, SVT)
Nifedipine	X	X	
Amlodipine	X	X	
Nicardipine	X	X	
Felodipine		X	
Verapamil, diltiazem	X	X	X

Complications

SIDE/ADVERSE EFFECTS	NURSING INTERVENTIONS/CLIENT EDUCATION
Nifedipine	
Reflex tachycardia	• Monitor clients for an increased heart rate. • Administer a beta-adrenergic blocker (metoprolol [Lopressor]) to counteract tachycardia.
Peripheral edema	• Inform clients to observe for swelling in lower extremities and notify the provider if this occurs. • Administer a diuretic to control edema.
Acute toxicity resulting in hypotension, bradycardia, AV block and ventricular tachydysrhythmias	• Monitor the client's vital signs and ECG. Gastric lavage and cathartic may be indicated. • Assist with emergency care as indicated.
Verapamil, diltiazem	
Orthostatic hypotension and peripheral edema	• Monitor the client's blood pressure, edema, and weight daily. • Instruct clients to observe for swelling in the lower extremities, and notify the provider if it occurs. • Administer a diuretic to control edema. • Instruct clients about the signs of orthostatic hypotension (lightheadedness, dizziness). If these occur, advise clients to sit or lie down. Instruct clients to change positions slowly.
Constipation (primarily verapamil)	• Advise clients to increase intake of high fiber food and oral fluids, if not restricted.
Suppression of cardiac function (bradycardia, heart failure)	• Monitor the client's ECG, pulse rate, and rhythm. • Advise clients to observe for suppression of cardiac function (slow pulse, activity intolerance), and to notify the provider if these occur. Tell clients the provider may discontinue the medication.
Dysrhythmias (QRS complex is widened and QT interval is prolonged)	• Monitor the client's vital signs and ECG.
Acute toxicity resulting in hypotension, bradycardia, AV block and ventricular tachydysrhythmias.	• Monitor the client's vital signs and ECG. Gastric lavage and cathartic may be indicated. • Assist with emergency care as indicated.

Contraindications/Precautions

- Pregnancy Risk Category C

- Use cautiously with women who are lactating.

- Use verapamil and diltiazem cautiously in clients receiving digoxin and beta-adrenergic blockers.

 • Use cautiously in older adults and clients who have kidney disorders, liver disorders, or mild to moderate heart failure.

- These medications are contraindicated in clients who have heart block, hypotension, bradycardia, aortic stenosis, or severe heart failure.

Interactions

MEDICATION/FOOD INTERACTIONS	NURSING INTERVENTIONS/CLIENT EDUCATION
Nifedipine	
Use beta-adrenergic blockers such as metoprolol (Lopressor) to decrease reflex tachycardia	• Monitor clients for excessive slowing of heart rate.
Consuming grapefruit juice and nifedipine can lead to toxicity.	• Monitor clients for signs of decrease in blood pressure, increase in heart rate, and flushing. • Advise clients to avoid drinking grapefruit juice.
Verapamil, diltiazem	
Verapamil can increase digoxin (Lanoxin) levels, increasing the risk of digoxin toxicity. Digoxin can cause an additive effect and intensify AV conduction suppression.	• Monitor digoxin levels to maintain therapeutic range between 0.5 to 2.0 ng/mL. • Monitor vital signs for bradycardia
Consuming grapefruit juice and verapamil or diltiazem can lead to toxicity.	• Monitor clients for signs of constipation, a decrease in blood pressure, a decrease in heart rate, and AV block. • Advise clients to avoid drinking grapefruit juice.

Nursing Administration

- Advise clients not to chew or crush sustained-release tablets.

- Advise clients who have angina to record pain frequency, intensity, duration, and location. Instruct clients to notify the provider if attacks increase in frequency, intensity, and/or duration.

- Show clients how to monitor blood pressure and heart rate, as well as keep a blood pressure record.

MEDICATION CLASSIFICATION: ALPHA-ADRENERGIC BLOCKERS (SYMPATHOLYTICS)

- Select Prototype Medication – Prazosin (Minipress)
- Other Medication – Doxazosin mesylate (Cardura)

Purpose

- Expected Pharmacological Action
  - Selective alpha$_1$ blockade results in:
    - Venous and arterial dilation
    - Smooth muscle relaxation of the prostatic capsule and bladder neck
- Therapeutic Uses
  - Primary hypertension
  - Use doxazosin (Cardura) to decrease symptoms of benign prostatic hypertrophy (BPH), which include urgency, frequency, and dysuria.

Complications

SIDE/ADVERSE EFFECTS	NURSING INTERVENTIONS/CLIENT EDUCATION
First-dose orthostatic hypotension	<ul><li>Start treatment with low dosage of medication.</li><li>Give first dose at bedtime. Monitor blood pressure for 2 hr after the initiation of treatment, if given during the day.</li><li>Instruct clients to avoid activities requiring mental alertness for the first 12 to 24 hr.</li><li>Instruct clients to change positions slowly and to lie down if feeling dizzy, lightheaded, or faint.</li></ul>

Contraindications/Precautions

- Pregnancy Risk Category C
- Contraindicated in clients with hypersensitivity to medication

Interactions

MEDICATION/FOOD INTERACTIONS	NURSING INTERVENTIONS/CLIENT EDUCATION
Antihypertensive medications may have an additive hypotensive effect	<ul><li>Instruct clients to observe for signs of hypotension (dizziness, lightheadedness, faintness).</li><li>Instruct clients to lie down if these symptoms occur, and to change positions slowly.</li></ul>
NSAIDs and clonidine may decrease the antihypertensive effects of prazosin.	<ul><li>Advise clients to avoid OTC NSAIDs.</li></ul>

Nursing Administration

- Obtain baseline blood pressure and heart rate.

- Instruct clients that the medication can be taken with food.

- Recommend that clients take the initial dose at bedtime to decrease "first-dose" hypotensive effect.

MEDICATION CLASSIFICATION: CENTRALLY ACTING ALPHA$_2$ AGONISTS

- Select Prototype Medication – Clonidine (Catapres)   *lowering high blood pressure*

- Other Medications – Guanfacine HCl (Tenex), methyldopa (Aldomet) *to prevent strokes*

Purpose

- Expected Pharmacological Action

  o These medications act within the CNS to decrease sympathetic outflow resulting in decreased stimulation of the adrenergic receptors (both alpha and beta receptors) of the heart and peripheral vascular system.

    ▪ Decrease in sympathetic outflow to the myocardium results in bradycardia and decreased cardiac output (CO).

    ▪ Decrease in sympathetic outflow to the peripheral vasculature results in vasodilation, which leads to decreased blood pressure.

- Therapeutic Uses

  o Primary hypertension (administered alone, with a diuretic, or with another antihypertensive agent)

  o Severe cancer pain (administered parenterally by epidural infusion)

  o Investigational use

    ▪ Migraine headache

    ▪ Flushing from menopause

    ▪ Management of ADHD and Tourette's syndrome

    ▪ Management of withdrawal symptoms from alcohol, tobacco, and opioids

Complications

SIDE/ADVERSE EFFECTS	NURSING INTERVENTIONS/CLIENT EDUCATION
Drowsiness and sedation	• Advise clients that drowsiness will diminish as use of medication continues. • Advise clients to avoid activities that require mental alertness until symptoms subside.
Dry mouth	• Advise clients to adhere to the medication regimen. • Reassure clients that symptoms usually resolve in 2 to 4 weeks. • Encourage clients to chew gum or suck on hard candy, and to sip small amounts of water or suck on ice chips.
Rebound hypertension	• Advise clients not to discontinue treatment without consulting the provider. • Reinforce to clients how to slowly taper dosage over 2 to 4 days.

 Contraindications/Precautions

- Clonidine is Pregnancy Risk Category C.

- Avoid use during lactation.

- This medication is contraindicated for clients taking anticoagulant medications.

- Avoid use of transdermal patch on affected skin in scleroderma and systemic lupus erythematosus (SLE).

- Use cautiously in clients with cerebrovascular disease, recent MI, diabetes mellitus, major depressive disorder, or chronic renal failure.

Interactions

MEDICATION/FOOD INTERACTIONS	NURSING INTERVENTIONS/CLIENT EDUCATION
Antihypertensive medications may have an additive hypotensive effect.	• Instruct clients to observe for signs of hypotension (dizziness, lightheadedness, faintness). • Instruct clients to lie down if feeling dizzy, lightheaded, or faint, and change positions slowly.
Concurrent use of prazosin (Minipress), MAOIs, and tricyclic antidepressants can counteract the antihypertensive effect of clonidine.	• Monitor clients for therapeutic effect. • Monitor blood pressure. • Avoid concurrent use.
Additive CNS depression can occur with concurrent use of other CNS depressants, such as alcohol.	• Advise clients of additive CNS depression with alcohol, and encourage clients to avoid use.

Nursing Administration

- Administer medication by oral or transdermal route. Medication is also available for epidural administration.

- Instruct clients that medication is usually administered twice a day in divided doses and to take larger dose at bedtime to decrease the occurrence of daytime sleepiness.

- Inform clients to apply a transdermal patch every 7 days. Advise clients to apply patch on hairless, intact skin on torso or upper arm.

MEDICATION CLASSIFICATION: BETA-ADRENERGIC BLOCKERS (SYMPATHOLYTICS)

- Select Prototype Medications:

  - Cardioselective: Beta$_1$

    - Metoprolol (Lopressor)

    - Atenolol (Tenormin)

    - Metoprolol succinate (Toprol XL)

    - Esmolol HCL (Brevibloc)

  - Nonselective: (Beta$_1$ and Beta$_2$)

    - Propranolol (Inderal)

    - Nadolol (Corgard)

    - Labetalol (Normodyne)

Purpose

- Expected Pharmacological Action

  - In cardiac conditions, the primary effects of beta-adrenergic blockers are a result of beta$_1$-adrenergic blockade in the myocardium and in the electrical conduction system of the heart.

    - Decreased heart rate (negative chronotropic [rate] action)

    - Decreased myocardial contractility (negative inotropic [force] action)

    - Decreased rate of conduction through the AV node

    - Reduced peripheral vascular resistance

- Therapeutic Uses

  - Primary hypertension (exact mechanism unknown – may be related to long-term use causing reduction in peripheral vascular resistance)

  - Angina, tachydysrhythmias, heart failure and myocardial infarction.

  - Other uses may include:

    - Treatment of hyperthyroidism, migraine headache, stage fright, pheochromocytoma, and glaucoma

Complications

SIDE/ADVERSE EFFECTS	NURSING INTERVENTIONS/CLIENT EDUCATION
Beta₁ Blockade: metoprolol, propranolol	
Bradycardia	• Monitor the client's pulse and if below 60/min, hold medication, and notify the provider. • Use cautiously in clients with diabetes. This medication can mask tachycardia, an early sign of low blood glucose level in clients with diabetes. Advise clients to monitor blood glucose level to detect hypoglycemia.
Decreased cardiac output	• Use cautiously with clients in heart failure. • Advise clients to observe for signs of worsening heart failure (shortness of breath, edema, fatigue) and to notify the provider.
AV block	• Obtain a baseline ECG and monitor.
Orthostatic hypotension	• Advise clients to sit or lie down if experiencing dizziness or faintness and to change positions slowly.
Rebound myocardium excitation	• Advise clients not to stop taking beta-adrenergic blockers abruptly, but to follow the provider's instructions. • Reinforce to clients how to slowly taper dosage over 1 to 2 weeks.
Beta₂ Blockade: propranolol	
Bronchoconstriction	• Contraindicated in clients with asthma.
Glycogenolysis is inhibited	• Clients with diabetes rely on the breakdown of glycogen into glucose to manage low blood glucose (can happen with insulin overdose). • In addition, a decreased heart rate can further mask symptoms of impending low blood glucose level. Clients with diabetes should be administered a beta₁ selective agent.

 Contraindications/Precautions

- Beta-adrenergic blockers are contraindicated in clients with AV block and sinus bradycardia.

- Nonselective beta-adrenergic blockers are contraindicated in clients with asthma, bronchospasm, and heart failure.

- Use cardioselective beta-adrenergic blockers cautiously in clients with heart failure, asthma, bronchospasm, diabetes, a history of severe allergies, and depression.

Interactions

MEDICATION/FOOD INTERACTIONS	NURSING INTERVENTIONS/CLIENT EDUCATION
Beta$_1$ Blockade: metoprolol, propranolol	
Calcium channel blockers (CCB): verapamil (Calan) and diltiazem (Cardizem) intensify the effects of beta-adrenergic blockers • Decreased heart rate • Decreased myocardial contractility • Decreased rate of conduction through the AV node	• Monitor ECG and blood pressure. • Monitor clients closely if taking a CCB and beta-adrenergic blocker concurrently. Notify the provider for possible reduction of dose. • Instruct clients to take pulse rate and report symptoms of bradycardia (dizziness, fatigue, faintness) to the provider.
Concurrent use of antihypertensive medications with beta-adrenergic blockers can intensify the hypotensive effect of both medications.	• Monitor clients for a drop in blood pressure. • Instruct clients to check blood pressure and to report changes to the provider.
Beta$_2$ Blockade: propranolol	
Insulin – Prevents glycogenolysis (Same as above)	• Inform clients that insulin dosage may need to be adjusted when using propranolol.

Nursing Administration

- Administer medications orally, usually once or twice a day.

- Advise clients not to discontinue medication without consulting the provider.

- Advise clients to avoid sudden changes in position to prevent occurrence of orthostatic hypotension.

- Instruct clients not to crush or chew extended-release tablets.

- Show clients how to self-monitor heart rate and blood pressure at home on a daily basis.

Nursing Evaluation of Medication Effectiveness

- Depending on therapeutic intent, effectiveness may be evidenced by:

    o Absence of chest pain.

    o Absence of cardiac dysrhythmias.

    o Normotensive blood pressure readings.

    o Control of heart failure signs and symptoms.

APPLICATION EXERCISES

1. Propranolol (Inderal) is contraindicated for a client who has which of the following conditions?

    A. Asthma

    B. Diabetes

    C. Angina

    D. Dementia

2. A nurse is reinforcing teaching for a client who has a prescription for verapamil (Calan). Which of the following statements by the client indicates a need for further teaching?

    A. "I should increase the amount of fiber in my diet since the medication causes constipation."

    B. "I should eliminate grapefruit juice from my diet while taking verapamil."

    C. "I should decrease the amount of calcium in my diet while taking the medication."

    D. "I should take the medication with food if it causes an upset stomach."

3. A nurse is preparing to administer the first dose of a new prescription of captopril (Capoten) to a hospitalized client. What nursing interventions are necessary following the first dose of captopril?

4. A nurse is caring for a client with a prescription for nifedipine (Procardia) to treat angina pectoris. The nurse should plan to monitor the client for which of the following findings?

    A. Weight loss

    B. Reflex tachycardia

    C. Grand mal seizures

    D. Urinary Retention

5. A nurse is caring for a client on a medical unit who takes regular doses of propranolol (Inderal) for hypertension. Before administering the client's morning dose of propranolol, which of the following should the nurse plan to monitor? (Select all that apply.)

    _____ Urinary output

    _____ Pulse rate

    _____ Temperature

    _____ Blood pressure

    _____ Deep tendon reflexes

6. A nurse is caring for a client who has been taking clonidine (Catapres) for 1 week to treat hypertension. The client relates that she may stop taking the medication because it makes her mouth dry. What does the client need to know about this adverse effect?

APPLICATION EXERCISES ANSWER KEY

1. Propranolol (Inderal) is contraindicated for a client who has which of the following conditions?

    A. Asthma

    B. Diabetes

    C. Angina

    D. Dementia

    Propranolol is a nonselective beta-adrenergic blocker and blocks both $beta_1$ and $beta_2$ receptors. A blockade of $beta_2$ receptors in the lungs causes bronchoconstriction and is contraindicated in clients with asthma. Use propranolol cautiously with clients who have diabetes, but it is not contraindicated. Use propranolol to treat angina. It is not contraindicated in dementia.

     NCLEX® Connection: Pharmacological Therapies, Adverse Effects/Contraindications/Side Effects/Interactions

2. A nurse is reinforcing teaching for a client who has a prescription for verapamil (Calan). Which of the following statements by the client indicates a need for further teaching?

    A. "I should increase the amount of fiber in my diet since the medication causes constipation."

    B. "I should eliminate grapefruit juice from my diet while taking verapamil."

    C. "I should decrease the amount of calcium in my diet while taking the medication."

    D. "I should take the medication with food if it causes an upset stomach."

    There is no restriction on calcium intake when taking verapamil. The client should increase fiber and fluid intake to prevent constipation while taking verapamil. Grapefruit juice can increase blood levels of verapamil, increasing the risk of toxicity. Verapamil can be taken with food to prevent GI adverse effects.

     NCLEX® Connection: Pharmacological Therapies, Medication Administration

3. A nurse is preparing to administer the first dose of a new prescription of captopril (Capoten) to a hospitalized client. What nursing interventions are necessary following the first dose of captopril?

    A sudden drop in blood pressure may occur following the first administered dose of an ACE inhibitor, such as captopril, and orthostatic hypotension may cause injury to the client. The nurse should monitor the client's blood pressure for the first few hours and advise the client to move slowly from lying to sitting or standing positions during this time. If the client is at home, he should take the medication at bedtime and take care when arising. The nurse should be aware that this reaction is even more likely to occur if the client is concurrently taking a diuretic.

     NCLEX® Connection: Pharmacological Therapies, Adverse Effects/Contraindications/Side Effects/Interactions

4. A nurse is caring for a client with a prescription for nifedipine (Procardia) to treat angina pectoris. The nurse should plan to monitor the client for which of the following findings?

    A. Weight loss

    B. Reflex tachycardia

    C. Grand mal seizures

    D. Urinary Retention

Reflex tachycardia may occur with the administration of nifedipine. Many clients who take nifedipine are also prescribed a beta-adrenergic blocker to prevent reflex tachycardia. Weight gain and increased peripheral edema may occur with nifedipine use. Seizures and urinary retention are not expected adverse effects when taking the medication.

 NCLEX® Connection: Pharmacological Therapies, Adverse Effects/Contraindications/Side Effects/Interactions

5. A nurse is caring for a client on a medical unit who takes regular doses of propranolol (Inderal) for hypertension. Before administering the client's morning dose of propranolol, which of the following should the nurse plan to monitor? (Select all that apply.)

_____	Urinary output
X	**Pulse rate**
_____	Temperature
X	**Blood pressure**
_____	Deep tendon reflexes

Prior to administering propranolol, the nurse should monitor the client's pulse for bradycardia and blood pressure for hypotension. The nurse should withhold the medication and notify the provider for a pulse rate less than 60 bpm or a systolic BP less than 90 mm Hg. It is not necessary to monitor urinary output, temperature, and deep tendon reflexes before administering propranolol.

 NCLEX® Connection: Pharmacological Therapies, Medication Administration

6. A nurse is caring for a client who has been taking clonidine (Catapres) for 1 week to treat hypertension. The client relates that she may stop taking the medication because it makes her mouth dry. What does the client need to know about this adverse effect?

The client should know that xerostomia (dry mouth) decreases after 2 to 4 weeks of therapy with clonidine. The client may try sipping fluids, chewing gum, or sucking hard candy to minimize this adverse effect.

 NCLEX® Connection: Pharmacological Therapies, Adverse Effects/Contraindications/Side Effects/Interactions

UNIT 4	MEDICATIONS AFFECTING THE CARDIOVASCULAR SYSTEM
Chapter 21	Cardiac Glycosides and Heart Failure

 Overview

- Heart failure, cardiac failure, or pump failure results from the inability of the heart muscle to pump enough blood to supply the whole body.

- The different determinants of cardiac output such as heart rate, stroke volume, preload, and afterload are affected in heart failure.

- Inability to pump sufficient blood results in:

  o Decreased tissue perfusion as evidenced by fatigue, weakness, and activity intolerance

  o Pulmonary and systemic congestion or volume overload as evidenced by jugular venous distention, peripheral edema, and dyspnea.

- Diuretics, ACE inhibitors, angiotensin II receptor blockers (ARBs), and beta-adrenergic blockers are the medications of choice for treatment of heart failure. Cardiac glycosides are indicated if these medications are unable to control symptoms.

- Adrenergic agonists may be catecholamines or noncatecholamines and may be administered orally, by inhalation, IM and subcutaneous injection and intravenously. Use of these medications primarily takes place in critical care situations for situations such as shock and heart failure. One adrenergic agonist, epinephrine, has use for emergency care of anaphylaxis.

MEDICATION CLASSIFICATION: CARDIAC GLYCOSIDES

- Select Prototype Medication – Digoxin (Lanoxin, Lanoxicaps, and Digitek)

Purpose

- Expected Pharmacological Action

  o Increased myocardial contractility (positive inotropic effect)

    ▪ Increased force and efficiency of myocardial contraction improves the heart's effectiveness as a pump, improving stroke volume and cardiac output.

  o Decreased heart rate (negative chronotropic effect)

    ▪ At therapeutic levels, digoxin slows the rate of SA node depolarization and the rate of impulses through the conduction system of the heart.

    ▪ A decreased heart rate gives the ventricles more time to fill with blood coming from the atria, which leads to increased stroke volume and increased cardiac output.

- Therapeutic Uses
  - ○ Treatment of heart failure
  - ○ Dysrhythmias (atrial fibrillation)

Complications

SIDE/ADVERSE EFFECTS	NURSING INTERVENTIONS/CLIENT EDUCATION

• Dysrhythmias (caused by interfering with the electrical conduction in the myocardium)
• Cardiotoxicity leading to bradycardia
• Hypokalemia, increased serum digoxin levels, and heart disease increase the risk of developing digoxin-induced dysrhythmias.
	• Conditions that increase the risk of developing digoxin-induced dysrhythmias include hypokalemia, increased serum digoxin levels, and heart disease.
	• Monitor serum levels of K+ to maintain a level between 3.5 to 5.0 mEq/L.
	• Instruct clients to report signs of hypokalemia (nausea/vomiting, general weakness).
	• Instruct clients to consume high-potassium foods (spinach, bananas, potatoes).
	• Monitor the client's digoxin level.
	  ○ Therapeutic serum levels may vary but usually range from 0.5 to 2.0 ng/mL.
	  ○ Signs of toxicity may appear at levels less than 1.75 ng/mL.
	  ○ Clients with heart failure respond best with serum medication levels between 0.5 to 08 ng/mL.
	  ○ The provider should base the dosage on serum levels and client response to medication.
	• Show clients how to monitor pulse rate, and recognize and report changes (irregular rate, extra or skipped beats).

• Gastrointestinal effects include anorexia (usually the first sign) nausea, vomiting, and abdominal pain.	• Instruct clients to monitor for these side effects and to report to the provider.
• CNS effects include fatigue, weakness, vision changes (diplopia, blurred vision, yellow-green or white halos around objects).	• Instruct clients to monitor for these side effects and report to the provider if they occur.

Contraindications/Precautions

- Cardiac glycosides are Pregnancy Risk Category C.

- These agents are contraindicated in clients with disturbances in ventricular rhythm, including ventricular fibrillation, ventricular tachycardia, and second- and third-degree heart block.

- Use cautiously in clients who have hypokalemia, partial AV block, advanced heart failure, and renal insufficiency.

Interactions

MEDICATION/FOOD INTERACTIONS	NURSING INTERVENTIONS/CLIENT EDUCATION
• Thiazide diuretics, such as hydrochlorothiazide (HydroDIURIL), and loop diuretics, such as furosemide (Lasix), may lead to hypokalemia, which increases the risk of developing dysrhythmias	• Monitor K+ level and maintain between 3.5 to 5.0 mEq/L. • Manage and prevent hypokalemia by administering potassium supplements or a potassium-sparing diuretic.
• ACE inhibitors and ARBs increase the risk of hyperkalemia, which can lead to decreased therapeutic effects of digoxin.	• Use cautiously if these medications are used with potassium supplements or a potassium-sparing diuretic. • Maintain K+ between 3.5 to 5.0 mEq/L.
• Sympathomimetic medications such as dopamine (Intropin) complement the inotropic action of digoxin and increase the rate and force of heart muscle contraction. • These medications may be beneficial, but also may increase the risk of tachydysrhythmias.	• Monitor ECG.
• Concurrent use with quinidine increases the risk of digoxin toxicity.	• Avoid concurrent use.
• Verapamil (Calan) increases plasma levels of digoxin.	• Avoid concurrent use.

Nursing Administration

- Advise clients to take the medication as prescribed. If a dose is missed, the next dose should not be doubled.

- Check pulse rate and rhythm before administration of digoxin and record. Notify the provider if heart rate is less than 60/min in an adult, less than 70/min in children, and less than 90/min in infants.

- Administer digoxin at the same time daily.

- Monitor digoxin levels periodically during treatment and maintain therapeutic levels between 0.5 to 2.0 ng/mL to prevent digoxin toxicity.

- Instruct clients to avoid taking OTC medications to prevent adverse and side effects and medication interactions.

- Instruct clients to observe for symptoms of hypokalemia, such as muscle weakness, and to notify the provider if symptoms occur.

- Instruct clients to observe for symptoms of digoxin toxicity (anorexia, fatigue, weakness), and to notify the provider if symptoms occur.

- Assist with management of digoxin toxicity

   o Withhold digoxin and potassium-sparing medication immediately.

  o Monitor K+ levels. For levels less than 3.5 mEq/L, monitor clients receiving potassium intravenously or by mouth. Do not give any further K+ if the level is greater than 5.0 mEq/L.

  o Monitor clients receiving phenytoin (Dilantin) or lidocaine for dysrhythmias.

  o Monitor clients receiving atropine for bradycardia.

  o For excessive overdose, monitor clients receiving activated charcoal, cholestyramine, or Digibind can be used to bind digoxin and prevent absorption.

Nursing Evaluation of Medication Effectiveness

- Depending on therapeutic intent, effectiveness may be evidenced by:

  o Control of heart failure signs and symptoms.

  o Absence of cardiac dysrhythmias.

MEDICATION CLASSIFICATION: ADRENERGIC AGONISTS

- Select Prototype Medication

  o Catecholamines

    - Epinephrine hydrochloride (Adrenaline)

    - Dopamine (Intropin)

    - Dobutamine (Dobutrex)

- Other Medications

  o Isoproterenol – Catecholamine

  o Terbutaline – Noncatecholamine

Purpose

RECEPTORS	PHARMACOLOGICAL ACTION	THERAPEUTIC USE
Epinephrine		
Alpha₁	• Vasoconstriction	• Slows absorption of local anesthetics • Manages superficial bleeding • Increases blood pressure
Beta₁	• Increased heart rate • Increased myocardial contractility • Increased rate of conduction through the AV node	• Treatment of AV block and cardiac arrest
Beta₂	• Bronchodilation	• Asthma
Alpha and beta receptors	• Bronchodilation	• Anaphylaxis

Complications

SIDE/ADVERSE EFFECTS	NURSING INTERVENTIONS/CLIENT EDUCATION
Epinephrine	
Vasoconstriction from activation of alpha₁ receptors in the heart can lead to hypertensive crisis.	• Monitor clients receiving continuous cardiac monitoring. • Report changes in vital signs to the provider.
Beta₁ receptor activation in the heart can cause dysrhythmias. Beta₁ receptor activation also increases the workload of the heart and increases oxygen demand, leading to the development of angina.	• Monitor clients receiving continuous cardiac monitoring. • Report changes in vital signs to the provider. • Administer beta-adrenergic blocker.

 Contraindications/Precautions

- Epinephrine is Pregnancy Risk Category C.

- These medications are contraindicated in clients who have tachydysrhythmias and ventricular fibrillation.

- Use cautiously in clients who have hyperthyroidism, angina, history of myocardial infarction, hypertension, and diabetes.

Interactions

MEDICATION/FOOD INTERACTIONS	NURSING INTERVENTIONS/CLIENT EDUCATION
MAOIs prevent inactivation of epinephrine and therefore prolong the effects of epinephrine.	• Avoid use of MAOIs in clients receiving epinephrine.
Tricyclic antidepressants block uptake of epinephrine, which will prolong and intensify effects of epinephrine.	• Clients taking these medications concurrently may need a lowered dosage of epinephrine.

Nursing Administration

- Administer medication by IM, subcutaneous, inhalation or topical route.

- Monitor clients receiving medication by IV route.

- Provide instruction for clients in use of EpiPen. Instruct clients to seek medical care after use.

Nursing Evaluation of Medication Effectiveness

- Depending on therapeutic intent, effectiveness may be evidenced by:

  o Resolution of bronchospasm with no evidence of respiratory distress.

  o Stabilization of blood pressure.

APPLICATION EXERCISES

1. A nurse is monitoring serum electrolytes for a client prescribed digoxin (Lanoxin). The serum potassium is reported to be 2.8 mEq/L. What action should the nurse take? Why?

2. A nurse is reinforcing teaching to a client who is prescribed digoxin (Lanoxin). Which of the following should the nurse instruct the client to report to the provider? (Select all that apply.)

    _____ Fatigue

    _____ Constipation

    _____ Anorexia

    _____ Rash

    _____ Diplopia

3. A nurse is reinforcing teaching for a client who has a new prescription for digoxin (Lanoxin). Which of the following medications, which the client reports taking, should the nurse report to the provider because it is contraindicated when taken with digoxin?

    A. Potassium chloride

    B. Furosemide (Lasix)

    C. Quinidine sulfate

    D. Atorvastatin (Lipitor)

4. A nurse is reinforcing teaching to a client who has heart failure and takes digoxin (Lanoxin). The client tells the nurse that he sometimes forgets to take his medication and asks if he can just take a double dose of digoxin the next morning to make up for the missed dose. What is an appropriate response by the nurse?

APPLICATION EXERCISES ANSWER KEY

1. A nurse is monitoring serum electrolytes for a client prescribed digoxin (Lanoxin). The serum potassium is reported to be 2.8 mEq/L. What action should the nurse take? Why?

    The nurse should report the low level of potassium immediately to the provider as hypokalemia can result in fatal dysrhythmias. Digoxin works by binding to and inhibiting the enzyme Na+K+-ATPase. Potassium and digoxin compete for the same binding sites on this enzyme. With hypokalemia, digoxin has more opportunity to bind to Na+K+-ATPase and can lead to cardiotoxicity.

     NCLEX® Connection: Pharmacological Therapies, Adverse Effects/Contraindications/Side Effects/Interactions

2. A nurse is reinforcing teaching to a client who is prescribed digoxin (Lanoxin). Which of the following should the nurse instruct the client to report to the provider? (Select all that apply.)

X	**Fatigue**
____	Constipation
X	**Anorexia**
____	Rash
X	**Diplopia**

    Fatigue, anorexia, and diplopia are side effects indicating a possible digoxin toxicity. Constipation and rash are not side effects of digoxin toxicity.

     NCLEX® Connection: Pharmacological Therapies, Adverse Effects/Contraindications/Side Effects/Interactions

3. A nurse is reinforcing teaching for a client who has a new prescription for digoxin (Lanoxin). Which of the following medications, which the client reports taking, should the nurse report to the provider because it is contraindicated when taken with digoxin?

    A. Potassium chloride

    B. Furosemide (Lasix)

    C. Quinidine sulfate

    D. Atorvastatin (Lipitor)

    Quinidine sulfate and digoxin should not be taken concurrently as the result could be greatly increased digoxin levels and digoxin toxicity. The nurse should notify the provider about the client's report. Potassium chloride and furosemide are frequently taken concurrently with digoxin without adverse interactions. Taking atorvastatin does not cause an interaction with digoxin.

     NCLEX® Connection: Pharmacological Therapies, Adverse Effects/Contraindications/Side Effects/Interactions

4. A nurse is reinforcing teaching to a client who has heart failure and takes digoxin (Lanoxin). The client tells the nurse that he sometimes forgets to take his medication and asks if he can just take a double dose of digoxin the next morning to make up for the missed dose. What is an appropriate response by the nurse?

   Due to the narrow therapeutic range of digoxin and the high risk for toxicity, the client should not take a double dose of the medication the next day to attempt to make up for a missed dose.

 NCLEX® Connection: Pharmacological Therapies, Medication Administration

UNIT 4	MEDICATIONS AFFECTING THE CARDIOVASCULAR SYSTEM
Chapter 22	Angina

 Overview

- Anginal pain is a result of an imbalance between myocardial oxygen supply and demand. Use pharmacological management to prevent myocardial ischemia and pain as well as to prevent myocardial infarction and death.

- Use organic nitrates, beta-adrenergic blocking agents, calcium channel blockers, and ranolazine to treat anginal pain. In addition, clients with chronic stable angina should concurrently take an antiplatelet agent, such as aspirin or clopidogrel (Plavix), a cholesterol-lowering agent, and an ACE inhibitor to prevent myocardial infarction and death.

MEDICATION CLASSIFICATION: ORGANIC NITRATES

- Select Prototype Medication:

  - Nitroglycerin

    - Sublingual tablet: Nitrostat

    - Translingual spray: Nitrolingual

    - Transmucosal tablets: Nitrogard

    - Topical ointment: Nitro-Bid

    - Transderm patch: Nitro-Dur

    - Intravenous: Nitro-Bid IV

- Other Medications

  - Sublingual – Isosorbide dinitrate (Isordil)

  - Oral – Isosorbide mononitrate (Imdur)

Purpose

- Expected Pharmacological Action

  - In chronic stable exertional angina, nitroglycerin (NTG) dilates veins and decreases venous return (preload), which decreases cardiac oxygen demand.

  - In variant (Prinzmetal's or vasospastic) angina, nitroglycerin prevents or reduces coronary artery spasm, thus increasing oxygen supply.

- Therapeutic Uses

  o Treatment of acute angina attack

  o Prophylaxis of chronic stable angina or variant angina

Complications

SIDE/ADVERSE EFFECTS	NURSING INTERVENTIONS/CLIENT EDUCATION
Headache	• Instruct clients to use aspirin or acetaminophen to relieve pain. • Instruct clients to notify the provider if symptoms do not resolve in a few weeks. Tell clients the provider may reduce the dosage.
Orthostatic hypotension	• Advise clients to sit or lie down if experiencing dizziness or faintness. Elevate feet if possible. • Clients should avoid sudden changes of position and rise slowly.
Reflex tachycardia	• Monitor the client's vital signs. Report elevated heart rate to the provider. • Administer a beta-adrenergic blocker, such as metoprolol (Lopressor), to treat tachycardia.
Tolerance	• Instruct all clients that all long-acting forms of nitroglycerin should be taken with a medication-free period each day (usually 10 to 12 at night).

 Contraindications/Precautions

- Nitroglycerin is Pregnancy Risk Category C.

- This medication is contraindicated in clients with hypersensitivity to nitrates.

- Nitroglycerin is contraindicated in clients with traumatic head injury because the medication can increase intracranial pressure.

- Use cautiously in clients taking antihypertensive medications and clients who have renal or liver dysfunction.

Interactions

MEDICATION/FOOD INTERACTIONS	NURSING INTERVENTIONS/CLIENT EDUCATION
Use of alcohol can contribute to the hypotensive effect of nitroglycerin.	• Advise clients to avoid use of alcohol.
Antihypertensive medications, such as beta-adrenergic blockers, calcium channel blockers, and diuretics can contribute to hypotensive effect.	• Use nitroglycerin cautiously in clients receiving these medications.
Use of sildenafil (Viagra) and nitroglycerin can result in life-threatening hypotension.	• Instruct clients not to take sildenafil if prescribed nitroglycerin.

Nursing Administration

ROUTE	USE	CLIENT EDUCATION

Sublingual tablet and translingual spray
• Rapid onset
• Short duration
	• Treat acute attack
	• Prophylaxis of acute attack
		• Use this rapid-acting nitrate at the first sign of chest pain. Do not wait until pain is severe.
		• Use prior to activity that is known to cause chest pain, such as climbing a flight of stairs.
		• For sublingual tablet:
		  ○ Place the tablet under the tongue and allow it to dissolve.
		  ○ Store tablets in original bottles, and in a cool, dark place.
		  ○ Discard tablets after 24 months unless indicated on the package.
		• Spray translingual spray against oral mucosa. Client should not inhale spray.

Transmucosal • Rapid onset • Long duration	• Treat acute attack • Prophylaxis of acute attack • Long-term prophylaxis against anginal attacks	• Use this rapid-acting nitrate at the first sign of chest pain. Do not wait until pain is severe. • Use prior to activity that is known to cause chest pain, such as climbing a flight of stairs. • Do not chew or swallow the tablet, but place the tablet between the upper lip and gum, or between the cheek and gum to be dissolved, which takes 3 to 5 hr.
Sustained-release oral capsules • Slow onset • Long duration	• Long-term prophylaxis against anginal attacks	• Swallow capsules without crushing or chewing.

ROUTE	USE	CLIENT EDUCATION
Transdermal • Slow onset • Long duration	• Long-term prophylaxis against anginal attacks	• Apply at the same time once each day, preferably in the morning. Keep patch on for 12 to 14 hr each day. • Remove the patch at night to reduce the risk of developing tolerance to nitroglycerin. Be medication-free a minimum of 10 to 12 hr each day (usually at night). • Do not cut patches to ensure appropriate dosage. • Place the patch on a hairless area of skin (chest, back, or abdomen) and rotate sites to prevent skin irritation. • Wash skin with soap and water and dry thoroughly before applying new patch.
Topical ointment • Slow onset • Long duration	• Long-term prophylaxis against anginal attacks	• Remove the prior dose before a new dose is applied. Measure specific dose with applicator paper and spread over 2.5 to 3.5 inches of the paper. • Apply to a clean, hairless area of the body, and cover with clear plastic wrap. • Follow same guidelines for site selection as for transdermal patch. • Avoid touching ointment with the hands.

 View Media Supplement: Application of Nitroglycerin Transdermal Patch & Topical Ointment (Video)

- Treatment of Anginal Attack
  - Instruct clients to:
    - Stop activity.
    - Take a dose of rapid-acting nitroglycerin immediately.
    - Wait 5 min.
    - Call 911 or be driven to an emergency department if pain unrelieved.
    - Take another dose.
    - Wait 5 min.
    - Take another dose if pain unrelieved.

- Clients can take up to three doses at 5 min intervals.

- Advise clients not to stop taking long-acting nitroglycerin abruptly and follow the provider's instructions.

- Advise clients who have angina to record pain frequency, intensity, duration, and location. Notify the provider if attacks increase in frequency, intensity, and/or duration.

Nursing Evaluation of Medication Effectiveness

- Depending on therapeutic intent, effectiveness may be evidenced by:

  - Prevention of acute anginal attacks

  - Long-term management of stable angina

  - Control of perioperative blood pressure

  - Control of heart failure following acute MI

MEDICATION CLASSIFICATION: ANTIANGINAL AGENT

- Select Prototype Medication – Ranolazine (Ranexa)

Purpose

- Expected Pharmacological Action

  - Lowers cardiac oxygen demand and thereby improves exercise tolerance and decreases pain

- Therapeutic Uses

  - Chronic stable angina in combination with amlodipine (Norvasc), a beta-adrenergic blocker or an organic nitrate

Complications

SIDE/ADVERSE EFFECTS	NURSING INTERVENTIONS/CLIENT EDUCATION
QT prolongation	Monitor ECG
Elevated blood pressure in clients with renal disease.	Monitor blood pressure

 Contraindications/Precautions

- Ranolazine is contraindicated in clients who have QT prolongation or in clients taking other medications that can result in QT prolongation.

- This medication is contraindicated in clients who have liver dysfunction.

 - Use cautiously in older adult clients.

Interactions

MEDICATION/FOOD INTERACTIONS	NURSING INTERVENTIONS/CLIENT EDUCATION
Inhibitors of CYP3A4 can increase levels of ranolazine and lead to torsades de pointes. Agents include grapefruit juice, HIV protease inhibitors, macrolide antibiotics, azole antifungals and verapamil.	• Avoid concurrent use.
Quinidine and sotalol (Betapace) can further increase QT interval	• Avoid concurrent use.
Concurrent use of digoxin (Lanoxin) and simvastatin (Zocor) increases serum levels of digoxin and simvastatin.	• Monitor digoxin level. • Instruct clients to report muscle weakness.

Nursing Administration

- Administer as an extended release oral tablet, twice daily.

- Obtain baseline and monitor ECG for QT prolongation.

- Obtain baseline and monitor digoxin level with concurrent use.

Nursing Evaluation of Medication Effectiveness

- Depending on therapeutic intent, effectiveness may be evidenced by:

  o Prevention of acute anginal attacks

  o Long-term management of stable angina

(A) APPLICATION EXERCISES

1. A nurse is caring for a client who is prescribed isosorbide mononitrate (Imdur) for chronic stable angina. The nurse should plan to monitor the client for which of the following findings?

    A. Bradycardia

    B. Fever

    C. Hypertension

    D. Headache

2. A nurse is providing teaching to a client who is prescribed nitroglycerin (Nitrostat) for acute angina attacks. Place the following steps in the order in which the client should perform them

    _____ Call 911 if pain is unrelieved.

    _____ Take a dose of nitroglycerin.

    _____ Wait 5 min.

    _____ Stop activity.

3. A nurse is caring for a client who has angina pectoris and is prescribed a nitroglycerin patch (Nitro-Dur) once daily. Which of the following is true regarding the administration of transdermal nitroglycerin? (Select all that apply)

    _____ Apply the patch at the same time each morning.

    _____ Leave the patch in place for 24 hr before replacing.

    _____ Put the patch on a hairless area of skin.

    _____ Rotate the sites of administration with each application

    _____ Cut patches in half to allow for smaller doses of prescribed medication.

4. A nurse is caring for a client who is prescribed nitroglycerin in transmucosal rapid-acting tablets. Where should the nurse place one of the tablets during administration?

APPLICATION EXERCISES ANSWER KEY

1. A nurse is caring for a client who is prescribed isosorbide mononitrate (Imdur) for chronic stable angina. The nurse should plan to monitor the client for which of the following findings?

   A. Bradycardia

   B. Fever

   C. Hypertension

   D. Headache

   Headache is a side effect of all nitrate medications. Reflex tachycardia, rather than bradycardia may occur as an adverse effect, and a beta-adrenergic blocker may be prescribed to decrease pulse rate. Fever is not an adverse effect of isosorbide mononitrate. Orthostatic hypotension, rather than hypertension may occur and the nurse should advise the client to be careful when moving from lying down to sitting or standing.

 NCLEX® Connection: Pharmacological Therapies, Adverse Effects/Contraindications/Side Effects/Interactions

2. A nurse is providing teaching to a client who is prescribed nitroglycerin (Nitrostat) for acute angina attacks. Place the following steps in the order in which the client should perform them

   __4__ Call 911 if pain is unrelieved.

   __2__ Take a dose of nitroglycerin.

   __3__ Wait 5 min.

   __1__ Stop activity.

   When the client experiences an acute angina attack he should stop all activity, take a dose of nitroglycerin, and wait 5 min. If the pain is unrelieved, the client needs to call 911 or be driven to the closest emergency department. He can take up to two more doses of nitroglycerin at 5 min intervals.

 NCLEX® Connection: Pharmacological Therapies, Expected Actions/Outcomes

3. A nurse is caring for a client who has angina pectoris and is prescribed a nitroglycerin patch (Nitro-Dur) once daily. Which of the following is true regarding the administration of transdermal nitroglycerin? (Select all that apply)

   X   **Apply the patch at the same time each morning.**

         Leave the patch in place for 24 hr before replacing.

   X   **Put the patch on a hairless area of skin.**

   X   **Rotate the sites of administration with each application**

         Cut patches in half to allow for smaller doses of prescribed medication.

The nurse should apply the patch at the same time each morning, put the patch on a hairless area of skin, and rotate the sites of administration with each application. It is important to remove the transdermal patch each evening to leave the client a medication-free interval of 10 to 12 hr daily. This prevents tolerance to nitroglycerin. The patch should never be cut to deliver a smaller dose of medication. Nitro-Dur patches are available in a variety of doses.

 NCLEX® Connection: Pharmacological Therapies, Medication Administration

4. A nurse is caring for a client who is prescribed nitroglycerin in transmucosal rapid-acting tablets. Where should the nurse place one of the tablets during administration?

The nurse should place the transmucosal tablet between the upper lip and the gum, or in the buccal area (between the cheek and the gum). The nurse should allow the tablet to dissolve in place and instruct the client not to chew or swallow the tablet.

 NCLEX® Connection: Pharmacological Therapies, Medication Administration

UNIT 4	MEDICATIONS AFFECTING THE CARDIOVASCULAR SYSTEM
Chapter 23	Antilipemic Agents

 Overview

- Antilipemic agents work in different ways to help lower low-density lipoprotein (LDL cholesterol) levels, raise high-density lipoprotein (HDL cholesterol) levels, and possibly decrease very low-density lipoprotein (VLDL) levels. Use these medications along with lifestyle modifications such as regular activity, reduced cholesterol and fat, and diet and weight control.

- Prior to starting these medications, obtain baseline levels of total cholesterol, LDL cholesterol level, HDL cholesterol, and triglycerides (TGs). Monitor these blood values periodically throughout the course of therapy.

- In addition, obtain baseline liver and renal function tests and monitor periodically throughout the course of therapy.

- Classifications include:

  o Fibrates

  o HMG CoA reductase inhibitors (Statins)

  o Cholesterol absorption inhibitors

  o Bile-acid sequestrants

  o Nicotinic acid

MEDICATION CLASSIFICATION: FIBRATES

- Select Prototype Medication – Gemfibrozil (Lopid)

- Other Medications – Fenofibrate (TriCor, Lofibra), clofibrate (Atromid-S)

Purpose

- Expected Pharmacological Action

  o Decrease in triglyceride levels (increase in VLDL excretion for clients unable to lower triglyceride levels with lifestyle modification)

  o Increase in HDL levels by promoting production of precursors to HDLs

- Therapeutic Uses

  o Reduction of plasma triglycerides (VLDL)

  o Increased levels of HDL

Complications

SIDE/ADVERSE EFFECTS	NURSING INTERVENTIONS/CLIENT EDUCATION
Gastrointestinal (GI) distress (nausea, abdominal pain, and diarrhea)	• Usually mild and self-limiting
Gallbladder stones (right upper quadrant pain, fat intolerance, bloating)	• Advise clients to observe for symptoms of gallbladder disease (right upper quadrant pain, fat intolerance, bloating). • Advise clients to notify the provider if symptoms occur.
Myopathy (muscle tenderness, pain)	• Obtain baseline creatine kinase (CK) level. • Monitor CK levels periodically during treatment. • Monitor symptoms of muscle aches, pain, and tenderness, and notify the provider if symptoms occur. • Withhold medication if CK levels are elevated.
Hepatotoxicity (anorexia, vomiting, nausea, jaundice)	• Obtain baseline liver function tests and monitor periodically. • Advise clients to observe for symptoms of liver dysfunction and notify the provider if symptoms occur. • Withhold medication if liver function tests are abnormal.

 Contraindications/Precautions

- Pregnancy Risk Category C

- Contraindicated in clients with liver disorders, severe renal dysfunction, and gallbladder disease

Interactions

MEDICATION/FOOD INTERACTIONS	NURSING INTERVENTIONS/CLIENT EDUCATION
With concurrent use, warfarin (Coumadin) increases the risk of bleeding	• Obtain the client's baseline and INR, and perform periodic monitoring. • Advise clients to report signs of bleeding (bruising, bleeding gums), and notify the provider if symptoms occur. • Tell clients the provider may decrease the dosage.
Concurrent use with statins increases the risk of myopathy.	• Obtain baseline (CK) level. • Monitor CK levels periodically during treatment. • Advise clients to report symptoms of muscle aches and pain, • Avoid concurrent use.
Bile acid sequestrants such as cholestyramine interfere with absorption.	• Advise clients to take gemfibrozil 1 hr before or 4 hr after taking bile sequestrants.

Nursing Administration

- Administer by oral route.

- Advise clients to take medication 30 min prior to breakfast and dinner.

MEDICATION CLASSIFICATION: HMG COA REDUCTASE INHIBITORS (STATINS)

- Select Prototype Medication – Atorvastatin (Lipitor)

- Other Medications:

  o   Simvastatin (Zocor)

  o   Lovastatin (Mevacor)

  o   Pravastatin sodium (Pravachol)

  o   Rosuvastatin (Crestor)

  o   Fluvastatin (Lescol, Lescol XL)

Purpose

- Expected Pharmacological Action

  o   Decrease manufacture of LDL cholesterol

  o   Decrease manufacture of very low-density lipoproteins (VLDL)

  o   Increase manufacture of high-density lipoproteins (HDL)

  o   Besides affecting lipid levels, other beneficial effects include: promotion of vasodilation, decrease in plaque site inflammation, and decreased risk of thromboembolism.

- Therapeutic Uses

  o   Primary hypercholesterolemia

  o   Prevention of coronary events

  o   Protection against MI and stroke for clients with diabetes

  o   Increasing levels of HDL in clients with primary hypercholesterolemia

Complications

SIDE/ADVERSE EFFECTS	NURSING INTERVENTIONS/CLIENT EDUCATION
• Hepatotoxicity (anorexia, vomiting, nausea, jaundice, increase in serum transaminase)	• Obtain the client's baseline liver function. • Monitor liver function tests after 12 weeks and then every 6 to 12 months. • Advise clients to observe for symptoms of liver dysfunction and notify the provider if symptoms occur. • Advise clients to avoid alcohol. • Tell clients the provider may discontinue the medication if liver function tests are abnormal.
• Myopathy (muscle aches, pain, and tenderness) • May progress to myositis, or rhabdomyolysis.	• Obtain baseline CK level. • Monitor CK levels while on treatment periodically. • Advise clients to report symptoms. • Tell clients the provider may discontinue the medication if CK levels are elevated.
• Peripheral neuropathy (weakness, numbness, tingling, and pain in the hands and feet)	• Advise clients to observe for signs and symptoms, and to notify the provider if symptoms occur.

 Contraindications/Precautions

- Statins are Pregnancy Risk Category X.

- These medications are contraindicated in clients who have hepatitis induced by viral infection or alcohol.

- Avoid use of rosuvastatin for clients of Asian descent.

 • Use cautiously in older adult clients, clients in debilitated condition, and those with chronic renal disease.

Interactions

MEDICATION/FOOD INTERACTIONS	NURSING INTERVENTIONS/CLIENT EDUCATION
Fibrates (gemfibrozil, fenofibrate) and ezetimibe (Zetia) increase the risk of myopathy	• Obtain baseline CK level. • Monitor the client's CK levels periodically during treatment. • Tell clients the provider may discontinue the medication if CK levels are elevated.
Medications that suppress CYP3A4, such as erythromycin and ketoconazole, can increase levels of statins when taken concurrently.	• Atorvastatin, lovastatin, and simvastatin should be avoided. • Level of statin may need to be decreased. • Advise clients to inform the provider of all medications currently taken.
Grapefruit juice suppresses CYP3A4 and can increase levels of statins.	• Advise clients to limit the amount of grapefruit juice consumed each day. Clients should not drink more than 240 mL (8 oz) a day.

Nursing Administration

- Administer statins by oral route.

- Instruct clients to take lovastatin with evening meal. Tell clients to take other statins with or without food, but evening dosing is best.

- Administer atorvastatin or fluvastatin to clients with renal insufficiency.

- Advise clients to obtain baseline cholesterol levels, HDL, LDL, and triglycerides, and monitor periodically while taking the medication.

- Advise clients to obtain baseline liver, renal function tests, and monitor periodically during treatment.

MEDICATION CLASSIFICATION: CHOLESTEROL ABSORPTION INHIBITOR

- Select Prototype Medication – Ezetimibe (Zetia)

Purpose

- Expected Pharmacological Action

  o Ezetimibe inhibits absorption of cholesterol secreted in the bile and from food.

- Therapeutic Uses

  o As an adjunct with dietary medications to help lower LDL cholesterol

  o Use alone or in combination with a statin medication.

Complications

SIDE/ADVERSE EFFECTS	NURSING INTERVENTIONS/CLIENT EDUCATION
Hepatitis (anorexia, vomiting, nausea, jaundice)	• Obtain the client's baseline liver function. • Advise clients to observe for symptoms of liver dysfunction and notify the provider if symptoms occur. • Advise clients to avoid alcohol. • Tell clients the provider may discontinue the medication if liver function tests are abnormal.
Myopathy (muscle aches and pains)	• Obtain baseline CK level. • Monitor CK levels while on treatment periodically. • Advise clients to notify the provider if symptoms occur. • Tell clients the provider may discontinue the medication if CK levels are elevated.

 Contraindications/Precautions

- Ezetimibe is Pregnancy Risk Category X.

- Use cautiously in women who are breastfeeding.

- This medication is contraindicated in clients who have renal dysfunction.

- Use caution in clients with liver disease.

Interactions

MEDICATION/FOOD INTERACTIONS	NURSING INTERVENTIONS/CLIENT EDUCATION
Bile acid sequestrants, such as cholestyramine, interfere with absorption.	• Advise clients to take ezetimibe 1 hr before or 4 hr after taking bile sequestrants.
Statins, such as atorvastatin, can increase the risk of liver dysfunction and/or myopathy.	• Obtain baseline liver function tests and monitor periodically. Advise clients to report signs of liver damage to the provider, who may discontinue the medication. • Advise clients to notify the provider of symptoms such as muscle aches and pains. • Tell clients the provider may discontinue the medication if CK levels are elevated.
Concurrent use with fibrates, such as gemfibrozil, increases the risk of gallstone development and myopathy.	• Avoid concurrent use.
Levels of ezetimibe can be increased with concurrent use of cyclosporine.	• Monitor clients for side effects (liver damage, myopathy).

Nursing Administration

- Advise clients to obtain baseline cholesterol levels, HDL, LDL, and triglyceride, and monitor periodically while taking the medication.

- Advise clients to obtain baseline liver, renal function tests, and monitor periodically during treatment.

- Advise clients to follow a low-fat/low-cholesterol diet and to get involved in a regular exercise regimen.

- Inform clients that this medication can be taken in a fixed-dose combination with simvastatin as Vytorin.

MEDICATION CLASSIFICATION: BILE-ACID SEQUESTRANTS

- Select Prototype Medication– Colesevelam (Welchol)

- Other Medications – Cholestyramine (Questran), colestipol (Colestid)

Purpose

- Expected Pharmacological Action

  o Decrease in LDL cholesterol

- Therapeutic Use

  o As adjunct with a HMG CoA reductase inhibitor, such as atorvastatin, and with dietary measures to lower cholesterol levels

Complications

SIDE/ADVERSE EFFECTS	NURSING INTERVENTIONS/CLIENT EDUCATION
Cholestyramine and colestipol may cause GI distress and decrease absorption of fat-soluble vitamins.	• Administer vitamin supplements.
Constipation (less with colesevelam)	• Advise clients to increase the intake of high-fiber food and oral fluids, if not restricted.

 Contraindications/Precautions

- These medications are contraindicated in clients with biliary disease.

- Avoid use in clients with elevated VLDL.

Interactions

MEDICATION/FOOD INTERACTIONS	NURSING INTERVENTIONS/CLIENT EDUCATION
Cholestyramine and colestipol form complexes with digoxin (Lanoxin), warfarin (Coumadin), thiazides, and tetracyclines that interfere with absorption.	• Advise clients to take other medications 1 hr before or 4 hr after taking bile sequestrants. • Advise clients to inform the provider of all medications currently taken.

Nursing Administration

- Instruct clients to take colesevelam tablets with food or water.

- Instruct clients not to crush or chew colestipol tablets. Clients should take tablets 30 min before a meal.

- Advise clients to use an adequate amount of fluid (4 to 8 oz) to dissolve the medication when taking powder formulation of cholestyramine and colestipol. This will prevent irritation or impaction of the esophagus.

OTHER MEDICATIONS: NICOTINIC ACID, NIACIN (NIACOR, NIASPAN)

Purpose

- Expected Pharmacological Action

  o Decrease in LDL cholesterol and triglyceride levels

  o Increase in HDL cholesterol

- Therapeutic Uses

  o For clients at risk for pancreatitis and elevated triglyceride levels

  o To lower elevated LDL cholesterol and triglycerides, and to raise HDL levels (Niaspan)

Complications

SIDE/ADVERSE EFFECTS	NURSING INTERVENTIONS/CLIENT EDUCATION
GI distress	• Usually self-limiting. Advise client to take with food.
Facial flushing	• Advise client to take aspirin 30 min before each dose. May be less with extended release formation.
Hyperglycemia	• Monitor blood glucose levels
Hepatotoxicity (anorexia, vomiting, nausea, jaundice)	• Obtain baseline liver function tests and monitor periodically. • Advise clients to observe for symptoms of liver dysfunction and notify the provider if symptoms occur. • Tell clients the provider may discontinue the medication if liver function tests are abnormal.
Hyperuricemia	• Monitor kidney function, BUN, and creatinine, I&O. • Encourage adequate fluid intake of 2 to 3 L of water each day from food and beverage sources. • Administer allopurinol if uric acid level is elevated.

Ⓢ Contraindications/Precautions

- Contraindicated in clients with liver disease and gout

Nursing Administration

- Administer by oral route, either in pill or liquid form. Pill may be standard form or time-released.

- Administer standard form three times a day with or after meals.

- Administer time-released formulations once in the evening.

- Advise clients that dosage is much larger than dosage when taken as vitamin supplement.

Nursing Evaluation of Medication Effectiveness

- Depending on therapeutic intent, effectiveness may be evidenced by:

  ○ Decreased LDL cholesterol level

  ○ Decreased triglyceride (VLDL) levels

  ○ Increased HDL levels

  ○ Absence of cardiovascular events such as stroke, MI, thrombosis

APPLICATION EXERCISES

1. A nurse is reinforcing teaching to a client who is prescribed lovastatin (Mevacor). Which of the following should be included in the teaching?

    A. Take the medication with the evening meal.

    B. Change position slowly when rising from a chair.

    C. Maintain a steady intake of green leafy vegetables.

    D. Consume no more than 1 L of fluid/day.

2. A nurse is caring for a client who has received a prescription for gemfibrozil (Lopid). The nurse should know that which of the following lab values should be reviewed before the client begins taking the medication? (Select all that apply)

    _____ RBC count

    _____ Liver function tests

    _____ WBC count

    _____ Serum electrolytes

    _____ Creatine kinase (CK)

3. A nurse is reinforcing teaching for a client who has been prescribed Ezetimibe (Zetia) for some time and now has a new prescription for cholestyramine (Questran). Both medications are to be taken once daily. How should the nurse advise the client to take these two medications in order to prevent an interaction?

4. A nurse is reinforcing teaching for a client who is to begin taking a new prescription for niacin (Niacor). The nurse should instruct the client to expect which of the following?

    A. Facial flushing

    B. Frontal headache

    C. Blurred vision

    D. Dry mouth

5. Match each of the following cholesterol-lowering medications with its classification below:

    _____ Ezetimibe (Zetia)   A. Cholesterol absorption inhibitor

    _____ Colesevelam HCL (Welchol)   B. HMG COA reductase inhibitor (statin)

    _____ Gemfibrozil (Lopid)   C. Bile acid sequestrant

    _____ Atorvastatin (Lipitor)   D. Fibrate

APPLICATION EXERCISES ANSWER KEY

1. A nurse is reinforcing teaching to a client who is prescribed lovastatin (Mevacor). Which of the following should be included in the teaching?

    A. Take the medication with the evening meal.

    B. Change position slowly when rising from a chair.

    C. Maintain a steady intake of green leafy vegetables.

    D. Consume no more than 1 L of fluid/day.

    Instruct the client to take lovastatin with the evening meal to increase absorption. Changing positions slowly may be necessary when taking an antihypertensive. Maintaining a steady intake of green leafy vegetables would be important if taking warfarin. There is no indication for fluid restriction with statins.

     NCLEX® Connection: Pharmacological Therapies, Medication Administration

2. A nurse is caring for a client who has received a prescription for gemfibrozil (Lopid). The nurse should know that which of the following lab values should be reviewed before the client begins taking the medication? (Select all that apply)

_____	RBC count
X	**Liver function tests**
_____	WBC count
_____	Serum electrolytes
X	**Creatine kinase (CK)**

    Check the client's liver function and creatine kinase (CK) levels before beginning the prescription for gemfibrozil. If baseline liver enzymes are elevated, hepatotoxicity may be present and would be a contraindication to beginning a fibrate medication. A baseline CK is obtained since myopathy is a possible adverse reaction to gemfibrozil. Monitor both laboratory values throughout therapy with the medication. It is not necessary to check the other laboratory values before the client begins taking gemfibrozil.

     NCLEX® Connection: Pharmacological Therapies, Medication Administration

3. A nurse is reinforcing teaching for a client who has been prescribed Ezetimibe (Zetia) for some time and now has a new prescription for cholestyramine (Questran). Both medications are to be taken once daily. How should the nurse advise the client to take these two medications in order to prevent an interaction?

    Ezetimibe should be taken 2 hr before or 4 hr following the cholestyramine. If taken together, the cholestyramine can decrease absorption of the ezetimibe.

     NCLEX® Connection: Pharmacological Therapies, Medication Administration

4. A nurse is reinforcing teaching for a client who is to begin taking a new prescription for niacin (Niacor). The nurse should instruct the client to expect which of the following?

    A. Facial flushing

    B. Frontal headache

    C. Blurred vision

    D. Dry mouth

    Facial flushing occurs within a few minutes after taking Niacor. It can be prevented by taking aspirin 325 mg 30 min before the Niacor is ingested. The flushing usually decreases after several weeks. Clients who are prescribed the extended-release niacin (Niaspan) may have a much less intense flushing response. Headache, blurred vision, and dry mouth are not expected side effects of niacin.

 NCLEX® Connection: Pharmacological Therapies, Adverse Effects/Contraindications/Side Effects/Interactions

5. Match each of the following cholesterol-lowering medications with its classification below:

A	Ezetimibe (Zetia)	A. Cholesterol absorption inhibitor
C	Colesevelam HCL (Welchol)	B. HMG COA reductase inhibitor (statin)
D	Gemfibrozil (Lopid)	C. Bile acid sequestrant
B	Atorvastatin (Lipitor)	D. Fibrate

 NCLEX® Connection: Pharmacological Therapies, Expected Actions/Outcomes

UNIT 5: MEDICATIONS AFFECTING THE HEMATOLOGIC SYSTEM

- Medications Affecting Coagulation
- Growth Factors

NCLEX® CONNECTIONS

When reviewing the chapters in this section, keep in mind the relevant sections of the NCLEX® outline, in particular:

CLIENT NEEDS: PHARMACOLOGICAL THERAPIES

Relevant topics/tasks include:
- Adverse Effects/Contraindications/Side Effects/Interactions
  - Monitor anticipated interactions among client prescribed medications and fluids.
- Expected Actions/Outcomes
  - Monitor client use of medications over time.
- Medication Administration
  - Administer medication by oral route.

UNIT 5	MEDICATIONS AFFECTING THE HEMATOLOGIC SYSTEM
Chapter 24	Medications Affecting Coagulation

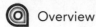 Overview

- Use pharmaceutical agents to modify coagulation in order to prevent clot formation or break apart an already formed clot. These medications work in the blood to alter the clotting cascade, prevent platelet aggregation, or dissolve a clot.

- The goal of medications that alter coagulation is to increase circulation and perfusion, decrease pain and prevent further tissue damage.

- Medications include oral and parenteral anticoagulants, antiplatelet medications, and thrombolytic agents. Thrombolytic agents include streptokinase (Streptase), alteplase (Activase, tPA), tenecteplase (TNKase), and reteplase (Retavase)

MEDICATION CLASSIFICATION: ANTICOAGULANTS/PARENTERAL

- Select Prototype Medication – Heparin

- Low molecular weight heparins (LMWH):

    o Select Prototype Medication – Enoxaparin (Lovenox)

    o Other Medications – Dalteparin (Fragmin), tinzaparin (Innohep)

- Activated factor X (Xa) inhibitor:

    o Select Prototype Medication – Fondaparinux (Arixtra)

Purpose

- Expected Pharmacological Action

    o Parenteral anticoagulants prevent clotting by inactivation of thrombin formation and factor Xa, resulting in inhibition of the formation of fibrin.

- Therapeutic Uses

    o Heparin, LMWH, fondaparinux sodium

        ▪ In conditions necessitating prompt anticoagulant activity (evolving stroke, pulmonary embolism, massive deep venous thrombosis)

        ▪ As an adjunct for clients having open heart surgery or renal dialysis

        ▪ As low-dose therapy for prophylaxis against postoperative venous thrombosis (for example, hip/knee replacement surgery, abdominal surgery)

- o Heparin, LMWH
  - In conjunction with thrombolytic therapy when treating an acute myocardial infarction
- o Heparin
  - Treatment of disseminated intravascular coagulation

Administration

- These medications cannot be absorbed by the intestinal tract and must be given by subcutaneous injection or IV infusion:
  - o Heparin – Subcutaneously every 12 hr, continuous or intermittent IV bolus infusion
  - o Enoxaparin, dalteparin sodium, tinzaparin – Subcutaneously every 12 hr for 2 to 8 days
  - o Fondaparinux sodium – Subcutaneously every 12 hr for 5 to 9 days

Complications

SIDE/ADVERSE EFFECTS	NURSING INTERVENTIONS/CLIENT EDUCATION
Heparin sodium	
Hemorrhage secondary to heparin overdose (increased heart rate, decreased blood pressure, bruising, bleeding gums, petechiae, hematomas, black tarry stools)	• Monitor vital signs. • Advise clients to report signs of bleeding. • In the case of heparin overdose, stop heparin and assist with the administration of protamine sulfate. • Monitor activated partial thromboplastin time (aPTT). Keep value at 1.5 to 2 times the baseline (60 to 80 seconds).
Heparin-induced thrombocytopenia (low platelet count and increased development of thrombi – mediated by antibody development)	• Monitor the client's platelet count periodically throughout treatment, especially in the first month. • Stop heparin if platelet count is less than 100,000/mm^3.
Hypersensitivity reactions (chills, fever, urticaria)	• Administer a small test dose prior to the administration of heparin.
Toxicity/overdose	• Assist with administration of protamine sulfate IV bolus, which binds with heparin and forms a heparin-protamine complex that has no anticoagulant properties. • Administer protamine sulfate slowly by IV bolus, no faster than 20 mg/min or 50 mg in 10 min.

SIDE/ADVERSE EFFECTS	NURSING INTERVENTIONS/CLIENT EDUCATION
Enoxaparin and fondaparinux	
Hemorrhage	• Monitor vital signs • Advise clients to observe for signs and symptoms of bleeding, such as increased heart rate, decreased blood pressure, bruising, petechiae, hematomas, black tarry stools. • Monitor platelet count. Instruct clients to avoid aspirin.
Neurologic damage from hematoma formed during spinal or epidural anesthesia	• In clients with spinal or epidural anesthesia – Check insertion site for signs of hematoma formation, such as redness or swelling. Monitor sensation and movement of lower extremities. Notify provider of abnormal findings.
Thrombocytopenia, as evidenced by low platelet count	• Monitor platelets. Discontinue medication for platelet count less than 100,000/mm³.
Toxicity/overdose (enoxaparin)	• Assist with administration of protamine sulfate IV bolus.

 Contraindications/Precautions

- Parenteral anticoagulants are contraindicated in clients with low platelet counts (thrombocytopenia) or uncontrollable bleeding.

- Do not use these medications during or following surgeries of the eye(s), brain, or spinal cord; lumbar puncture; or regional anesthesia.

- Use cautiously in clients who have hemophilia, increased capillary permeability, dissecting aneurysm, peptic ulcer disease, severe hypertension, hepatic or renal disease, or threatened abortion.

Interactions

MEDICATION/FOOD INTERACTIONS	NURSING INTERVENTIONS/CLIENT EDUCATION
Anti-platelet agents such as aspirin, NSAIDs, and other anticoagulants may increase risk for bleeding.	• Avoid concurrent use when possible. • Monitor carefully for evidence of bleeding. • Take precautionary measures to avoid injury (limit venipunctures and injections).

Nursing Administration

- Heparin:

  o Obtain the client's baseline vital signs.

  o Obtain baseline and monitor complete blood count (CBC) and platelet count.

○ Read label carefully. Heparin is dispensed in units and in different concentrations.

○ Check dosages with another nurse before administration.

○ Monitor aPTT every 4 to 6 hr until appropriate dose is determined, then monitor daily.

○ For subcutaneous injections, use a 20-to-22 gauge needle to withdraw medication from the vial. Then, change the needle to a smaller needle (25 or 26 gauge, 1/2 to 5/8 inch long).

○ Administer deep subcutaneous injections in the abdomen ensuring a distance of 2 inches from the umbilicus. Do not aspirate.

○ Apply pressure for 1 to 2 min after the injection. Rotate and record injection sites.

○ Instruct clients to monitor for bleeding gums, nose bleeds, and signs of bleeding (bruising, abdominal pain, coffee-ground emesis, and tarry stools).

○ Instruct clients not to take over-the-counter NSAIDs, aspirin, or medications containing salicylates.

○ Advise clients to use an electric razor for shaving and a soft toothbrush.

- Enoxaparin/fondaparinux

○ No monitoring is required. Therefore, these medications are acceptable for home use.

○ Provide instruction regarding correct self-administration. Medications may be available in pre-filled syringes.

○ For subcutaneous injections, use a 20-to-22 gauge needle to withdraw medication from the vial. Then, change to a small needle (25 or 26 gauge, 1/2 to 5/8 inch long).

○ Administer subcutaneous injections in the abdomen, ensuring a distance of 2 inches from the umbilicus. Do not aspirate.

○ Apply pressure for 1 to 2 min after the injection. Rotate and record injection sites.

○ Instruct clients to monitor for signs of bleeding such as bruising, bleeding gums, abdominal pain, nose bleeds, coffee-ground emesis, and tarry stools.

○ Instruct clients not to take over-the-counter NSAIDs, aspirin, or medications containing salicylates.

○ Advise clients to use an electric razor for shaving and a soft toothbrush.

Nursing Evaluation of Medication Effectiveness

- Depending on therapeutic intent, effectiveness may be evidenced by the following:

○ Heparin

  ▪ Client aPTT levels of 60 to 80 seconds

○ Heparin, enoxaparin, and fondaparinux sodium

  ▪ No development or no further development of venous thrombi or emboli

MEDICATION CLASSIFICATION: ANTICOAGULANT/ORAL

- Select Prototype Medication – Warfarin (Coumadin)

Purpose

- Expected Pharmacological Action

  o Oral anticoagulants antagonize vitamin K, thereby preventing the synthesis of four coagulation factors: factor VII, IX, X, and prothrombin.

- Therapeutic Uses

  o Treatment of venous thrombosis

  o Treatment of thrombus formation in clients who have atrial fibrillation or prosthetic heart valves

  o Prevention of recurrent myocardial infarction, transient ischemic attacks

Complications

SIDE /ADVERSE EFFECTS	NURSING INTERVENTIONS/CLIENT EDUCATION
Hemorrhage (increased heart rate, decreased blood pressure, bruising, bleeding gums, petechiae, hematomas, black tarry stools)	<ul><li>Monitor the client's vital signs.</li><li>Advise clients to observe for signs and symptoms of bleeding.</li><li>Obtain baseline (PT) (11-12.5 seconds) and monitor levels of PT and International Normalized Ratio (INR) periodically.</li><li>In the case of a warfarin overdose, discontinue administration of warfarin, and administer vitamin K (Mephyton).</li></ul>
Hepatitis	<ul><li>Monitor liver enzymes. Check for jaundice.</li></ul>
Toxicity/overdose	<ul><li>Administer vitamin K to promote synthesis of coagulation factors VII, IX, X, and prothrombin.</li><li>Administer vitamin K slowly by IV bolus, in a diluted solution to prevent anaphylactoid-type reaction.</li><li>Use oral or subcutaneous route whenever possible.</li><li>If vitamin K cannot control bleeding, monitor clients receiving fresh frozen plasma or whole blood.</li></ul>

(S) Contraindications/Precautions

- Oral anticoagulants fall into Pregnancy Risk Category X due to high risk of fetal hemorrhage, fetal death, and CNS defects. Advise clients to notify the provider if they become pregnant during warfarin therapy. If anticoagulation is needed during pregnancy, heparin can be safely used.

- Use is contraindicated in clients with low platelet counts (thrombocytopenia) or uncontrollable bleeding.

- Use is contraindicated during or following surgeries of the eye(s), brain, or spinal cord; lumbar puncture; or regional anesthesia.

- Use is contraindicated in clients with vitamin K deficiencies, liver disorders, and alcoholism due to the additive risk of bleeding.

- Use cautiously in clients who have hemophilia, dissecting aneurysm, peptic ulcer disease, severe hypertension, or threatened abortion.

Interactions

MEDICATION/FOOD INTERACTIONS	NURSING INTERVENTIONS/CLIENT EDUCATION
Concurrent use of heparin, aspirin, acetaminophen, nonaspirin antiplatelets, glucocorticoids, sulfonamides, and parenteral cephalosporins increases effects of warfarin, which increases the risk for bleeding.	• Avoid concurrent use if possible. • Instruct clients to observe for inclusion of aspirin in over-the-counter medications. • If used concurrently, monitor clients carefully for signs of bleeding and increased prothrombin time (PT), INR, and aPTT levels. • Tell clients the provider may adjust the dosage.
Concurrent use of phenobarbital, carbamazepine (Tegretol), phenytoin (Dilantin), oral contraceptives, and vitamin K decreases anticoagulant effects	• Avoid concurrent use if possible. • If used concurrently, monitor clients carefully for reduced PT and INR levels. • Medication dosage should be adjusted accordingly.
Foods high in vitamin K, such as dark green leafy vegetables (lettuce, cooked spinach), cabbage, broccoli, brussel sprouts, mayonnaise, canola, and soybean oil may decrease anticoagulant effects with excessive intake	• Provide clients with a list of foods high in vitamin K. • Instruct clients to maintain a consistent intake of vitamin K to avoid sudden fluctuations that could affect the action of warfarin.

Nursing Administration

- Administration is usually oral, once daily.

- Obtain the client's baseline vital signs.

- Monitor PT levels (therapeutic level 18 to 24 seconds, or 1.5 to 2 times the normal value) and INR levels (therapeutic levels 2 to 3 for most clients). INR levels are the most accurate. Withhold dose and notify the provider if these levels exceed therapeutic ranges.

- Obtain baseline and monitor CBC, platelet count, and Hct levels.

- Instruct clients that anticoagulant effects may take 8 to 12 hr and full therapeutic effect is not achieved for 3 to 5 days. For clients in the hospital setting, explain the need for continued heparin infusion when starting oral warfarin.

- Advise clients that anticoagulation effects can persist for up to 5 days following discontinuation of medication because of long half-life.

- Advise clients to avoid alcohol and over-the-counter and non-prescription medications to prevent adverse effects and medication interactions, such as risk of bleeding.

- Advise clients to employ nonpharmacological measures to avoid development of thrombi, including avoiding sitting for prolonged periods of time, not wearing constricting clothing, and elevating and moving legs when sitting.

- Advise clients to wear a medical alert bracelet indicating warfarin use.

- Be prepared to administer vitamin K for warfarin overdose.

- Advise clients to record dosage, route, and time of warfarin administration on a daily basis.

- Plan for frequent PT monitoring for clients who are prescribed medications that interact with warfarin. The client is at greatest risk for harm when the interacting medication is being deleted or added. Frequent PT monitoring will allow for dosage adjustments as necessary.

- Advise clients to notify the provider regarding warfarin use.

- Advise clients to use a soft-bristle toothbrush to prevent gum bleeding.

Nursing Evaluation of Medication Effectiveness

- Depending on therapeutic intent, effectiveness may be evidenced by:

  o PT 1.5 to 2 times control

  o INR of 2 to 3 for treatment of acute myocardial infarction, atrial fibrillation, pulmonary embolism, venous thrombosis, and/or tissue heart valves

  o INR of 3 to 4.5 for mechanical heart valve or recurrent systemic embolism

  o No development or no further development of venous thrombi

MEDICATION CLASSIFICATION: ANTIPLATELETS

- Antiplatelet/salicylic

  o Select Prototype Medication – Aspirin (Ecotrin)

- Antiplatelet/glycoprotein inhibitors

  o Select Prototype Medication – Abciximab (ReoPro)

  o Other Medications – Eptifibatide (Integrilin), tirofiban (Aggrastat)

- Antiplatelet/ADP inhibitors:
  - Select Prototype Medications – Clopidogrel (Plavix)
  - Other Medications – Ticlopidine (Ticlid)
- Antiplatelet/arterial vasodilator:
  - Select Prototype Medication – Pentoxifylline (Trental)
  - Other Medications – Dipyridamole (Persantine), cilostazol (Pletal)

Purpose

- Expected Pharmacological Action
  - Antiplatelets prevent platelets from clumping together by inhibiting enzymes and factors that normally lead to arterial clotting.
  - Antiplatelet medications inhibit platelet aggregation at the onset of the clotting process. These medications alter bleeding time.
- Therapeutic Uses
  - Primary prevention of acute myocardial infarction
  - Prevention of reinfarction in clients following an acute myocardial infarction
  - Prevention of reocclusion following coronary stenting
  - Prevention of stroke
  - Acute coronary syndromes (abciximab, tirofiban, eptifibatide)
  - Intermittent claudication (cilostazol, pentoxifylline, dipyridamole)

Route of administration

  - Aspirin – Oral
  - Abciximab – IV
  - Clopidogrel – Oral
  - Pentoxifylline – Oral

Complications

SIDE/ADVERSE EFFECTS	NURSING INTERVENTIONS/CLIENT EDUCATION
Aspirin	
GI effects (nausea, vomiting, dyspepsia)	• Advise clients to use enteric-coated tablets and to take aspirin with food. • Concurrent use of a proton pump inhibitor, such as omeprazole (Prilosec), may be appropriate.
Hemorrhagic stroke	• Advise clients to observe for signs of weakness, dizziness, and headache, and to notify the provider if symptoms occur.
Prolonged bleeding time, thrombocytopenia	• Monitor bleeding time. • Advise clients to monitor for bleeding and to report to the provider.
Tinnitus, hearing loss	• Monitor for hearing loss. • If symptoms occur, withhold dose and notify the provider.
Abciximab	
Hypotension and bradycardia	• Monitor heart rate and blood pressure.
Prolonged bleeding time, thrombocytopenia, bleeding from cardiac catheterization site	• Monitor bleeding time. • Advise clients to monitor for bleeding and to report to the provider. • Apply pressure to cardiac catheter access site.
Clopidogrel	
Prolonged bleeding time, thrombocytopenia	• Monitor bleeding time. • Advise clients to monitor for bleeding and to report to the provider. • Apply pressure to cardiac catheter access
Pentoxifylline	
Dyspepsia, nausea, vomiting	• Take with food. • Do not crush or chew medication. • Monitor hydration if GI upset occurs.

 Contraindications/Precautions

- Aspirin

  o Aspirin is Pregnancy Risk Category D in the third trimester.

  o Use is contraindicated in clients with bleeding disorders and thrombocytopenia.

  o Use cautiously in clients with peptic ulcer disease and severe renal and/or hepatic disorders. Do not give to children or adolescents with fever or recent chickenpox.

 o Use with caution in older adults.

- Abciximab

  - Abciximab is Pregnancy Risk Category C.

  - Contraindications include clients with bleeding disorders, thrombocytopenia, recent stroke, AV malformation, aneurysm, uncontrolled hypertension, and recent major surgery.

  - Use cautiously in clients with peptic ulcer disease and severe renal and/or hepatic disorders.

- Clopidogrel

  - Clopidogrel is Pregnancy Risk Category B.

  - Contraindications include clients with bleeding disorders, thrombocytopenia, peptic ulcer disease, and intracranial bleed.

  - Use cautiously in clients with peptic ulcer disease and severe renal and/or hepatic disorders. Clients who are breastfeeding should not take this medication.

- Pentoxifylline

  - Pentoxifylline is Pregnancy Risk Category C.

  - Use is contraindicated in clients who have bleeding disorders or retinal or cerebral bleeds.

Interactions

MEDICATION/FOOD INTERACTIONS	NURSING INTERVENTIONS/CLIENT EDUCATION
Aspirin	
Concurrent use of other medications that enhance bleeding (NSAIDs, heparin, warfarin, thrombolytics, antiplatelets) increases risk for bleeding.	• Advise clients to avoid concurrent use. • If used concurrently, monitor clients carefully for signs of bleeding.
Urine acidifiers (ammonium chloride) may increase aspirin levels.	• Monitor for aspirin toxicity (hearing loss, tinnitus).
Concurrent use of aspirin may reduce hypertensive action of beta-adrenergic blockers.	• Monitor blood pressure.
Corticosteroids may increase aspirin excretion and decrease aspirin effects. These medications may increase risk for GI bleed.	• Monitor for decreased aspirin effectiveness. • Monitor for gastric bleed (coffee-ground emesis and tarry or bloody stools).
Caffeine may increase aspirin absorption.	• Monitor for toxicity.
Abciximab	
Concurrent use of other medications that enhance bleeding (NSAIDs, heparin, warfarin, thrombolytics, antiplatelets) increases risk for bleeding.	• Advise clients to avoid concurrent use. • If used concurrently, monitor the client carefully for signs of bleeding.

MEDICATION/FOOD INTERACTIONS	NURSING INTERVENTIONS/CLIENT EDUCATION
Clopidogrel	
Concurrent use of other medications that enhance bleeding (NSAIDs, heparin, warfarin, thrombolytics, antiplatelets) increases risk for bleeding.	• Advise clients to avoid concurrent use. • If used concurrently, monitor clients carefully for signs of bleeding.
Pentoxifylline	
Concurrent use of anticoagulants increases risk for bleeding.	• Monitor PT and INR. Clients may require reduced dosage.
Pentoxifylline may increase levels of theophylline.	• Monitor theophylline level. Clients may require reduced dosage.

Nursing Administration

- Remind clients to take low-dose aspirin (81 mg) to prevent strokes, myocardial infarctions, and reinfarction.

- Administer 325 mg during initial acute episode of myocardial infarction.

- Advise clients to notify the provider for signs and symptoms of bleeding.

Nursing Evaluation of Medication Effectiveness

- Depending on therapeutic intent, effectiveness may be evidenced by:

  o Absence of arterial thrombosis, adequate tissue perfusion, and blood flow without occurrence of abnormal bleeding.

APPLICATION EXERCISES

1. A nurse is monitoring a client who has a venous thrombus in her leg and is receiving a continuous IV infusion of heparin. Discuss the use of laboratory values to monitor the effectiveness of heparin.

2. A nurse is preparing to administer heparin 5,000 units subcutaneously to a surgical client. Which of the following steps should the nurse take when administering the medication?

    _____ Draw up the heparin with a 28 gauge, 3/8 inch needle.

    _____ Administer the heparin with a 26 gauge, 1/2 inch needle.

    _____ Administer the heparin in the client's abdomen at least 2 inches from the umbilicus.

    _____ Aspirate for blood after inserting the syringe into the client's tissue.

    _____ Hold gentle pressure at injection site for 1 to 2 min after administering the medication.

3. A nurse is caring for a client who takes a daily dose of warfarin (Coumadin). The client begins vomiting blood. Which of the following medications should the nurse prepare to give to reverse the effects of warfarin?

    A. Vitamin K

    B. Atropine sulfate

    C. Protamine sulfate

    D. Calcium gluconate

4. A nurse is caring for a client who has been taking a daily dose of warfarin for the past two weeks following an acute myocardial infarction. The client's most recent INR is 1 to 2. If the client has been taking the warfarin as prescribed, the nurse should expect which of the following changes to the client's prescription?

    A. The warfarin will be continued at the same dose.

    B. The warfarin will be discontinued.

    C. The warfarin dosage will be increased.

    D. The warfarin dosage will be decreased.

5. When caring for a client taking aspirin to reduce the risk for a myocardial infarction, the nurse should monitor for which of the following adverse effects? (Select all that apply)

    _____ Petechiae

    _____ Hypertension

    _____ Tinnitus

    _____ Bruising

    _____ Bradycardia

    _____ Black stools

APPLICATION EXERCISES ANSWER KEY

1. A nurse is monitoring a client who has a venous thrombus in her leg and is receiving a continuous IV infusion of heparin. Discuss the use of laboratory values to monitor the effectiveness of heparin.

   Use an activated partial thromboplastin time (aPTT) to evaluate the effects of heparin. The value should be kept at 1.5 to 2 times the baseline (30 to 40 seconds), usually 60 to 80 seconds.

    NCLEX® Connection: Pharmacological Therapies, Expected Actions/Outcomes

2. A nurse is preparing to administer heparin 5,000 units subcutaneously to a surgical client. Which of the following steps should the nurse take when administering the medication?

   _____ Draw up the heparin with a 28 gauge, 3/8 inch needle.

   __X__ **Administer the heparin with a 26 gauge,1/2 inch needle.**

   __X__ **Administer the heparin in the client's abdomen at least 2 inches from the umbilicus.**

   _____ Aspirate for blood after inserting the syringe into the client's tissue.

   __X__ **Hold gentle pressure at injection site for 1 to 2 min after administering the medication.**

   The nurse should change needles to a 25 to 26 gauge, 1/2 in to 5/8 inch needle after drawing up the heparin to prevent tracking heparin into the client's tissue during needle insertion. The preferred site to administer subcutaneous heparin is in the client's abdomen, at least 2 inches from the umbilicus. After injecting the medication and removing the needle from the skin, hold gentle pressure at the injection site for 1 to 2 min to prevent bruising. The nurse should use a larger (20-to-22 gauge) needle to draw up the medication, and should not aspirate after inserting the syringe into the client's tissue.

    NCLEX® Connection: Pharmacological Therapies, Medication Administration

3. A nurse is caring for a client who takes a daily dose of warfarin (Coumadin). The client begins vomiting blood. Which of the following medications should the nurse prepare to give to reverse the effects of warfarin?

   A. Vitamin K

   B. Atropine sulfate

   C. Protamine sulfate

   D. Calcium gluconate

   Administer vitamin K to reverse warfarin (Coumadin) toxicity. Protamine sulfate reverses the effects of heparin sodium. Use atropine sulfate to reverse bradycardia caused by beta-adrenergic blockers. Use calcium gluconate to treat magnesium sulfate toxicity.

    NCLEX® Connection: Pharmacological Therapies, Expected Actions/Outcomes

4. A nurse is caring for a client who has been taking a daily dose of warfarin for the past two weeks following an acute myocardial infarction. The client's most recent INR is 1 to 2. If the client has been taking the warfarin as prescribed, the nurse should expect which of the following changes to the client's prescription?

    A. The warfarin will be continued at the same dose.

    B. The warfarin will be discontinued.

    C. The warfarin dosage will be increased.

    D. The warfarin dosage will be decreased.

If the client has been taking the warfarin as prescribed, the nurse may expect the warfarin dosage to be increased by the provider. The INR for a client who has had an acute myocardial infarction should be 2 to 3, so the client's INR has not yet reached the recommended range. The nurse should not expect that the warfarin will be continued at the same dose, decreased, or discontinued. It is the nurse's responsibility to inform the provider of the results of the INR.

 NCLEX® Connection: Pharmacological Therapies, Expected Actions/Outcomes

5. When caring for a client taking aspirin to reduce the risk for a myocardial infarction, the nurse should monitor for which of the following adverse effects? (Select all that apply)

__X__	**Petechiae**
_____	Hypertension
__X__	**Tinnitus**
__X__	**Bruising**
_____	Bradycardia
__X__	**Black stools**

Aspirin may cause prolonged bleeding time and thrombocytopenia. Monitor the client for signs of bleeding, such as petechiae, bruising, and bloody or black, tarry stools. Tinnitus is a symptom of aspirin toxicity. Hypertension and bradycardia are not adverse effects of aspirin.

 NCLEX® Connection: Pharmacological Therapies, Adverse Effects/Contraindications/Side Effects/Interactions

UNIT 5	MEDICATIONS AFFECTING THE HEMATOLOGIC SYSTEM
Chapter 25	Growth Factors

 Overview

- Blood cells and platelets are produced in the body by the biological process known as hematopoiesis. In the body, this process is naturally controlled by hormones, also known as hematopoietic growth factors.

- Genetically engineered products are available for therapeutic purposes, which include:

  ○ Replacement of neutrophils and platelets after chemotherapy

  ○ Hastening of bone marrow function after a bone marrow transplant

  ○ Increase in RBC production for clients with chronic renal failure

- There are 3 groups of hematopoietic growth factors:

  ○ Erythropoietic growth factors

    ▪ Biological name – Erythropoietin

  ○ Leukopoietic growth factors

    ▪ Biological name

      □ Granulocyte colony stimulating factor (G-CSF)

      □ Granulocyte-macrophage colony-stimulating factor (GM-CSF)

  ○ Thrombopoietic growth factor

    ▪ Interleukin-11

MEDICATION CLASSIFICATION: ERYTHROPOIETIC GROWTH FACTORS

- Select Prototype Medication – Epoetin alfa (Epogen, Procrit)

- Other Medications:

  ○ Darbepoetin alfa (Aranesp) – Long-acting erythropoietin

  ○ Methoxy polyethylene glycol (MGEG)-epoetin beta (Mircera) – Very long-acting erythropoietin

Purpose

- Expected Pharmacological Action

    o Hematopoietic growth factors act on the bone marrow to increase production of red blood cells.

- Therapeutic Uses

    o Anemia related to chronic renal failure, use of zidovudine (Retrovir) in clients with HIV infection, chemotherapy, and elective surgery if significant blood loss is expected.

    o May be an alternative to packed RBC transfusions for surgical clients.

Complications

SIDE/ADVERSE EFFECTS	NURSING INTERVENTIONS/CLIENT EDUCATION
Hypertension secondary to elevations in Hct level in clients with chronic renal failure.	• Monitor the client's Hgb levels and blood pressure, and if elevated, administer antihypertensive medications.
Increased risk for a cardiovascular event (MI, stroke, cardiac arrest) with an increase in Hgb above 12 g/dL or more than 1 g in 2 weeks	• Administer a decreased dosage when these limits are reached. Resume therapy when Hgb drops to acceptable level, but with a reduced dosage.

 Contraindications/Precautions

- Use is contraindicated in clients with uncontrolled hypertension.

- Use is contraindicated in clients with certain cancers because of possible increase in tumor growth.

- Use is contraindicated prior to vascular or cardiac surgery.

- Risk for deep vein thrombosis is higher in preoperative clients taking erythropoietic growth factors. Prophylactic use of anticoagulants decreases this risk.

Nursing Administration

- Obtain the client's baseline blood pressure. In clients with chronic renal failure, control hypertension before the start of treatment.

- Administer by subcutaneous injection. Monitor clients receiving medication by IV bolus injection.

- Do not agitate the vial of medication. Use each vial for one dose and do not put the needle back into the vial when withdrawing the medication.

- Do not mix medication with any other medication in syringe.

- Follow dosing as prescribed; usually 3 times/week, but may be once a week with some types of chemotherapy.

- Monitor the client's iron levels and take measures to ensure an iron level within the expected reference range. RBC growth is dependent upon adequate quantities of iron, folic acid, and vitamin B_{12}. Without adequate levels of these, erythropoietin is significantly less effective.

- Monitor the client's Hgb and Hct twice a week until target range is reached.

- Epoetin alfa should not be agitated and should not be combined with other medications.

- The longer-acting forms are administered less frequently (weekly or monthly), but may be prescribed for clients with chronic renal failure only.

Nursing Evaluation of Medication Effectiveness

- Depending on therapeutic intent, effectiveness may be evidenced by:

  o Hgb level of 10 to 12 g/dL and Hct of 40%

MEDICATION CLASSIFICATION: LEUKOPOIETIC GROWTH FACTORS

- Select Prototype Medication – Filgrastim (Neupogen)

- Other Medication – Pegfilgrastim (Neulasta)

Purpose

- Expected Pharmacological Action

  o Stimulates the bone marrow to increase production of neutrophils

- Therapeutic Use

  o Decreases the risk of infection in clients with neutropenia, such as from cancer

Complications

SIDE/ADVERSE EFFECTS	NURSING INTERVENTIONS/CLIENT EDUCATION
Bone pain	• Monitor clients for symptoms and notify the provider. • Administer acetaminophen or opioid analgesic.
Leukocytosis	• Monitor CBC two times per week during treatment. • Decrease dose or interrupt treatment if WBC is greater than 100,000/mm^3.

 Contraindications/Precautions

- This medication is contraindicated in clients who are sensitive to Escherichia coli protein.

- Use cautiously in clients with cancer of the bone marrow.

Nursing Administration

- Administer filgrastim by subcutaneous infusion, or subcutaneous injection. Monitor clients receiving intermittent IV bolus or continuous IV infusion.

- Do not agitate the vial of medication. Use each vial for one dose and do not combine with other medications. Do not put the needle back into the vial when withdrawing the medication.

- Monitor CBC two times per week.

Nursing Evaluation of Medication Effectiveness

- Depending on therapeutic intent, effectiveness may be evidenced by:

  o Absence of infection

  o In chemotherapy for cancer treatment, an absolute neutrophil count increase to greater than 10,000/mm³ after the chemotherapeutic-induced nadir (the peak of chemotherapeutic cell destruction, usually occurring 10 to 14 days after administration)

MEDICATION CLASSIFICATION: GRANULOCYTE MACROPHAGE COLONY STIMULATING FACTOR

- Select Prototype Medication – Sargramostim (Leukine)

Purpose

- Expected Pharmacological Action

  o This medication acts on the bone marrow to increase production and function of white blood cells (neutrophils, monocytes, macrophages, eosinophils).

- Therapeutic uses

  o Hastens bone marrow function after bone marrow transplant

  o Treatment of failed bone marrow transplant

Complications

SIDE/ADVERSE EFFECTS	NURSING INTERVENTIONS/CLIENT EDUCATION
Diarrhea, weakness, rash, malaise, and bone pain	- Monitor clients for symptoms and notify the provider if they occur. - Administer acetaminophen.
Leukocytosis, thrombocytosis	- Monitor CBC two times per week during treatment. - Reduce dose or interrupt treatment for WBC greater than 50,000 mm³, absolute neutrophil count greater than 20,000 mm³, or platelets greater than 500,000 mm³.

Contraindications/Precautions

- Use is contraindicated in clients allergic to yeast products.

- Use cautiously in clients with heart disease, hypoxia, peripheral edema, or pleural or pericardial effusion.

- Use cautiously in clients with cancer of the bone marrow.

Nursing Administration

- Monitor clients receiving IV infusion.

- Obtain baseline CBC, differential, and platelet count. Monitor periodically during treatment.

Nursing Evaluation of Medication Effectiveness

- Depending on therapeutic intent, effectiveness may be evidenced by:

  o Absence of infection

  o WBC and differential within expected reference ranges

MEDICATION CLASSIFICATION: THROMBOPOIETIC GROWTH FACTORS

- Select Prototype Medication – Oprelvekin (Interleukin-11, Neumega)

Purpose

- Expected Pharmacological Action

  o Increases the production of platelets

- Therapeutic Uses

  o Decreases thrombocytopenia and the need for platelet transfusions in clients receiving chemotherapy.

Complications

SIDE/ADVERSE EFFECTS	NURSING INTERVENTIONS/CLIENT EDUCATION
Fluid retention (peripheral edema, dyspnea on exertion)	• Monitor the client's I&O. • If symptoms occur, stop the medication and notify the provider.
Cardiac dysrhythmias (tachycardia, atrial fibrillation, atrial flutter)	• Use cautiously in clients with a history of cardiac dysrhythmias. • Monitor the client's vital signs, heart rate, and rhythm. • If symptoms occur, stop the medication and notify the provider.

SIDE/ADVERSE EFFECTS	NURSING INTERVENTIONS/CLIENT EDUCATION
Conjunctival injection, transient blurring of vision, papilledema	• Advise clients to observe for symptoms, and if symptoms occur, stop the medication and notify the provider.
Allergic reactions, possible anaphylaxis	• Observe clients carefully for allergic reactions; stop the medication and notify the provider if symptoms occur.

 Contraindications/Precautions

- These medications are generally contraindicated in clients who have cancer of the bone marrow, because they may stimulate tumor growth.

- Use cautiously in clients with heart failure and pleural effusion.

Nursing Administration

- Obtain the client's baseline CBC, platelet count, and electrolytes.

- Do not agitate vial of oprelvekin and do not combine with other medications.

- Administer oprelvekin once daily by subcutaneous injection until platelet count reaches prescribed level.

Nursing Evaluation of Medication Effectiveness

- Depending on therapeutic intent, effectiveness may be evidenced by:

  ○ Platelet count greater than 50,000/mm^3

APPLICATION EXERCISES

1. A client has been receiving daily doses of oprelvekin (Interleukin-11). Which laboratory value should the nurse monitor to determine the effectiveness of the medication?

2. Which of the following interventions should the nurse implement when preparing to administer filgrastim (Neupogen) for the first time to a client who has undergone a bone marrow transplant?

   A. Administer intramuscularly in a large muscle mass to prevent injury.

   B. Give orally with a meal or snack to prevent severe gastrointestinal upset.

   C. Shake vial gently to mix well before withdrawing dose.

   D. Discard vial after removing one dose of the medication.

3. A nurse is caring for a client who has been receiving epoetin alfa (Epogen) three times a week for several weeks. At a visit to the clinic, the client's Hgb has increased from 7 g/dL to 8.5 g/dL in the past week. Which of the following actions should the nurse expect to take regarding today's dose of epoetin alfa?

   A. To increase today's dose.

   B. To administer the ordered dose.

   C. To withhold today's dose.

   D. To discontinue the medication.

4. A nurse is monitoring a client who is receiving sargramostim (Leukine) following a bone marrow transplant. For which of the following adverse reactions should the nurse monitor the client?

   A. Constipation

   B. Bone pain

   C. Insomnia

   D. Hair loss

APPLICATION EXERCISES ANSWER KEY

1. A client has been receiving daily doses of oprelvekin (Interleukin-11). Which laboratory value should the nurse monitor to determine the effectiveness of the medication?

   The nurse should plan to monitor the client's thrombocyte count. The expected outcome for oprelvekin is an increased thrombocyte count greater than 50,000/mm3.

 NCLEX® Connection: Pharmacological Therapies, Expected Actions/Outcomes

2. Which of the following interventions should the nurse implement when preparing to administer filgrastim (Neupogen) for the first time to a client who has undergone a bone marrow transplant?

   A. Administer intramuscularly in a large muscle mass to prevent injury.

   B. Give orally with a meal or snack to prevent severe gastrointestinal upset.

   C. Shake vial gently to mix well before withdrawing dose.

   D. Discard vial after removing one dose of the medication.

   Filgrastim is dispensed in a vial meant for single-dose use and the nurse should discard any unused portion. Administer the medication by subcutaneous and IV routes only, so neither oral nor IM administration is appropriate. Do not shake the vial before withdrawal, as it may damage the medication.

 NCLEX® Connection: Pharmacological Therapies, Medication Administration

3. A nurse is caring for a client who has been receiving epoetin alfa (Epogen) three times a week for several weeks. At a visit to the clinic, the client's Hgb has increased from 7 g/dL to 8.5 g/dL in the past week. Which of the following actions should the nurse expect to take regarding today's dose of epoetin alfa?

   A. To increase today's dose.

   B. To administer the ordered dose.

   C. To withhold today's dose.

   D. To discontinue the medication.

   The nurse should expect the provider to withhold the dose to eliminate today's dose of epoetin alfa since a rapid rise in Hgb may precipitate a myocardial infarction or other cardiac event. The dose of epoetin alfa is usually decreased or interrupted when the Hgb reaches 12 g/dL or if it increases by more than 1 g/dL in 2 weeks. The nurse should not expect the dose to increase or remain the same. The nurse should not expect the medication to be discontinued at this time, since the target Hgb (usually 10 to 12 g/dL) has not been reached.

 NCLEX® Connection: Pharmacological Therapies, Expected Actions/Outcomes

4. A nurse is monitoring a client who is receiving sargramostim (Leukine) following a bone marrow transplant. For which of the following adverse reactions should the nurse monitor the client?

    A. Constipation

    B. Bone pain

    C. Insomnia

    D. Hair loss

    Bone pain is an adverse reaction of sargramostim. Other possible adverse reactions include diarrhea, rash, fatigue, and malaise. Constipation, insomnia, and hair loss are not adverse reactions seen during sargramostim therapy.

 NCLEX® Connection: Pharmacological Therapies, Adverse Effects/Contraindications/Side Effects/Interactions

UNIT 6: MEDICATIONS AFFECTING THE GASTROINTESTINAL SYSTEM AND NUTRITION

- Peptic Ulcer Disease

- Gastrointestinal Disorders

- Vitamins, Minerals, and Supplements

NCLEX® CONNECTIONS

When reviewing the chapters in this section, keep in mind the relevant sections of the NCLEX® outline, in particular:

CLIENT NEEDS: PHARMACOLOGICAL THERAPIES

Relevant topics/tasks include:
- Adverse Effects/Contraindications/Side Effects/Interactions
  - Monitor and document client side effects to medications.
- Expected Actions/Outcomes
  - Reinforce education to client regarding medications.
- Medication Administration
  - Administer medication by gastrointestinal tube.

UNIT 6	MEDICATIONS AFFECTING THE GASTROINTESTINAL SYSTEM AND NUTRITION
Chapter 26	Peptic Ulcer Disease

 Overview

- Pharmacological management of peptic ulcer disease (PUD) addresses the imbalance between gastric mucosal defenses and antagonistic factors such as *H. pylori* infection, NSAIDs, and secretions including gastric acid and pepsin.

- Therapeutic management outcomes include:

  o Lessening of symptoms

  o Encouragement of healing

  o Decreased risk of complications

  o Stopping reoccurrence

- Only antibiotics alter the disease process. All other medications make an environment that is conducive to healing.

- The groups of medications used in the management of PUD include:

  o Antibiotics

  o Antisecretory agents

  o Mucosal protectants

  o Antacids

MEDICATION CLASSIFICATION: ANTIBIOTICS

- Select Prototype Medications:

  o Amoxicillin (Amoxil)

  o Bismuth (Pepto-Bismol)

  o Clarithromycin (Biaxin)

  o Metronidazole (Flagyl)

  o Tetracycline (Achromycin V)

Purpose

- Expected Pharmacological Action

  o Eradication of *H. pylori* bacteria

- Therapy should include:

  o Combination of 2 or 3 antibiotics for 14 days

MEDICATION CLASSIFICATION: HISTAMINE$_2$-RECEPTOR ANTAGONISTS

- Select Prototype Medication: ranitidine (Zantac)

- Other Medications:

  o Nizatidine (Axid)

  o Famotidine (Pepcid)

  o Cimetidine (Tagamet)

Purpose

- Expected Pharmacological Action

  o Histamine$_2$-receptor antagonists suppress the secretion of gastric acid by selectively blocking H$_2$ receptors in parietal cells lining the stomach.

- Therapeutic Uses

  o Gastric and peptic ulcers, GERD, and hypersecretory conditions, such as Zollinger-Ellison syndrome.

  o Use in conjunction with antibiotics to treat ulcers caused by *H. pylori*.

Complications

SIDE/ADVERSE EFFECTS	NURSING INTERVENTIONS/CLIENT EDUCATION
Cimetidine can block androgen receptors, resulting in decreased libido and impotence.	• Inform clients of these possible effects. Side effects reverse when medication is stopped.
Cimetidine can cause CNS effects (lethargy, depression, confusion).	• These effects are seen more often in an older adult with kidney or liver dysfunction. • Avoid use in older adults.

- Ranitidine, nizatidine, and famotidine have few adverse effects and interactions.

 Contraindications/Precautions

- These medications are Pregnancy Risk Category B.

 H$_2$-receptor antagonists decrease gastric acidity, which promotes bacterial colonization of the stomach and the respiratory tract. Use cautiously in clients who are at a high risk for pneumonia, such as clients who have COPD.

Interactions

MEDICATION/FOOD INTERACTIONS	NURSING INTERVENTIONS/CLIENT EDUCATION
Cimetidine can inhibit medication-metabolizing enzymes and thus increase the levels of warfarin (Coumadin), phenytoin (Dilantin), theophylline (Theolair), and lidocaine.	• In clients taking warfarin, monitor for signs of bleeding. • Monitor PT and INR levels, and administer adjusted warfarin dosages accordingly. • In clients taking phenytoin, theophylline, and lidocaine, monitor serum levels and administer adjusted dosages accordingly.
Concurrent use of antacids can decrease absorption of histamine$_2$-receptor antagonists	• Advise clients not to take an antacid 1 hr before or after taking a histamine$_2$-receptor antagonist.

Nursing Administration

- Monitor clients receiving cimetidine, ranitidine, and famotidine by IV route for acute situations.

- Advise clients to practice good nutrition. Suggest eating six small meals rather than three large meals a day.

- Inform clients that adequate rest and reduction of stress can promote healing.

- Instruct clients to avoid smoking, because smoking can delay healing.

- Encourage clients to avoid aspirin and other NSAIDs unless taking low-dose aspirin therapy for prevention of cardiovascular disease.

- If alcohol exacerbates symptoms, advise clients to stop drinking.

- Recognize that availability of these medications OTC may discourage clients from seeking appropriate health care. Encourage clients to see the provider if symptoms persist.

- Recognize that the medication regimen can be complex, often requiring clients to take two to three different medications for an extended period of time. Encourage clients to adhere to the medication regimen and provide support.

- Instruct clients to take ranitidine with or without food

- Instruct clients that treatment of PUD is usually started as an oral dose twice a day until the ulcer is healed, followed by a maintenance dose, which is usually taken once a day at bedtime.

- Instruct clients to notify the provider for any sign of obvious or occult gastrointestinal (GI) bleeding, such as coffee-ground emesis.

MEDICATION CLASSIFICATION: PROTON PUMP INHIBITOR

- Select Prototype Medication: omeprazole (Prilosec)

- Other Medications:

    o Pantoprazole (Protonix)

    o Lansoprazole (Prevacid)

    o Rabeprazole sodium (AcipHex)

    o Esomeprazole (Nexium)

Purpose

- Expected Pharmacological Action

    o Proton pump inhibitors reduce gastric acid secretion by irreversibly inhibiting the enzyme that produces gastric acid.

    o Proton pump inhibitors reduce basal and stimulated acid production.

- Therapeutic Uses

    o Gastric and peptic ulcers, GERD, and hypersecretory conditions, such as Zollinger-Ellison syndrome.

Complications

- Insignificant side effects and adverse effects with short-term treatment

- Low incidence of headache, diarrhea, and nausea/vomiting

- Decreases gastric acid pH, which promotes bacterial colonization of the stomach and the respiratory tract. Use cautiously in clients who are at high risk for pneumonia, such as clients who have COPD.

- Risk of thrombophlebitis with IV administration of pantoprazole. Monitor the client's IV site for signs of inflammation (redness, swelling, local pain) and ensure the IV site is changed if indicated.

Contraindications/Precautions

- These medications are Pregnancy Risk Category C.

- Use cautiously with children and women who are breastfeeding.

- Contraindicated for clients who are hypersensitive to medication.

- Long-term use of proton pump inhibitors increases the risk of gastric cancer and osteoporosis.

Interactions

MEDICATION/FOOD INTERACTIONS	NURSING INTERVENTIONS/CLIENT EDUCATION
Digoxin (Lanoxin) levels may be increased when used concurrently with omeprazole.	• Monitor digoxin levels carefully if prescribed concurrently.
Absorption of ketoconazole (formerly Nizoral), itraconazole (Sporanox), and atazanavir (Reyataz) is extremely decreased when taken concurrently with proton pump inhibitors.	• Avoid concurrent use. If necessary to administer concurrently, separate medication administration by 2 to 12 hr.

Nursing Administration

- Instruct clients not to crush, chew, or break sustained-release capsules.

- Tell clients they can sprinkle the contents of the capsule over food to facilitate swallowing.

- Instruct clients to take omeprazole once a day prior to eating in the morning.

- Encourage clients to avoid alcohol and irritating medications, such as NSAIDs.

- Instruct clients that active ulcers should be treated for 4 to 6 weeks.

- Instruct clients to notify the provider for any sign of obvious or occult GI bleeding, such as coffee-ground emesis.

MEDICATION CLASSIFICATION: MUCOSAL PROTECTANT

- Select Prototype Medication: sucralfate (Carafate)

Purpose

- Expected Pharmacological Action

  ○ The acidic environment of the stomach and duodenum changes sucralfate into a thick substance that adheres to an ulcer. This protects the ulcer from further injury that may be caused by acid and pepsin.

  ○ This viscous substance can stick to the ulcer for up to 6 hr.

- Therapeutic Uses

  ○ Treatment of acute duodenal ulcers and maintenance therapy.

  ○ Investigational use of sucralfate includes gastric ulcers and GERD.

Complications

- To prevent constipation, encourage clients to increase dietary fiber and drink at least 1,500 mL/day if fluids are not restricted.

- Sucralfate has no systemic effects.

Contraindications/Precautions

- Pregnancy Risk Category B

- Contraindicated in clients who are hypersensitive to the medication

Interactions

MEDICATION/FOOD INTERACTIONS	NURSING INTERVENTIONS/CLIENT EDUCATION
Sucralfate may interfere with the absorption of phenytoin, digoxin, warfarin, and ciprofloxacin.	• Instruct clients to maintain a 2-hr interval between these medications and sucralfate to minimize this interaction.
Antacids interfere with the absorption of sucralfate.	• Advise clients to avoid taking an antacid within 30 min of sucralfate.

Nursing Administration

- Assist clients with the medication regimen.

- Instruct clients to take the medication on an empty stomach.

- Instruct clients to take sucralfate four times a day, 1 hr before meals, and again at bedtime.

- Instruct clients to break or dissolve the medication in water, but not to crush or chew the tablet.

- Encourage clients to complete the course of treatment.

MEDICATION CLASSIFICATION: ANTACIDS

- Select Prototype Medication: aluminum hydroxide (Amphojel)

- Other Medications:

  o Aluminum carbonate

  o Magnesium hydroxide (Milk of Magnesia)

  o Sodium bicarbonate

Purpose

- Expected Pharmacological Action

  o Antacids neutralize gastric acid and inactivate pepsin.

  o Mucosal protection can occur through the antacid's ability to stimulate the production of prostaglandins.

- Therapeutic Uses

  o Management of PUD by promoting healing and relieving pain.

  o Symptomatic relief for clients who have GERD.

Complications

SIDE/ADVERSE EFFECTS	NURSING INTERVENTIONS/CLIENT EDUCATION
Aluminum and calcium compounds cause constipation, whereas magnesium compounds cause diarrhea.	• Advise clients to alternate these compounds to offset intestinal effects and normalize bowel function. • If a client has difficulty managing bowel function, recommend the use of a combination product. This product contains aluminum hydroxide, magnesium hydroxide, and simethicone.
Antacids containing sodium can result in fluid retention.	• Reinforce to clients who have hypertension or heart failure to avoid antacids that contain sodium.
Aluminum hydroxide can lead to hypophosphatemia.	• Monitor the client's phosphate level.
Magnesium compounds can lead to toxicity in clients who have renal impairment.	• Reinforce to clients who have renal impairment to avoid antacids that contain magnesium.

 Contraindications/Precautions

- Antacids are Pregnancy Risk Category C.

- Antacids are contraindicated for clients who have GI perforation or obstruction.

- Use cautiously in clients who have abdominal pain.

Interactions

MEDICATION/FOOD INTERACTIONS	NURSING INTERVENTIONS/CLIENT EDUCATION
Aluminum compounds bind to warfarin and tetracycline, interfering with absorption.	• Reinforce to clients to take these medications 1 hr apart.

Nursing Administration

- Instruct clients to chew the tablets thoroughly and then drink at least 8 oz of water or milk.

- Reinforce to clients to shake liquid formulations to ensure even dispersion of the medication.

- Recognize adherence is difficult for clients because of the frequency of administration. Medication is administered seven times a day: 1 hr and 3 hr after meals, and again at bedtime. Encourage adherence by reinforcing the intended effect of the antacid, such as relief of pain and healing of the ulcer.

- Instruct clients to take all medications at least 1 hr before or after taking an antacid.

MEDICATION CLASSIFICATION: PROSTAGLANDIN E ANALOG

- Select Prototype Medication: misoprostol (Cytotec)

Purpose

- Expected Pharmacological Action

  o Prostaglandin E analog acts as an endogenous prostaglandin in the GI tract to decrease acid secretion, increase the secretion of bicarbonate and protective mucus, and promote vasodilation to maintain submucosal blood flow. These actions all serve to prevent gastric ulcers.

- Therapeutic Uses

  o Prevention of gastric ulcers in clients taking long-term NSAIDs.

  o Induction of labor by causing cervical ripening.

Complications

SIDE/ADVERSE EFFECTS	NURSING INTERVENTIONS/CLIENT EDUCATION
Diarrhea and abdominal pain	• Instruct clients to notify the provider of symptoms of diarrhea or abdominal pain. • Tell clients the provider may need to reduce the dosage.
Women may experience dysmenorrhea and spotting.	• Instruct clients to notify the provider if dysmenorrhea and spotting occur. • The provider may discontinue the medication.

 Contraindications/Precautions

- Pregnancy Risk Category X

Nursing Administration

- Reinforce to clients to take misoprostol with meals and at bedtime.

Nursing Evaluation of Medication Effectiveness

- Depending on therapeutic intent, effectiveness may be evidenced by:

  o Reduced frequency or absence of GERD symptoms (heartburn, bloating, belching)

  o Absence of GI bleeding

  o Healing of gastric and duodenal ulcers

  o No reoccurrence of ulcer

APPLICATION EXERCISES

1. A nurse is reinforcing teaching for a client who has peptic ulcer disease on how to properly self-administer ranitidine (Zantac). Which of the following client statements indicates effective teaching by the nurse?

    A. "I should call my doctor if my stools look black and sticky."

    B. "I will take ranitidine regularly until my burning symptoms disappear."

    C. "I need to take ranitidine on an empty stomach."

    D. "I can take ibuprofen if I have minor aches and pains."

2. A nurse is reinforcing teaching for a client who is newly diagnosed with peptic ulcer disease and has prescriptions for several different medications. The nurse should recognize that which of the following medications is used as a mucosal protectant to promote healing of the ulcer?

    A. Bismuth (Pepto-Bismol)

    B. Sucralfate (Carafate)

    C. Ranitidine hydrochloride (Zantac)

    D. Metronidazole (Flagyl)

3. A nurse is caring for a client who has a prescription for sucralfate (Carafate) PO to treat peptic ulcer disease. The client states he also takes an antacid several times daily. When reinforcing teaching about sucralfate, what instructions should the nurse include?

4. A nurse is monitoring a client who has peptic ulcer disease and chronic bronchitis and is prescribed omeprazole (Prilosec). Why should the nurse plan to monitor this particular client carefully?

5. A nurse is reinforcing teaching for a client who has a prescription for misoprostol (Cytotec) to treat an ulcer caused by taking NSAIDs for arthritis pain. For which of the following should the nurse instruct the client to monitor and report to the provider?

    A. Headache

    B. Diarrhea

    C. Nasal congestion

    D. Rash

APPLICATION EXERCISES ANSWER KEY

1. A nurse is reinforcing teaching for a client who has peptic ulcer disease on how to properly self-administer ranitidine (Zantac). Which of the following client statements indicates effective teaching by the nurse?

   A. "I should call my doctor if my stools look black and sticky."
   B. "I will take ranitidine regularly until my burning symptoms disappear."
   C. "I need to take ranitidine on an empty stomach."
   D. "I can take ibuprofen if I have minor aches and pains."

   Clients need to notify the provider if signs of GI bleeding develop. Symptom relief does not indicate ulcer healing. Clients can take ranitidine without regard to food. Clients who have PUD should avoid NSAIDs, such as ibuprofen, due to the risk of bleeding.

    NCLEX® Connection: Pharmacological Therapies, Adverse Effects/Contraindications/Side Effects/Interactions

2. A nurse is reinforcing teaching for a client who is newly diagnosed with peptic ulcer disease and has prescriptions for several different medications. The nurse should recognize that which of the following medications is used as a mucosal protectant to promote healing of the ulcer?

   A. Bismuth (Pepto-Bismol)
   B. Sucralfate (Carafate)
   C. Ranitidine hydrochloride (Zantac)
   D. Metronidazole (Flagyl)

   Sucralfate (Carafate) is a mucosal protectant which coats the ulcer and promotes healing. Bismuth and metronidazole are antibiotics which are prescribed to kill *H. pylori* bacteria. More than one antibiotic is prescribed to prevent the development of resistance. Ranitidine is an H$_2$-receptor antagonist prescribed to suppress the secretion of gastric acid.

    NCLEX® Connection: Pharmacological Therapies, Expected Actions/Outcomes

3. A nurse is caring for a client who has a prescription for sucralfate (Carafate) PO to treat peptic ulcer disease. The client states he also takes an antacid several times daily. When reinforcing teaching about sucralfate, what instructions should the nurse include?

   Antacids interfere with the absorption of sucralfate (Carafate) and the client should allow at least a 30 min interval between sucralfate and the antacid.

    NCLEX® Connection: Pharmacological Therapies, Medication Administration

4. A nurse is monitoring a client who has peptic ulcer disease and chronic bronchitis and is prescribed omeprazole (Prilosec). Why should the nurse plan to monitor this particular client carefully?

   Omeprazole promotes bacterial growth in the stomach due to its action of decreasing gastric acid pH. The nurse should monitor any client who is at an increased risk for pneumonia, such as a client who has chronic bronchitis, for respiratory infection.

 NCLEX® Connection: Pharmacological Therapies, Adverse Effects/Contraindications/Side Effects/Interactions

5. A nurse is reinforcing teaching for a client who has a prescription for misoprostol (Cytotec) to treat an ulcer caused by taking NSAIDs for arthritis pain. For which of the following should the nurse instruct the client to monitor and report to the provider?

   A. Headache

   B. Diarrhea

   C. Nasal congestion

   D. Rash

   Diarrhea is a common dose-related adverse effect of misoprostol. Reinforce to the client to notify the provider if diarrhea occurs. Headache, nasal congestion, and rash are not expected adverse effects of misoprostol.

 NCLEX® Connection: Pharmacological Therapies, Adverse Effects/Contraindications/Side Effects/Interactions

UNIT 6	MEDICATIONS AFFECTING THE GASTROINTESTINAL SYSTEM AND NUTRITION

Chapter 27   Gastrointestinal Disorders

 Overview

- The medications in this section affect some aspect of the gastrointestinal (GI) tract to treat or prevent nausea/vomiting, motion sickness, diarrhea, constipation, or to treat GERD by increasing gastric motility.

- Medications include antiemetics, laxatives, antidiarrheals, prokinetic agents, and medications for irritable bowel syndrome.

MEDICATION CLASSIFICATION: ANTIEMETICS

- Select Prototype Medications:

    o   Glucocorticoid: dexamethasone (Decadron)

    o   Substance P/Neurokinin$_1$ antagonist: aprepitant (Emend)

    o   Serotonin antagonists: ondansetron (Zofran), granisetron (Kytril);

    o   Dopamine antagonists: prochlorperazine (Compazine), metoclopramide (Reglan), promethazine (Phenergan)

    o   Cannabinoid: dronabinol (Marinol)

    o   Anticholinergic: scopolamine (Transderm Scop)

    o   Antihistamines: dimenhydrinate (Dramamine), hydroxyzine (Vistaril)

    o   Benzodiazepines: lorazepam (Ativan), diazepam (Valium)

Purpose

EXPECTED PHARMACOLOGICAL ACTION	THERAPEUTIC USES
Glucocorticoid: dexamethasone	
The antiemetic mechanism of dexamethasone is unknown.	• Use dexamethasone in combination with other antiemetics to treat chemotherapy-induced nausea and vomiting (CINV). • Administer by PO or IV.

EXPECTED PHARMACOLOGICAL ACTION	THERAPEUTIC USES
Substance P/neurokinin₁ antagonist: aprepitant	
Aprepitant inhibits substance P/neurokinin₁ in the brain.	• For best results, use in combination with a glucocorticoid or serotonin antagonist. • Use for chemotherapy-induced nausea and vomiting (CINV). • Extended duration of action makes it effective for immediate use and delayed response.
Serotonin antagonist: ondansetron	
Ondansetron prevents emesis by blocking the serotonin receptors in the chemoreceptor trigger zone (CTZ), and antagonizing the serotonin receptors on the afferent vagal neurons that travel from the upper GI tract to the CTZ.	• Ondansetron prevents emesis related to chemotherapy, radiation therapy, and postoperative recovery. • Can be administered PO or IV.
Dopamine antagonist: prochlorperazine (a subset of phenothiazine)	
Antiemetic effects of prochlorperazine result from blockade of dopamine receptors in the CTZ.	• Prochlorperazine prevents emesis related to chemotherapy, opioids, and postoperative recovery. • Can be administered PO or IV.
Cannabinoid: dronabinol	
Antiemetic mechanism of dronabinol is unknown.	• Use dronabinol to control CINV and to increase appetite in clients who have AIDS. • Administer PO.
Anticholinergic: scopolamine	
Scopolamine interferes with the transmission of nerve impulses traveling from the vestibular apparatus of the inner ear to the vomiting center (VC) in the brain.	• Scopolamine treats motion sickness. • Administer topical, PO, or subcutaneously.
Antihistamine: muscarinic	
Muscarinic and histaminergic receptors in nerve pathways that connect the inner ear and VC are blocked by dimenhydrinate.	• Dimenhydrinate treats motion sickness. • Can be administered PO, IM or IV.

Complications

SIDE/ADVERSE EFFECTS	NURSING INTERVENTIONS/CLIENT EDUCATION
Substance P/neurokinin₁ antagonist: aprepitant	
Fatigue, diarrhea, dizziness, possible liver damage	• Treat headache with nonopioid analgesics. • Monitor stool pattern.

SIDE/ADVERSE EFFECTS	NURSING INTERVENTIONS/CLIENT EDUCATION
Serotonin antagonist: ondansetron	
Headache, diarrhea, dizziness	• Treat headache with nonopioid analgesics. • Monitor stool pattern.
Dopamine antagonists	
Extrapyramidal symptoms (EPS) (restlessness, anxiety, spasms of face and neck)	• Advise clients to stop the medication and inform the provider if EPS occur. • Administer an anticholinergic medication, such as diphenhydramine (Benadryl), to treat symptoms.
Hypotension	• Monitor clients receiving antihypertensive medications for low blood pressure.
Sedation	• Inform clients of the potential for sedation. • Advise clients to avoid activities that require alertness, such as driving.
Anticholinergic effects (dry mouth, urinary hesitancy, retention, constipation)	• Instruct clients to increase fluid and fiber intake. • Instruct clients to increase physical activity by engaging in regular exercise. • Tell clients to suck on hard candy, sip on fluids, or chew gum to help relieve dry mouth. • Administer a stimulant laxative, such as senna (Senokot), to counteract a decrease in bowel motility, or stool softeners, such as docusate sodium (Colace), to prevent constipation. • Advise clients to void every 4 hr.
Cannabinoid: dronabinol	
Potential for dissociation, dysphoria	• Avoid using in clients who have mental health disorders.
Hypotension, tachycardia, drowsiness	• Use cautiously in clients who have cardiovascular disorders. • Do not combine with CNS depressants, alcohol, or sedatives.
Anticholinergic: scopolamine and Antihistamines: dimenhydrinate	
Sedation	• Inform clients of the potential for sedation. • Advise clients to avoid activities that require alertness, such as driving.
Anticholinergic effects (dry mouth, urinary retention, constipation)	• Provide instructions to reduce anticholinergic effects (increase fluids and fiber, chew gum, sip on fluids, void on a regular basis).

Contraindications/Precautions

- Use dopamine antagonists cautiously, if at all, with children and older adults due to the increased risk of EPS.

- Use dopamine antagonists, antihistamines, and anticholinergic antiemetics cautiously in clients who have urinary retention or obstruction, asthma, and narrow angle glaucoma.

Interactions

MEDICATION/FOOD INTERACTIONS	NURSING INTERVENTIONS/CLIENT EDUCATION
CNS depressants, such as opioids and alcohol, can intensify CNS depression of antiemetics.	• Advise clients that CNS depression is more likely and to avoid activities that require mental alertness.
Concurrent use of antihypertensives can intensify hypotensive effects of antiemetics.	• Advise clients to sit or lie down if symptoms of lightheadedness or dizziness occur. Clients should avoid sudden changes in position by moving slowly from a lying to a sitting or standing position. • Provide assistance with ambulation as needed.
Concurrent use of anticholinergic medications (antihistamines) can intensify anticholinergic effects of antiemetics.	• Provide instructions to reduce anticholinergic effects (increase fluids and fiber, chew gum, sip on fluids, void on a regular basis).

Nursing Administration

- Collect data regarding cause of nausea and vomiting and inform provider to facilitate appropriate antiemetic.

- When a client is receiving a chemotherapy agent that causes severe nausea, combining three antiemetics and administering them prior to chemotherapy is more effective than treating nausea that is already occurring.

Nursing Evaluation of Medication Effectiveness

- Depending on therapeutic intent, effectiveness may be evidenced by:

  o Absence of nausea and vomiting.

MEDICATION CLASSIFICATION: LAXATIVES

- Select Prototype Medications:

  o Psyllium (Metamucil)

  o Docusate sodium (Colace)

     ○   Bisacodyl (Dulcolax)

     ○   Magnesium hydroxide (Milk of Magnesia)

   • Other Medications: senna (Senokot), lactulose

Purpose

EXPECTED PHARMACOLOGICAL ACTION	THERAPEUTIC USES
Bulk-forming laxative: psyllium	
Bulk-forming laxatives soften fecal mass and increase bulk, which is identical to the action of dietary fiber.	• Decrease diarrhea in clients who have diverticulosis and irritable bowel syndrome (IBS). • Control stool for clients who have an ileostomy or colostomy. • Promote defecation in older adults who have a decrease in peristalsis due to age-related changes in the GI tract.
Surfactant laxative: docusate sodium	
Surfactant laxatives lower surface tension of the stool to allow penetration of water.	• Constipation related to pregnancy or opioid use • Prevention of painful elimination for clients who have hemorrhoids or an episiotomy • Prevention of straining (cerebral aneurysm or post MI) • Decreases the risk of fecal impaction in immobile clients and promotes defecation in older adults who have decreased peristalsis due to age-related changes in the GI tract
Stimulant laxative: bisacodyl	
Stimulant laxatives result in stimulation of intestinal peristalsis.	• Client preparation prior to surgery or diagnostic tests (colonoscopy) • Short-term treatment of constipation caused by high-dose opioid use
Osmotic laxative: magnesium hydroxide	
Osmotic laxatives draw water into the intestine to increase the mass of stool, stretching musculature, which results in peristalsis.	• Low dose – Prevent painful elimination (clients who have episiotomy or hemorrhoids) • High dose – Client preparation prior to surgery or diagnostic tests (colonoscopy) • Rapid evacuation of the bowel after ingestion of poisons or following antihelminthic therapy to rid the body of dead parasites

Complications

SIDE/ADVERSE EFFECTS	NURSING INTERVENTIONS/CLIENT EDUCATION
GI irritation	• Instruct clients not to crush or chew enteric-coated tablets.
Rectal burning sensation, leading to proctitis	• Discourage clients from using bisacodyl suppositories on a regular basis.
Laxatives with magnesium salts, such as magnesium hydroxide, can lead to accumulation of toxic levels of magnesium.	• Advise clients who have renal dysfunction to read labels carefully and to avoid laxatives that contain magnesium.
Laxatives with sodium salts, such as sodium phosphate, place clients at risk for sodium absorption and fluid retention.	• Advise clients who have heart disease or hypertension to read labels carefully and to avoid laxatives that contain sodium.
Osmotic diuretics can cause dehydration.	• Monitor I&O. • Monitor for signs of dehydration (dry mouth and poor skin turgor). • Encourage clients to increase fluid intake to 2 to 3 L/day from food and beverage sources.

 Contraindications/Precautions

- Laxatives are contraindicated in clients who have fecal impaction, bowel obstruction, and acute surgical abdomen to prevent perforation.

- Laxatives are contraindicated in clients who have nausea, cramping, and abdominal pain.

- These medications are contraindicated in clients who have ulcerative colitis and diverticulitis with the exception of bulk-forming laxatives.

- Use cautiously during pregnancy and lactation.

Interactions

MEDICATION/FOOD INTERACTIONS	NURSING INTERVENTIONS/CLIENT EDUCATION
Milk and antacids can destroy enteric coating of bisacodyl.	• Instruct clients to take bisacodyl at least 1 hr apart from these medications.

Nursing Administration

- Obtain a complete history of laxative use and provide teaching as appropriate.

- Remind clients that chronic laxative use can lead to fluid and electrolyte imbalances.

- To promote defecation and resumption of normal bowel function, instruct clients to increase high-fiber foods in daily diet, such as bran, fresh fruits and vegetables, and increased amounts of fluids. Recommend at least 2 to 3 L/day from beverages and food sources.

- Encourage clients to maintain a regular exercise regimen to improve bowel function.

- Instruct clients to take bulk-forming and surfactant laxatives with a glass of water.

Nursing Evaluation of Medication Effectiveness

- Depending on therapeutic intent, effectiveness may be evidenced by:

  o Return to regular bowel function.

  o Evacuation of bowel in preparation for surgery or diagnostic tests.

MEDICATION CLASSIFICATION: ANTIDIARRHEALS

- Select Prototype Medication: diphenoxylate plus atropine (Lomotil)

- Other Medications: loperamide (Imodium), difenoxin (Motofen)

Purpose

- Expected Pharmacological Action

  o Antidiarrheals activate opioid receptors in the GI tract to decrease intestinal motility and to increase the absorption of fluid and sodium in the intestine.

- Therapeutic Uses

  o Use specific antidiarrheal agents to treat the underlying cause of diarrhea. For example, antibiotics can be used to treat diarrhea caused by a bacterial infection.

  o Use nonspecific antidiarrheal agents for symptomatic treatment of diarrhea (decrease in frequency and fluid content of stool).

Complications

- At recommended doses for diarrhea, diphenoxylate does not affect the CNS system.

- At high doses, clients may experience typical opioid effects, such as euphoria or CNS depression. However, the addition of atropine, which has unpleasant adverse effects (blurred vision, dry mouth, urinary retention, constipation, tachycardia) in Lomotil discourages ingestion of doses higher than those prescribed.

Contraindications/Precautions

- There is an increased risk of megacolon in clients who have inflammatory bowel disorders. This could lead to a serious complication, such as perforation of the bowel.

Interactions

- Alcohol or other CNS depressants can enhance CNS depression.

Nursing Administration

- Administer initial dose of diphenoxylate plus atropine, 4 mg; follow each loose stool with additional dose of 2 mg, but do not exceed 16 mg/day.

- Advise clients who have diarrhea to drink small amounts of a commercial oral rehydration solution to maintain electrolyte balance for the first 24 hr.

- Advise clients to avoid drinking plain water because it does not contain necessary electrolytes that have been lost in the stool.

- Advise clients to avoid caffeine. Caffeine exacerbates diarrhea by increasing GI motility.

- Clients who have severe cases of diarrhea may be hospitalized for management of dehydration.

- Management of dehydration should include monitoring of weight, I&O, and vital signs. A hypotonic solution, such as 0.45% sodium chloride may be prescribed.

Nursing Evaluation of Medication Effectiveness

- Depending on therapeutic intent, effectiveness may be evidenced by:

  o Return of normal bowel pattern as evidenced by decrease in frequency and fluid volume of stool.

MEDICATION CLASSIFICATION: PROKINETIC AGENTS

- Select Prototype Medication: metoclopramide (Reglan)

Purpose

- Expected Pharmacological Action

  o Metoclopramide controls nausea and vomiting by blocking dopamine and serotonin receptors in the CTZ.

  o Metoclopramide augments action of acetylcholine, which causes an increase in upper GI motility.

- Therapeutic Uses

  o Control of postoperative and chemotherapy-induced nausea and vomiting

  o Management of GERD and gastroparesis

Complications

SIDE/ADVERSE EFFECTS	NURSING INTERVENTIONS/CLIENT EDUCATION
Extrapyramidal symptoms (EPS) (restlessness, anxiety, spasms of face and neck)	• Administer an antihistamine, such as diphenhydramine, to minimize extrapyramidal symptoms.
Sedation	• Inform clients of the potential for sedation. • Advise clients to avoid activities that require alertness, such as driving.
Diarrhea	• Monitor the client's bowel function and for signs of dehydration.

 Contraindications/Precautions

- Contraindicated in clients who have GI perforation, GI bleeding, bowel obstruction, and hemorrhage

- Contraindicated in clients who have a seizure disorder due to increased risk of seizures

- Use cautiously in children and older adults due to the increased risk for EPS.

Interactions

MEDICATION/FOOD INTERACTIONS	NURSING INTERVENTIONS/CLIENT EDUCATION
Concurrent use of alcohol and other CNS depressants increases the risk of seizures and sedation.	• Advise clients to avoid the use of alcohol. • Use cautiously with other CNS depressants.
Opioids and anticholinergics decrease the effects of metoclopramide.	• Advise clients to avoid using opioids and medications with anticholinergic effects.

Nursing Administration

- Monitor clients for CNS depression and EPS.

- Administer via oral route. Monitor clients receiving medication via IV route.

Nursing Evaluation of Medication Effectiveness

- Depending on therapeutic intent, effectiveness may be evidenced by:

  o Absence of nausea and vomiting

MEDICATION CLASSIFICATION: MEDICATIONS FOR IRRITABLE BOWEL SYNDROME WITH DIARRHEA (IBS-D)

- Select Prototype Medication: alosetron (Lotronex)

Purpose

- Expected Pharmacological Action

    o Selective blockade of 5-HT3 receptors, which innervate the viscera and result in increased firmness in stool and decrease in urgency and frequency of defecation

- Therapeutic Uses

    o For female clients who have had irritable bowel syndrome with diarrhea that has lasted more than 6 months and has been resistant to conventional management

Complications

SIDE/ADVERSE EFFECTS	NURSING INTERVENTIONS/CLIENT EDUCATION
Constipation, which may result in GI toxicity, such as ischemic colitis, bowel obstruction, impaction or perforation.	• Administer medication only to clients who meet specific criteria and are willing to sign a treatment agreement. • Instruct clients to note rectal bleeding, bloody diarrhea, or abdominal pain, and report to the provider. Tell clients the provider will discontinue the medication.

 Contraindications/Precautions

- Contraindicated for clients who have chronic constipation, history of bowel obstruction, Crohn's disease, ulcerative colitis, impaired intestinal circulation, or thrombophlebitis

Interactions

MEDICATION/FOOD INTERACTIONS	NURSING INTERVENTIONS/CLIENT EDUCATION
Medications that induce cytochrome P450 enzymes, such as phenobarbital, may decrease levels of alosetron.	Monitor the effectiveness of medication.

Nursing Administration

- Instruct clients that symptoms should resolve within 1 to 4 weeks but will return 1 week after medication is discontinued.

- Instruct clients that dosage will start as once a day and may be increased to BID.

Nursing Evaluation of Medication Effectiveness

- Depending on therapeutic intent, effectiveness may be evidenced by:

  o Relief of diarrhea, decrease in urgency and frequency of defecation.

MEDICATION CLASSIFICATION: MEDICATIONS FOR IRRITABLE BOWEL SYNDROME WITH CONSTIPATION (IBS-C)

- Select Prototype Medication: lubiprostone (Amitiza)

Purpose

- Expected Pharmacological Action

  o Increases fluid secretion in the intestine to promote intestinal motility by acting as an antagonist at 5-HT$_2$ receptors

- Therapeutic Uses

  o Irritable bowel syndrome with constipation

  o Chronic constipation

Complications

SIDE/ADVERSE EFFECTS	NURSING INTERVENTIONS/CLIENT EDUCATION
Diarrhea	Monitor frequency of stools. Notify provider if severe diarrhea occurs.
Nausea	Instruct clients to take the medication with food and water.

 Contraindications/Precautions

- Pregnancy Risk Category C

- Contraindicated for clients who have a history of bowel obstruction, Crohn's disease, ulcerative colitis, or diverticulitis

Interactions

- No significant interactions

Nursing Administration

- Instruct clients to take the medication with food and water to decrease nausea.

- Instruct clients to take the medication BID.

Nursing Evaluation of Medication Effectiveness

- Depending on therapeutic intent, effectiveness may be evidenced by:

  - Relief of constipation

MEDICATION CLASSIFICATION: 5-AMINOSALICYLATES

- Select Prototype Medication: sulfasalazine (Azulfidine)

- Other Medications:

  - 5-aminosalicylates: mesalamine (Asacol, Rowasa)

  - Glucocorticoids: hydrocortisone

  - Immunosuppressants: azathioprine (Imuran)

  - Immunomodulators: infliximab (Remicade)

  - Antibiotics: metronidazole (Flagyl)

Purpose

- Expected Pharmacological Action

  - Decrease inflammation by inhibiting prostaglandin synthesis.

- Therapeutic Uses

  - Inflammatory bowel disease: Crohn's disease, ulcerative colitis

Complications

SIDE/ADVERSE EFFECTS	NURSING INTERVENTIONS/CLIENT EDUCATION
Blood disorders including agranulocytosis, hemolytic and macrocytic anemia	Monitor the client's complete blood count.
Nausea, fever, rash	Instruct clients to report symptoms to provider.

Contraindications/Precautions

- These medications are Pregnancy Risk Category B

- These medications are contraindicated in clients who have sensitivity to sulfonamides, salicylates, and/or thiazide diuretics.

- Use cautiously with older adults and in clients who have liver or kidney disease or blood dyscrasias.

Interactions

- No significant interactions.

Nursing Administration

- Administer in four divided oral doses throughout the day.

Nursing Evaluation of Medication Effectiveness

- Depending on therapeutic intent, effectiveness may be evidenced by:
  - o Decreased bowel inflammation
  - o Return to normal bowel function

APPLICATION EXERCISES

1. For which of the following clients is a laxative indicated? (Select all that apply.)

    _____ A young adult female who is postpartum following a vaginal delivery with an episiotomy

    _____ A young adult male who has constipation and periumbilical pain

    _____ A young adult client affected by IBS

    _____ An older adult client who has limited mobility and minor bowel incontinence

    _____ An older adult client preparing for a colonoscopy

2. A nurse is caring for a surgical client who has been prescribed aprepitant (Emend) PO to prevent postoperative nausea and vomiting. For which of the following should the nurse monitor the client?

    A. Diarrhea

    B. Hypotension

    C. Sedation

    D. Tachycardia

3. A nurse is preparing to administer prochlorperazine (Compazine) to an adult client who is experiencing nausea and vomiting. Which of the following current medications taken by the client earlier in the day may interact with the prochlorperazine to cause the intensification of an adverse effect?

    A. Ibuprofen (Motrin)

    B. Ranitidine (Zantac)

    C. Digoxin (Lanoxin)

    D. Metoprolol (Lopressor)

4. A nurse is preparing to administer sodium phosphate (Fleet Phospho-Soda) liquid osmotic laxative to a client who is undergoing bowel preparation for a colonoscopy. The nurse should understand that sodium phosphate may exacerbate what client condition?

5. A nurse is caring for a client who has a new prescription for sulfasalazine (Azulfidine) to treat ulcerative colitis. Which of the following laboratory values should the nurse plan to monitor while the client is taking sulfasalazine?

    A. Blood glucose level

    B. Complete blood count (CBC)

    C. Blood urea nitrogen (BUN)

    D. T_3 and T_4 levels

APPLICATION EXERCISES ANSWER KEY

1. For which of the following clients is a laxative indicated? (Select all that apply.)

    __X__ **A young adult female who is postpartum following a vaginal delivery with an episiotomy**

    _____ A young adult male who has constipation and periumbilical pain

    __X__ **A young adult client affected by IBS**

    _____ An older adult client who has limited mobility and minor bowel incontinence

    __X__ **An older adult client preparing for a colonoscopy**

    Laxatives will prevent straining until the episiotomy heals. Bulk-forming laxatives can provide relief of diarrhea for clients who have IBS. Use laxatives for bowel cleansing prior to diagnostic procedures of the gastrointestinal tract. Appendicitis can begin in the periumbilical area before progressing to the right lower quadrant. The older adult may be experiencing fecal impaction and a laxative could cause perforation.

     NCLEX® Connection: Pharmacological Therapies, Expected Actions/Outcomes

2. A nurse is caring for a surgical client who has been prescribed aprepitant (Emend) PO to prevent postoperative nausea and vomiting. For which of the following should the nurse monitor the client?

    A. Diarrhea

    B. Hypotension

    C. Sedation

    D. Tachycardia

    Diarrhea is a possible adverse effect of aprepitant for which the nurse should monitor the client. Hypotension, sedation, and tachycardia are not expected adverse effects of aprepitant.

     NCLEX® Connection: Pharmacological Therapies, Adverse Effects/Contraindications/Side Effects/Interactions

3. A nurse is preparing to administer prochlorperazine (Compazine) to an adult client who is experiencing nausea and vomiting. Which of the following current medications taken by the client earlier in the day may interact with the prochlorperazine to cause the intensification of an adverse effect?

    A. Ibuprofen (Motrin)

    B. Ranitidine (Zantac)

    C. Digoxin (Lanoxin)

    D. Metoprolol (Lopressor)

Metoprolol and other antihypertensive medications can intensify the adverse effects of hypotension, which may be seen when prochlorperazine is administered. Ibuprofen, ranitidine, and digoxin do not interact with prochlorperazine and do not intensify possible adverse effects of prochlorperazine.

 NCLEX® Connection: Pharmacological Therapies, Adverse Effects/Contraindications/Side Effects/Interactions

4. A nurse is preparing to administer sodium phosphate (Fleet Phospho-Soda) liquid osmotic laxative to a client who is undergoing bowel preparation for a colonoscopy. The nurse should understand that sodium phosphate may exacerbate what client condition?

Sodium laxatives can increase the risk for worsening of heart failure or hypertension. They can create fluid retention caused by increased serum sodium in a client who has an underlying heart condition.

 NCLEX® Connection: Pharmacological Therapies, Adverse Effects/Contraindications/Side Effects/Interactions

5. A nurse is caring for a client who has a new prescription for sulfasalazine (Azulfidine) to treat ulcerative colitis. Which of the following laboratory values should the nurse plan to monitor while the client is taking sulfasalazine?

    A. Blood glucose level

    B. Complete blood count (CBC)

    C. Blood urea nitrogen (BUN)

    D. T_3 and T_4 levels

The nurse should monitor the client's CBC because sulfasalazine can cause agranulocytosis or severe anemias. It is not necessary to monitor the glucose level, BUN, and thyroid function while a client takes sulfasalazine.

 NCLEX® Connection: Pharmacological Therapies, Adverse Effects/Contraindications/Side Effects/Interactions

UNIT 6	MEDICATIONS AFFECTING THE GASTROINTESTINAL SYSTEM AND NUTRITION

Chapter 28   Vitamins, Minerals, and Supplements

 Overview

- Various vitamins and minerals described in this section affect production of RBCs and help prevent various types of anemia.

- Potassium and magnesium regulate body fluid volume. Supplements of these substances prevent multiple serious conditions.

- Categories of medications include:

  o Vitamins, including vitamin B_{12} and folic acid

  o Iron supplements

  o Potassium and magnesium supplements

  o Various herbal supplements

MEDICATION CLASSIFICATION: IRON PREPARATIONS

- Select Prototype Medications:

  o Oral – Ferrous sulfate (Feosol)

  o Parenteral – Iron dextran (INFeD)

- Other Medications:

  o Oral – Ferrous gluconate (Fergon), ferrous fumarate (Ferro-Sequels)

  o Parenteral – Iron sucrose (Venofer), sodium-ferric gluconate complex (SFGC) (Ferrlecit)

Purpose

- Expected Pharmacological Action

  o Iron preparations provide iron needed for RBC development and oxygen transport to cells. During times of increased growth (in growing children or during pregnancy) or when RBCs are in high demand (after blood loss), the need for iron may be greatly increased. Iron is poorly absorbed by the body, so clients must ingest relatively large amounts of oral iron to increase Hgb and Hct levels.

- Therapeutic Uses

  o Iron-deficiency anemia

  o Use iron sucrose and SFGC only for clients who are undergoing long-term hemodialysis and are deficient in iron.

  o Prevention of iron-deficiency anemia for clients who are at an increased risk, such as pregnant women, infants, and children.

  o Parenteral forms should only be used in clients who are unable to take oral medications. IV route is preferred.

Complications

SIDE/ADVERSE EFFECTS	NURSING INTERVENTIONS/CLIENT EDUCATION
GI distress (nausea, constipation, heartburn)	• If intolerable, administer medication with food, but this greatly reduces absorption. • May need to reduce dosage. • Monitor the client's bowel pattern and intervene as appropriate. Advise clients that these side effects usually resolve with continued use.
Teeth staining (liquid form)	• Teach clients to dilute liquid iron with water or juice, drink with a straw, and rinse mouth after swallowing.
Staining of skin and other tissues with IM injections	• Give IM doses deep IM using Z-track technique. • Avoid this route if possible.
Anaphylaxis risk with parenteral administration	• Monitor clients who are receiving IV iron preparations. • Be prepared with life-support equipment.
Hypotension, which may progress to circulatory collapse with parenteral administration	• Monitor vital signs when administering parenteral iron.
Fatal iron toxicity in children can occur when an overdose of iron (2 to 10 g) is ingested (severe GI symptoms, shock, acidosis, liver and heart failure).	• Use the chelating agent, deferoxamine (Desferal), to treat toxicity.

 Contraindications/Precautions

- Contraindicated for clients with:

  o Previous hypersensitivity to iron

  o Hemolytic anemia, peptic ulcer disease, and severe liver disease

Interactions

MEDICATION/FOOD INTERACTIONS	NURSING INTERVENTIONS/CLIENT EDUCATION
Coadministration of antacids or tetracyclines reduces absorption of iron.	• Advise clients to separate use by at least 2 hr.

Nursing Administration

- Instruct clients to take iron on an empty stomach such as 1 hr before meals to maximize absorption. Stomach acid increases absorption.

- Instruct clients to take with food if GI adverse effects occur. This may increase adherence to therapy even though absorption is also decreased.

- Instruct clients to space doses at approximately equal intervals throughout the day to most efficiently increase RBC production. Inform clients to anticipate a harmless dark green or black color of stool.

- Reinforce to clients to dilute liquid iron with water or juice, drink with a straw, and rinse the mouth after swallowing.

- Instruct clients to increase water and fiber intake (unless contraindicated), and to maintain an exercise program to counter the constipation effects.

- Advise clients that therapy may last 1 to 2 months. Usually, dietary intake will be sufficient after Hgb levels return to appropriate level.

- Encourage concurrent intake of appropriate quantities of foods high in iron (liver, egg yolks, muscle meats, yeast).

Nursing Evaluation of Medication Effectiveness

- Depending on therapeutic intent, effectiveness may be evidenced by the following:

  o Increase in reticulocyte count is expected by at least 1 week after beginning iron therapy.

  o Increase in Hgb of 2 g/dL is expected one month after beginning therapy (fatigue and pallor subside or client reports increased energy level, client's skin and mucous membrane color no longer demonstrate pallor).

MEDICATION CLASSIFICATION: VITAMIN B$_{12}$

- Select Prototype Medication: vitamin B$_{12}$ (Cyanocobalamin)

- Other Medications: intranasal cyanocobalamin (Nascobal)

Purpose

- Expected Pharmacological Action

  o Vitamin B_{12} is necessary to convert folic acid from its inactive form to its active form. All cells rely on folic acid for DNA production.

- Therapeutic Uses

  o Treatment or prevention of vitamin B_{12} deficiency

  o Megaloblastic (macrocytic) anemia related to vitamin B_{12} deficiency

Complications

SIDE/ADVERSE EFFECTS	NURSING INTERVENTIONS/CLIENT EDUCATION
Hypokalemia secondary to the increased RBC production effects of vitamin B_{12}	• Monitor the client's potassium levels during the start of treatment. • Observe clients for findings of potassium deficiency (muscle weakness, abnormal cardiac rhythm). • Administer potassium supplements if indicated.

Contraindications/Precautions

- Use cautiously for clients who have heart disease, anemia, and pulmonary disease.

Interactions

MEDICATION/FOOD INTERACTIONS	NURSING INTERVENTIONS/CLIENT EDUCATION
Masking of signs of vitamin B_{12} deficiency with concurrent administration of folic acid	• Make sure that clients receive adequate doses of vitamin B_{12} when using folic acid.

Nursing Administration

- Obtain baseline vitamin B_{12}, Hgb, Hct, RBC, and reticulocyte counts. Monitor periodically.

- Monitor clients for signs of vitamin B_{12} deficiency, such as a beefy red tongue, pallor, neuropathy, oral ulcerations, bleeding, infection, and CNS injury.

- Administer cyanocobalamin intranasally, orally, or by IM or SC injection.

- Administer intranasal or parenteral preparations to clients who have malabsorption syndrome.

- Instruct clients to administer intranasal cyanocobalamin 1 hr before or after eating hot foods, which can cause the medication to be removed from nasal passages without being absorbed.

- Tell clients who have irreversible malabsorption syndrome (parietal cell atrophy or total gastrectomy) that they will need lifelong treatment, monthly injections, or intranasal preparations daily or weekly.

  ○ Encourage concurrent intake of appropriate quantities of foods high in vitamin B_{12}, such as dairy products for clients without impaired absorption.

  ○ B_{12} levels should be monitored every 3 to 6 months.

Nursing Evaluation of Medication Effectiveness

- Depending on therapeutic intent, effectiveness may be evidenced by:

  ○ Improvement of megaloblastic anemia as evidenced by increased reticulocyte count, absence of megaloblast in bone marrow, macrocytes in blood, and normal or increased Hgb and Hct levels.

  ○ Improvement of neurologic symptoms, such as absence of tingling sensation of hands and feet and numbness of extremities. Improvement may take months, and some clients will never attain full recovery.

MEDICATION CLASSIFICATION: FOLIC ACID

- Select Prototype Medication: folic acid

Purpose

- Expected Pharmacological Action

  ○ Folic acid is essential in the production of DNA and erythropoiesis (RBC, WBC, and platelets).

- Therapeutic Uses

  - Treatment of megaloblastic (macrocytic) anemia secondary to folic acid deficiency

  - Prevention of neural tube defects during pregnancy; therefore, it is needed in all women of child-bearing age who may become pregnant

  - Treatment of malabsorption syndrome, such as sprue

Interactions

MEDICATION/FOOD INTERACTIONS	NURSING INTERVENTIONS/CLIENT EDUCATION
Decreased folate levels with concurrent use of sulfonamides, sulfasalazine, or methotrexate	• Avoid concurrent use of these medications.

 Contraindications/Precautions

- Indiscriminate use of folic acid is inappropriate because of the risk of masking signs of vitamin B_{12} deficiency.

Nursing Administration

- Observe clients for signs and symptoms of megaloblastic anemia (pallor, easy fatigability, palpitations, paresthesias of hands or feet).

- Obtain the client's baseline folic acid levels, RBC and reticulocyte counts, Hgb and Hct levels. Monitor periodically.

- Advise clients who have a folic acid deficiency to concurrently increase intake of food sources of folic acid, such as green, leafy vegetables and liver. Monitor clients for risk factors, such as heavy alcohol use and child-bearing age.

Nursing Evaluation of Medication Effectiveness

- Depending on therapeutic intent, effectiveness may be evidenced by:

    o Folate level 6 to 15 mcg/mL

    o Return of RBC, reticulocyte count, and Hgb and Hct to levels within expected reference range

    o Improvement of anemia findings, such as absence of pallor, dyspnea, easy fatigability

    o Absence of neural tube defects in newborns

MEDICATION CLASSIFICATION: POTASSIUM SUPPLEMENTS

- Select Prototype Medication: potassium chloride (K-Dur, Slow-K)

- Other Medications:

    o Potassium gluconate (Kaon)

Purpose

- Expected Pharmacological Action

    o Potassium is essential for conducting nerve impulses, maintaining electrical excitability of muscle, and regulation of acid/base balance.

- Therapeutic Uses

    o Hypokalemia – Potassium less than 3.5 mEq/L

    o Potassium supplements:

    - For clients receiving diuretics resulting in potassium loss, such as furosemide (Lasix)

    - For clients with potassium loss due to excessive or prolonged vomiting, diarrhea, abuse of laxatives, intestinal drainage, and gastrointestinal (GI) fistulas, excessive sweating

Complications

SIDE/ADVERSE EFFECTS	NURSING INTERVENTIONS/CLIENT EDUCATION
GI distress and local GI ulceration (nausea, vomiting, diarrhea, abdominal discomfort, and esophagitis with oral administration)	• Instruct clients to take the medication with meals or a full glass of water to minimize GI discomfort and prevent ulceration. • Reinforce to clients not to dissolve the tablet in the mouth because oral ulceration will develop.
Hyperkalemia (potassium > 5.0 mEq/L)	• Monitor clients receiving IV potassium for signs of hyperkalemia (bradycardia, hypotension, ECG changes).

 Contraindications/Precautions

- Contraindicated for clients who have severe renal disease, hypoaldosteronism

Interactions

MEDICATION/FOOD INTERACTIONS	NURSING INTERVENTIONS/CLIENT EDUCATION
Concurrent use of potassium-sparing diuretics, such as spironolactone, or ACE inhibitors, such as lisinopril, increases the risk of hyperkalemia.	• Avoid concurrent use.

Nursing Administration

- Oral formulations
  - Mix powdered formulations in at least 4 oz (120 mL) of liquid.
  - Advise clients to take potassium chloride with a glass of water or with a meal to reduce the risk of adverse GI effects.
  - Instruct clients not to crush extended-release tablets.
  - Instruct clients to notify the provider if they have difficulty swallowing the pills. The provider may prescribe powder or sustained-release tablets that are easier to tolerate.
- IV administration
  - Check the IV site for local irritation, phlebitis, and infiltration. Report findings to charge nurse.
  - Monitor the client's I&O to ensure an adequate urine output of at least 30 mL/hr.

Nursing Evaluation of Medication Effectiveness

- Depending on therapeutic intent, effectiveness may be evidenced by:
  - Serum potassium level within expected reference range: 3.5 to 5.0 mEq/L

MEDICATION CLASSIFICATION: MAGNESIUM SULFATE

- Select Prototype Medication:

    ○ Parenteral – Magnesium sulfate

    ○ Oral – Magnesium gluconate, magnesium hydroxide

Purpose

- Expected Pharmacological Action

    ○ Magnesium activates many intracellular enzymes and plays a role in regulating skeletal muscle contractility and blood coagulation.

- Therapeutic Uses

    ○ Hypomagnesemia – Magnesium level less than 1.3 mEq/L.

    ○ Use oral preparations to prevent low magnesium levels.

    ○ Use parenteral (IM, IV) magnesium for clients who have severe hypomagnesemia.

    ○ Use IV magnesium sulfate to stop preterm labor.

Complications

SIDE/ADVERSE EFFECTS	NURSING INTERVENTIONS/CLIENT EDUCATION
Neuromuscular blockade and respiratory depression	• Monitor cardiac and neuromuscular status of clients receiving IV administration. • Monitor the client's serum magnesium levels.
Diarrhea	• Monitor the client's serum magnesium levels for magnesium loss from diarrhea. • Monitor the client's I&O and observe for signs of dehydration.

 Contraindications/Precautions

- Magnesium is Pregnancy Risk Category B

- Use cautiously with clients who have AV block, rectal bleeding, nausea/vomiting, and abdominal pain.

- Use cautiously with clients who have renal and/or cardiac disease.

Interactions

- Magnesium sulfate can decrease the absorption of tetracyclines.

- Monitor the therapeutic effect to determine if absorption has been affected.

Nursing Administration

- Monitor serum magnesium, calcium, and phosphorus.

- Monitor the client's blood pressure, heart rate, and respiratory rate when given intravenously.

- Check clients for depressed or absent deep tendon reflexes as a sign of toxicity.

- Monitor clients receiving calcium gluconate for magnesium sulfate toxicity.

- Instruct clients about dietary sources of magnesium (whole grain cereals; nuts; legumes; green, leafy vegetables; bananas).

Nursing Evaluation of Medication Effectiveness

- Depending on therapeutic intent, effectiveness may be evidenced by:

  o Serum magnesium levels within expected reference range: 1.3 to 2.1 mEq/L

HERBAL SUPPLEMENTS

 Overview

- There is wide use of herbal supplements but these agents are not regulated in the same way as conventional medications. Because different formulations are not standardized, it can be difficult to know which preparations may provide therapeutic effects.

HERBAL SUBSTANCE	ACTION	USES
Aloe, aloe vera (Aloe gel and Aloe latex)	• Antimicrobial, anti-inflammatory, and analgesic actions when applied topically to skin • Cathartic properties when ingested (Aloe latex)	• Soothes pain and heals the inflammation of burns (Aloe gel) • Softens skin • Laxative (Aloe latex)
Black cohosh	• Acts on the female reproductive system as an estrogen substitute; mechanism of action unknown	• Management of symptoms of menopause
Echinacea	• Stimulates the immune system, decreases inflammation and can treat viruses through phagocytosis; increases T-lymphocyte, tumor necrosis factor, and interferon production	• Oral form: prevents and treats the common cold; however research has not proven this • Topical forms: treats multiple skin disorders, wounds, and burns

HERBAL SUBSTANCE	ACTION	USES
Feverfew	• Possibly works by blocking a factor necessary to cause migraine • Stops release of arachidonic acid in thrombocytes and blocks platelet aggregation	• Can decrease the number and severity of migraine headaches but has not been found useful in treating an existing migraine

Garlic	• Garlic cells contain an amino acid which, when crushed, forms the enzyme allicin. This enzyme, along with another substance in garlic, has the following actions:
	  ○ Blocks cholesterol synthesis in the liver.
	  ○ Suppresses platelet aggregation and disrupts coagulation.
	  ○ Acts as a vasodilator.
		• Lowers total cholesterol, LDL, and triglycerides and slightly increases HDL
		• Can decrease both systolic (20 to 30 mm Hg) and diastolic blood pressure (10 to 15 mm Hg)

Ginger root	• By an unknown mechanism, ginger root acts on areas of the CNS that cause nausea. • Increases intestinal motility and gastric mucus production • Decreases GI spasms • Inhibits prostaglandins and leukotrienes to produce anti-inflammatory effects • Suppresses platelet aggregation	• Decreases nausea from morning sickness, motion sickness, and surgery • Can decrease the pain and stiffness of rheumatoid arthritis
Ginkgo biloba	• Promotes vasodilation throughout the body • Suppresses a substance that can increase platelet aggregation and bronchospasm	• Increases recall ability and mental processes by increasing blood flow in the brain; given to those who have dementia, including Alzheimer's disease • Erectile dysfunction in those who take SSRIs that cause impotence • Decreases pain in clients who have occlusive arterial disorders of the legs • May decrease risk of thrombosis and bronchospasm

HERBAL SUBSTANCE	ACTION	USES
Goldenseal	• Suppresses inflammation and may stimulate the immune system; works as an antiseptic; has bactericidal properties • Increases bile secretion	• Treats and prevents a wide variety of infections, including bacterial, fungal, and protozoal • Decreases gall bladder inflammation
Kava (Kava Kava)	• Actual actions unknown, but possibly acts on GABA receptors in CNS	• Insomnia, anxiety, and promotes muscle relaxation without decreasing ability to concentrate
Ma Huang (Ephedra sinica)	• May activate all alpha and beta adrenergic receptors to constrict arterioles, increase heart rate, cause bronchodilation, and suppress appetite • Stimulates CNS	• Relieves manifestations of colds, influenza, and allergies • Weight loss • Increases athletic abilities
St. John's Wort	• Affects serotonin, NE, dopamine, and GABA uptake to produce antidepressant effects	• Mild depression
Saw Palmetto	• Action unknown, but may reduce conversion of testosterone into dihydrotestosterone (DHT) in prostate	• Decreases symptoms of BPH
Valerian	• Increases GABA to prevent insomnia • May work in similar way to benzodiazepines	• Promotes sleep, with increased effect over time

HERBAL SUBSTANCE	ADVERSE REACTIONS AND PRECAUTIONS	INTERACTIONS	NURSING ADMINISTRATION
Aloe, Aloe vera (Aloe gel, Aloe Latex)	• Skin preparations: possible hypersensitivity • Laxative: possible fluid and electrolyte imbalances	• None known	• Inform clients about manifestations of fluid and electrolyte imbalance if using as a laxative.
Black cohosh	• GI distress, lightheadedness, headache, rash, weight gain • Contraindicated during the first two trimesters of pregnancy • Do not use for longer than 6 months due to lack of information regarding long-term effects	• Increases effects of antihypertensive medications • May increase effect of estrogen medications • Risk of hypoglycemia in clients taking hypoglycemic agents	• Question clients who take antihypertensives, hypoglycemic agents, or who may be pregnant, about possible use of black cohosh.
Echinacea	• Bitter taste • Mild GI symptoms or fever can occur. • Allergic reactions, especially in clients who are allergic to plants, such as ragweed or others in the daisy family	• With chronic use (more than 6 months), echinacea can decrease positive effects of medications for tuberculosis, HIV, or cancer.	• Question clients who have tuberculosis, cancer, HIV, lupus erythematosus, and rheumatoid arthritis about concurrent use and advise these clients to talk to the provider.
Feverfew	• Mild GI symptoms • Postfeverfew syndrome can occur, causing agitation, tiredness, inability to sleep, headache, joint discomfort. • Can cause allergic reactions in clients allergic to ragweed or echinacea.	• Can cause increased risk of bleeding in clients taking NSAIDs, heparin, warfarin.	• Question clients about concurrent use of NSAIDs, heparin, and warfarin.

HERBAL SUBSTANCE	ADVERSE REACTIONS AND PRECAUTIONS	INTERACTIONS	NURSING ADMINISTRATION
Garlic	• GI symptoms	• Increased risk of bleeding in clients taking NSAIDs, warfarin, and heparin. • Risk of hypoglycemia in clients taking hypoglycemic agents. • Decreases levels of saquinavir (Fortovase), a medication for HIV treatment.	• Question clients about concurrent use of NSAIDs, heparin, and warfarin. • Have clients inform the provider about all medications currently taking.
Ginger root	• Use cautiously in pregnancy because high doses may cause uterine spasms. • Adverse effects unknown, with potential CNS and cardiac problems with very large overdose.	• Increased risk of bleeding in clients taking NSAIDS, warfarin, and heparin	• Question clients about concurrent use of NSAIDs, heparin, and warfarin.
Ginkgo biloba	• Mild GI upset, headache, lightheadedness, which may be decreased by reducing dose	• May interact with medications that lower the seizure threshold, such as antihistamines, antidepressants, and antipsychotics. • Can interfere with coagulation.	• Question clients regarding history of seizures or use of medications that lower seizure threshold. • Question clients about concurrent use of NSAIDs, heparin, and warfarin.

HERBAL SUBSTANCE	ADVERSE REACTIONS AND PRECAUTIONS	INTERACTIONS	NURSING ADMINISTRATION
Goldenseal	• None at therapeutic or low doses; can stimulate the CNS and cause death from respiratory failure in large doses • Contraindicated during pregnancy, because it can stimulate the uterus.	• None known	• Question clients who are pregnant.
Kava (kava kava)	• Chronic use causes dry, flaky skin and jaundice. • Chronic use and large doses can cause liver damage, including severe liver failure.	• Can cause sedation when taken concurrently with CNS depressants.	• Question clients taking any CNS depressant, including alcohol, about use of kava. • Ask clients who have any liver condition about concurrent use.
Ma huang (Ephedra sinica)	• Because it contains ephedrine, ma huang can stimulate the cardiovascular system and, at high doses, can cause death from hypertension and dysrhythmias. • Stimulation of CNS may cause euphoria and, in high doses, psychosis.	• Interacts with any CNS stimulant to potentiate their effect. • May cause severe hypertension when taken with MAOI antidepressants. • Interacts with antihypertensive medications to decrease effect.	• Question clients carefully about other medications. • Products which include more than 10 mg per dose are forbidden to be sold in the U.S.

HERBAL SUBSTANCE	ADVERSE REACTIONS AND PRECAUTIONS	INTERACTIONS	NURSING ADMINISTRATION
St. John's wort	• Mild adverse effects, including dry mouth, lightheadedness, constipation, GI symptoms • Skin rash when exposed to sunlight	• Can cause serotonin syndrome when combined with other antidepressants, amphetamine, and cocaine • Decreases effectiveness of oral contraceptives, cyclosporine, warfarin, digoxin, calcium channel blockers, steroids, HIV protease inhibitors, and some cancer chemotherapy medications	• Encourage clients using St. John's wort to prevent prolonged sun exposure and use sunscreen.
Saw palmetto	• Few adverse effects; can cause mild GI effects • Precaution: Can decrease PSA, the marker used to detect prostate cancer	• Possible additive effects with finasteride (Proscar)	• Question male clients about use before they have PSA tests.
Valerian	• Can cause drowsiness, lightheadedness, depression • Risk of physical dependence • Precaution: Clients who have mental health disorders should use with caution • Should be avoided by pregnant and lactating women	• Not known if valerian potentiates effects of CNS depressants	• Warn clients taking valerian about possibility of drowsiness when operating motor vehicles and other equipment.

APPLICATION EXERCISES

1. A client who has an Hgb of 9 g/dL was started on iron therapy with oral ferrous sulfate (Feosol). Following 1 month of therapy, what should the nurse expect the client's Hgb level to be?

2. A nurse is caring for a group of clients in a community setting. Which of the following clients should the nurse recognize may benefit from folic acid therapy? (Select all that apply.)

   _____ A 12-year-old child who has iron-deficiency anemia

   _____ A 24-year-old woman who has no health problems

   _____ A 44-year-old man who has essential hypertension

   _____ A 50-year-old woman who has chronic alcohol abuse

   _____ A 55-year-old man who has type 2 diabetes mellitus

3. A nurse is caring for a client who has been prescribed potassium chloride (K-Dur) for a serum potassium level of 3.0 mEq/L. The client also has a new prescription for lisinopril (Zestril) to treat hypertension. The nurse should monitor the client for which of the following findings?

   A. Lisinopril toxicity

   B. Hyperkalemia

   C. Weight gain

   D. Bradycardia

4. A nurse is reinforcing teaching to a client who has a vitamin B_{12} deficiency and a new prescription for intranasal cyanocobalamin (Nascobal) inserted into one nostril once a week. What instruction should the nurse give the client about the administration of the medication?

5. Match each herbal supplement below with an adverse reaction that can occur when taking the supplement:

   _____ Echinacea   A. Cardiac dysrhythmias

   _____ Valerian   B. Jaundice, liver damage

   _____ Kava Kava   C. Allergic reactions in clients allergic to ragweed

   _____ Ma Huang   D. Sedation, possible physical dependence

6. A nurse is collecting data from an older adult client who states she takes ginkgo biloba to help her memory. Which of the following from the client's health history is a contraindication to the use of ginkgo biloba?

   A. Peripheral arterial disease

   B. Migraine headaches

   C. Seizure disorder

   D. Osteoporosis

APPLICATION EXERCISES ANSWER KEY

1. A client who has an Hgb of 9 g/dL was started on iron therapy with oral ferrous sulfate (Feosol). Following 1 month of therapy, what should the nurse expect the client's Hgb level to be?

   The nurse should expect the Hgb to rise by 2 g/dL during the first month of therapy. After 1 month, the client's Hgb should be 11 g/dL.

 NCLEX® Connection: Pharmacological Therapies, Expected Actions/Outcomes

2. A nurse is caring for a group of clients in a community setting. Which of the following clients should the nurse recognize may benefit from folic acid therapy? (Select all that apply.)

_____	A 12-year-old child who has iron-deficiency anemia
__X__	**A 24-year-old woman who has no health problems**
_____	A 44-year-old man who has essential hypertension
__X__	**A 50-year-old woman who has chronic alcohol abuse**
_____	A 55-year-old man who has type 2 diabetes mellitus

   Women of child-bearing age who may become pregnant benefit from supplemental folic acid (400 mcg/day) to prevent neural tube defects in a developing fetus. Alcoholism is a frequent cause of deficient folic acid in the body; therefore, the client who has chronic alcohol abuse is likely to benefit from folic acid therapy. Iron-deficiency anemia, hypertension, and diabetes mellitus are not treated with folic acid therapy.

 NCLEX® Connection: Pharmacological Therapies, Expected Actions/Outcomes

3. A nurse is caring for a client who has been prescribed potassium chloride (K-Dur) for a serum potassium level of 3.0 mEq/L. The client also has a new prescription for lisinopril (Zestril) to treat hypertension. The nurse should monitor the client for which of the following findings?

   A. Lisinopril toxicity

   B. Hyperkalemia

   C. Weight gain

   D. Bradycardia

   The nurse should monitor the client for hyperkalemia. ACE inhibitors, such as lisinopril, can increase potassium levels. If the client is concurrently taking a potassium supplement, the risk for hyperkalemia is even higher. The client is not at risk for lisinopril toxicity when taking both medications concurrently. Weight gain and bradycardia are not expected findings for a client taking lisinopril or potassium supplements.

 NCLEX® Connection: Pharmacological Therapies, Adverse Effects/Contraindications/Side Effects/Interactions

4. A nurse is reinforcing teaching to a client who has a vitamin B_{12} deficiency and a new prescription for intranasal cyanocobalamin (Nascobal) inserted into one nostril once a week. What instruction should the nurse give the client about the administration of the medication?

   Reinforce to the client not to administer intranasal cyanocobalamin within 1 hr after eating hot foods or liquids. This can increase nasal secretions and thus decrease the amount of medication absorbed.

 NCLEX® Connection: Pharmacological Therapies, Medication Administration

5. Match each herbal supplement below with an adverse reaction that can occur when taking the supplement:

C	Echinacea	A. Cardiac dysrhythmias
D	Valerian	B. Jaundice, liver damage
B	Kava Kava	C. Allergic reactions in clients allergic to ragweed
A	Ma Huang	D. Sedation, possible physical dependence

 NCLEX® Connection: Pharmacological Therapies, Adverse Effects/Contraindications/Side Effects/Interactions

6. A nurse is collecting data from an older adult client who states she takes ginkgo biloba to help her memory. Which of the following from the client's health history is a contraindication to the use of ginkgo biloba?

   A. Peripheral arterial disease

   B. Migraine headaches

   C. Seizure disorder

   D. Osteoporosis

   Ginkgo biloba can cause seizures, particularly in clients who may have a lower seizure threshold due to medications, such as decongestants, antihistamines, and some medications for depression or psychosis. Clients who have a history of seizures should not take ginkgo biloba. Pain from peripheral arterial disease may be helped by taking ginkgo biloba. Migraine headaches and hypertension are not affected by ginkgo biloba.

 NCLEX® Connection: Pharmacological Therapies, Adverse Effects/Contraindications/Side Effects/Interactions

UNIT 7: MEDICATIONS AFFECTING THE REPRODUCTIVE SYSTEM

- Medications Affecting the Reproductive Tract

NCLEX® CONNECTIONS

When reviewing the chapters in this section, keep in mind the relevant sections of the NCLEX® outline, in particular:

CLIENT NEEDS: PHARMACOLOGICAL THERAPIES

Relevant topics/tasks include:
- Adverse Effects/Contraindications/Side Effects/Interactions
  - Monitor and document client response to management of medication side effects including prescribed, over-the-counter, and herbal supplements.
- Expected Actions/Outcomes
  - Reinforce client teaching on actions and therapeutic effects of medications and pharmacological interactions.
- Medication Administration
  - Reinforce client teaching on client self-administration of medications.

UNIT 7	MEDICATIONS AFFECTING THE REPRODUCTIVE SYSTEM
Chapter 29	Medications Affecting the Reproductive Tract

 Overview

- Medications that affect the reproductive system include hormones that stimulate puberty, such as estrogen and progesterone in females and testosterone in males. Hormonal deficiency (male or female) or prevention of pregnancy in women (oral contraceptives) are other uses for hormones.

- Medications to treat benign prostatic hyperplasia (BPH) include 5-alpha reductase inhibitors and alpha$_1$-adrenergic antagonists. Medications to treat erectile dysfunction include the phosphodiesterase type 5 (PDE5) inhibitors.

MEDICATION CLASSIFICATION: ESTROGENS

- Select Prototype Medications: conjugated equine estrogens (Premarin)

- Other Medications: estradiol (Estrace), estradiol hemihydrate (Vagifem)

Purpose

- Expected Pharmacological Action

  o Estrogens are hormones needed for growth and maturation of the female reproductive tract and secondary sex characteristics. Estrogens block bone resorption and reduce low-density lipoprotein (LDL) levels. At high levels, estrogens suppress the release of a follicle-stimulating hormone (FSH) needed for conception.

- Therapeutic Uses

  o Contraception

  o Hormone replacement therapy (HRT) – replacement of estrogen to control symptoms (mood changes, hot flashes)

  o Prevention of postmenopausal osteoporosis

  o Treatment of dysfunctional uterine bleeding

  o Treatment of prostate cancer

  o Female hypogonadism (Turner's Syndrome)

- Route of administration: oral, transdermal, and intravaginal

Complications

SIDE/ADVERSE EFFECTS	NURSING INTERVENTIONS/CLIENT EDUCATION
Endometrial and ovarian cancers when prolonged estrogen is the only postmenopausal therapy	• Instruct clients to report persistent vaginal bleeding. • Advise clients to have a yearly pelvic exam.
Potential risk for estrogen-dependent breast cancer in postmenopausal women	• Rule out estrogen-dependent breast cancer prior to starting therapy. • Encourage regular self-breast examinations and mammograms.
Embolic events (MI, pulmonary embolism, DVT, cerebrovascular accident)	• Encourage clients to avoid all nicotine products. • Monitor clients for pain, swelling, warmth, or erythema of lower legs.

Ⓢ Contraindications/Precautions

- These medications are Pregnancy Risk Category X.

- These medications are contraindicated for clients who have:

  o Client or family history of heart disease

  o Abnormal vaginal bleeding that is undiagnosed

  o Breast or estrogen-dependent cancer

  o History or risk of thromboembolic disease

- Use cautiously during breastfeeding because estrogens decrease quantity and quality of milk and may be excreted in breast milk.

- Use cautiously in prepubescent girls. If administered, monitor bone growth, and check periodically for early epiphyseal plate closure.

Interactions

MEDICATION/FOOD INTERACTIONS	NURSING INTERVENTIONS/CLIENT EDUCATION
Estrogens can reduce the effectiveness of warfarin (Coumadin).	• If used concurrently, monitor client PT and INR. • Warfarin doses may need to be adjusted.
Concurrent use of phenytoin (Dilantin) can increase the risk of phenytoin toxicity.	• Monitor clients for signs of phenytoin toxicity (nystagmus, sedation, ataxia, cognitive impairment, diplopia).
Corticosteroids can increase effects of estrogen.	• Monitor for increased estrogen effects.

MEDICATION/FOOD INTERACTIONS	NURSING INTERVENTIONS/CLIENT EDUCATION
Estrogen may alter effects of tamoxifen.	• Do not use together.
Smoking increases risk for thrombophlebitis.	• Advise clients not to smoke.

Nursing Administration

- Inform clients who have had a hysterectomy that they will only receive estrogen for HRT.

- Instruct clients to take the medication at the same time each day (at bedtime).

- Instruct clients to apply estrogen patches to the skin of the trunk.

- Inject IM forms deep in a large muscle mass. Rotate injection sites.

- Instruct clients to report dysmenorrhea, amenorrhea, breakthrough bleeding, and/or breast changes.

- Encourage clients to perform monthly breast self-examinations and schedule annual gynecologic and breast examinations with the provider.

- Advise clients to notify the provider of any swelling or redness in legs, shortness of breath, or chest pain.

- Discontinue prior to knee or hip surgery or any surgical procedures that may cause extensive immobilization.

Nursing Evaluation of Medication Effectiveness

- Depending on therapeutic intent, effectiveness may be evidenced by:

  o No evidence of conception

  o Relief of postmenopausal symptoms (hot flashes, mood changes)

  o No evidence of postmenopausal osteoporosis

  o Reduction in dysfunctional uterine bleeding and endometriosis

  o Decrease in spread of prostate cancer

MEDICATION CLASSIFICATION: PROGESTINS

- Select Prototype Medications: medroxyprogesterone acetate (Provera)

- Other Medications: norethindrone (Micronor), megestrol acetate (Megace)

Purpose

- Expected Pharmacological Action

  o Progesterone replacement

- Therapeutic Uses

  o Combine with estrogen during HRT to prevent estrogen stimulation of the endometrium, which can lead to endometrial hyperplasia and cancer.

  o Dysfunctional uterine bleeding due to hormonal imbalance

  o Amenorrhea due to hormonal imbalance

  o Endometriosis

- Routes of administration: oral, IM, subcutaneous, transdermal, and intravaginal

Complications

SIDE/ADVERSE EFFECTS	NURSING INTERVENTIONS/CLIENT EDUCATION
Breast cancer	• Encourage regular self-breast examinations and mammograms.
Thromboembolic events (MI, pulmonary embolism, thrombophlebitis, cerebrovascular accident)	• Discourage clients from smoking. • Monitor clients for pain, swelling, warmth, or erythema of lower legs. • Advise client to notify the provider of chest pain or shortness of breath.
Breakthrough bleeding, amenorrhea, and breast tenderness	• Instruct clients to report abnormal vaginal bleeding.
Edema	• Monitor the client's blood pressure, I&O, and weight gain.
Jaundice (yellow skin and sclera)	• Monitor liver enzymes.
Migraine headaches	• Notify the provider of severe headache.

 Contraindications/Precautions

- This medication is Pregnancy Risk Category X.

- This medication is contraindicated in clients who have:

  o Undiagnosed vaginal bleeding

  o History of thromboembolic disease, cardiovascular, or cerebrovascular disease

  o History of breast cancer

- Use cautiously in clients who have diabetes, seizures disorders, and migraine headaches.

Interactions

MEDICATION/FOOD INTERACTIONS	NURSING INTERVENTIONS/CLIENT EDUCATION
Use of carbamazepine (Tegretol), phenobarbital (Luminal), phenytoin (Dilantin), and rifampin (Rifadin) can decrease contraceptive effectiveness.	• Advise clients to use alternative contraceptives during concurrent use of these medications.
Bromocriptine (Parlodel) can cause amenorrhea.	• Do not use together.
Smoking increases risk for thrombophlebitis.	• Advise clients not to smoke.

Nursing Administration

- Inform clients who have not had a hysterectomy that they will receive estrogen and progestin for HRT.

- Instruct clients to anticipate withdrawal bleeding 3 to 7 days after stopping the medication.

- Instruct clients to stop taking the medication immediately if pregnancy is suspected. Instruct clients to delay conception for 3 months following use.

Nursing Evaluation of Medication Effectiveness

- Depending on therapeutic intent, effectiveness may be evidenced by:

  o Restoration of hormonal balance with control of uterine bleeding (regular menstrual periods)

  o Restoration of menses

  o Decrease in endometrial hyperplasia in postmenopausal women receiving concurrent estrogen

  o Control of the spread of endometrial cancer

MEDICATION CLASSIFICATION: HORMONAL CONTRACEPTIVES

- Select Prototype Medications:

  o Combination oral contraceptives: ethinyl estradiol and norethindrone (Ovcon 35, Necon 1/35)

- Other Medications:

  o Transdermal patch: ethinyl estradiol and norelgestromin (Ortho Evra)

  o Vaginal contraceptive ring: ethinyl estradiol and etonogestrel (NuvaRing)

  o Parenteral: depot medroxyprogesterone acetate (DMPA) available as Depo-Provera for IM use and Depo-subQ for subcutaneous use

Purpose

- Expected Pharmacological Action

  o Oral contraceptives stop conception by preventing ovulation. They also thicken the cervical mucus and alter the endometrial lining to reduce the chance of fertilization.

- Therapeutic Uses

  o Pregnancy prevention

- Route of Administration

  o Oral, transdermal, intravaginal, IM, subcutaneous, and subdermal

Complications

SIDE/ADVERSE EFFECTS	NURSING INTERVENTIONS/CLIENT EDUCATION
Thromboembolic events (MI, pulmonary embolism, thrombophlebitis, cerebrovascular accident)	• Discourage clients from smoking. • Instruct clients to report warmth, edema, tenderness, and/or pain in lower legs.
Hypertension	• Monitor the client's blood pressure and report findings.
Breakthrough or abnormal uterine bleeding	• Instruct clients to record duration and frequency of breakthrough bleeding. • Evaluate clients for the possibility of pregnancy if two or more menstrual periods are missed.
Breast cancer	• Oral contraceptives can increase growth of a pre-existing breast cancer. Do not give to women who have breast cancer.

 Contraindications/Precautions

- These medications are Pregnancy Risk Category X.

- These medications are contraindicated for clients who have:

  o Client history of thrombophlebitis and cardiovascular events

  o Family history or risk factors for breast cancer

- Use cautiously in clients who are obese, who are greater than 35 years of age and smoke, and who have diabetes mellitus and hypercholesterolemia.

Interactions

MEDICATION/FOOD INTERACTIONS	NURSING INTERVENTIONS/CLIENT EDUCATION
Oral contraceptive effectiveness decreases with use of carbamazepine (Tegretol), phenobarbital (Luminal), phenytoin (Dilantin), and rifampin (Rifadin).	• Advise clients to use alternative contraceptives during concurrent use of these medications.
Oral contraceptives decrease the effects of warfarin (Coumadin) and oral hypoglycemics.	• Monitor the client's PT and INR levels and adjust warfarin dosages accordingly.

Nursing Administration

- Check for pregnancy prior to start of therapy.

- Instruct clients to take pills at the same time each day.

- Instruct clients to take medication for 21 days followed by 7 days of no medication (or inert pill). Begin the sequence on the fifth day after the onset of menses.

- For one missed dose, instruct clients to take two together at the next scheduled dose. For two missed doses, instruct the client to double up for 2 days. For three missed doses, because of an increased risk of ovulation and resulting pregnancy, instruct clients to use an additional form of birth control and to start a new cycle of medications after waiting 7 days.

- Encourage clients who smoke to quit.

- Advise client to report swelling or redness in legs, shortness of breath, or a severe headache.

Nursing Evaluation of Medication Effectiveness

- Depending on therapeutic intent, effectiveness may be evidenced by:

  o No evidence of conception

MEDICATION CLASSIFICATION: ANDROGENS

- Select Prototype Medications: testosterone (Andronaq-50, Testred)

- Other Medications: testolactone (Teslac), testosterone pellets (Testopel)

Purpose

- Expected Pharmacological Action

  o Development of sex traits in men and the production and maturation of sperm

  o Increase in skeletal muscle

  o Increase in synthesis of erythropoietin

- Therapeutic Uses

    o Hypogonadism in males

    o Delayed puberty in boys

    o Androgen replacement in testicular failure

    o Post menopausal breast cancer

- Route of administration: IM, transdermal, implantable pellets, buccal tablets

Complications

SIDE/ADVERSE EFFECTS	NURSING INTERVENTIONS/CLIENT EDUCATION
Androgenic effects: - In females these medications can cause irregularity or cessation of menses, hirsutism, weight gain, acne, lowering of voice, growth of clitoris, vaginitis, and baldness. - In males these medications can cause acne, priapism, increased facial and body hair, and penile enlargement.	- Advise clients of possible medication effects. - Advise women to report occurrence of these effects. - Tell clients the provider may discontinue the medication to prevent permanent changes.
Premature epiphyseal closure – Can reduce mature height in males.	- Monitor epiphysis with serial x-rays every 6 months.
Cholestatic hepatitis, jaundice	- Monitor for signs of jaundice. - Monitor liver enzymes.
Hypercholesterolemia – These medications can decrease high-density lipoproteins (HDL) and increase low-density lipoproteins (LDL).	- Monitor cholesterol levels. - Advise clients to adjust diet to reduce cholesterol levels.
Increase in growth of prostate cancer.	- Do not give to clients with prostate cancer. - Monitor for prostate cancer.
Edema from salt and water retention	- Instruct clients to monitor for weight gain and swelling of extremities and report to the provider. - Tell clients the provider may discontinue the medication or prescribe a diuretic.
High abuse potential	- Identify high-risk groups and educate regarding abuse potential and potential health risks.

Contraindications/Precautions

- These medications are Pregnancy Risk Category X.

- Androgens are contraindicated in men who have prostate or breast cancer, clients who have hypercalcemia, and older adult clients.

- Use cautiously in clients who have heart failure, hypertension, or renal or liver disease.

Interactions

MEDICATION/FOOD INTERACTIONS	NURSING INTERVENTIONS/CLIENT EDUCATION
Androgens can alter effects of oral anticoagulants.	• Monitor PT and INR.
Androgens can alter effects of hypoglycemic agents.	• Monitor blood glucose level and adjust dosages.
Concurrent use of androgens and hepatotoxic medications can increase risk for hepatotoxicity.	• Monitor liver enzymes. Check for jaundice.

Nursing Administration

- Inject into a large muscle and rotate injection sites.

- Monitor women for signs of masculinization (facial hair, baldness, deepened voice, acne).

- Advise clients to use a barrier method of birth control.

- Advise clients to reduce cholesterol in the diet.

- Advise clients at risk about abuse potential.

Nursing Evaluation of Medication Effectiveness

- Depending on therapeutic intent, effectiveness may be evidenced by the following:

  o Boys will experience puberty; men will have increased testosterone levels.

  o Women will experience a decrease in the progression of breast cancer in women.

MEDICATION CLASSIFICATION: 5-ALPHA REDUCTASE INHIBITORS

- Select Prototype Medications: finasteride (Proscar)

- Other Medications: dutasteride (Avodart)

Purpose

- Expected Pharmacological Action

  o Decreases usable testosterone and causes a reduction of the prostate size and increases hair growth.

- Therapeutic Uses

  o BPH

  o Male pattern baldness

- Route of administration: oral

Complications

SIDE/ADVERSE EFFECTS	NURSING INTERVENTIONS/CLIENT EDUCATION
Decreased libido, ejaculate amount	• Advise clients to notify the provider if adverse reactions occur.
Gynecomastia	• Advise clients to notify the provider if adverse reactions occur.

 Contraindications/Precautions

- These medications are Pregnancy Risk Category X.

- These medications are contraindicated in clients who have medication hypersensitivity.

- Use with caution in clients who have liver disease.

Interactions

- None significant

Nursing Administration

- Advise clients that therapeutic effects may take up to 6 months.

 - Advise pregnant women not to handle crushed or broken medication.

- Advise clients not to donate blood unless medication has been discontinued for at least 1 month.

Nursing Evaluation of Medication Effectiveness

- Depending on therapeutic intent, effectiveness may be evidenced by the following:

  o Prostate size is decreased and client is able to urinate effectively.

  o Prostate-specific antigen (PSA) levels have decreased from baseline.

  o Increased hair growth.

MEDICATION CLASSIFICATION: ALPHA₁-ADRENERGIC ANTAGONISTS

- Select Prototype Medication:

  - Selective alpha$_1$ receptor antagonist: tamsulosin (Flomax)

- Other Medications:

  - Selective alpha$_1$ receptor antagonist: silodosin (Rapaflo)

  - Nonselective alpha$_1$ receptor antagonists:

    - Alfuzosin (Uroxatral)

    - Terazosin (Hytrin)

    - Doxazosin (Cardura)

Purpose

- Expected Pharmacological Action

  - These agents decrease mechanical obstruction of the urethra by relaxing smooth muscles of the bladder neck and prostate.

  - Nonselective agents also affect blood vessels, resulting in lowered blood pressure. Use these agents for clients who have BPH and hypertension.

- Therapeutic Uses

  - Benign prostatic hyperplasia (BPH)

- Route of administration: oral

Complications

SIDE/ADVERSE EFFECTS	NURSING INTERVENTIONS/CLIENT EDUCATION
Hypotension, dizziness, nasal congestion, sleepiness, faintness (more likely with nonselective antagonists)	• Monitor blood pressure. • Advise clients to rise slowly from a sitting or lying position. • Advise clients not to drive or operate machinery when starting therapy or with change in dose until response is known.
Problems with ejaculation (failure, decreased volume)	• Advise clients of possible adverse effects.

 Contraindications/Precautions

- These agents are contraindicated in clients who have medication sensitivity.

- Do not combine these agents with antihypertensive medications.

- Use silodosin cautiously in clients who have renal impairment.

Interactions

MEDICATION/FOOD INTERACTIONS	NURSING INTERVENTIONS/CLIENT EDUCATION
Cimetidine (Tagamet) can decrease clearance of tamsulosin.	• Use together with caution.
Concurrent use of antihypertensives, PDE5 inhibitors, and nitroglycerin with nonselective agents can cause severe hypotension.	• Use with caution. Monitor blood pressure.
Concurrent use of erythromycin and HIV protease inhibitors (Ritonavir [Norvir]) will increase levels of alfuzosin and silodosin.	• Avoid concurrent use.

Nursing Administration

- Monitor blood pressure, especially at the start of therapy and with changes of dose.

- Advise clients to take medication daily as prescribed:

   o Tamsulosin – Take 30 min after a meal at the same time each day

   o Silodosin – Take with same meal each day

   o Alfuzosin – Take right after the same meal each day

   o Terazosin – Take at bedtime

   o Doxazosin – Take at same time each day

Nursing Evaluation of Medication Effectiveness

- Depending on therapeutic intent, effectiveness may be evidenced by:

   o Improved urinary flow with minimal adverse effects.

MEDICATION CLASSIFICATION: PHOSPHODIESTERASE TYPE 5 (PDE5) INHIBITORS

- Select Prototype Medications: sildenafil (Viagra)

- Other Medications: tadalafil (Cialis), vardenafil (Levitra)

Purpose

- Expected Pharmacological Action

   o Augments the effects of nitric oxide released during sexual stimulation, resulting in enhanced blood flow to the corpus cavernosum and penile erection.

- Therapeutic Uses

   o Erectile dysfunction

Complications

SIDE/ADVERSE EFFECTS	NURSING INTERVENTIONS/CLIENT EDUCATION
Priapism	• Instruct clients to notify the provider if erection lasts more than 4 hr.
Headache, flushing, dyspepsia	• Instruct clients to notify the provider who may discontinue the medication.

 ### Contraindications/Precautions

- These medications are contraindicated in clients taking any medications in the nitrate family, such as nitroglycerin.

- Use cautiously in clients who have cardiovascular disease (history within the last 6 months of myocardial infarction or cerebrovascular accident, resting hypotension or hypertension, heart failure, unstable angina).

Interactions

MEDICATION/FOOD INTERACTIONS	NURSING INTERVENTIONS/CLIENT EDUCATION
Organic nitrates, such as nitroglycerin (Nitrostat) and isosorbide dinitrate (Isordil), can lead to fatal hypotension.	• Avoid concurrent use.
Ketoconazole (Nizoral), erythromycin (E-Mycin), cimetidine, ritonavir, and grapefruit juice inhibit metabolism of sildenafil thereby, increasing plasma levels of medication.	• Use these cautiously in clients taking sildenafil.

Nursing Administration

- Administer by oral route.

- Instruct clients to take approximately 1 hr before sexual activity and to limit use to once a day.

Nursing Evaluation of Medication Effectiveness

- Depending on therapeutic intent, effectiveness may be evidenced by:

  o Erection sufficient for sexual intercourse

APPLICATION EXERCISES

1. A nurse is reinforcing teaching for a female client who is beginning a prescription of conjugated estrogens (Premarin) for symptoms of menopause. For which of the following should the nurse plan to monitor the client?

   A. Lower leg pain and swelling

   B. Shortened stature

   C. Vulvar and vaginal atrophy

   D. Weight loss

2. A nurse is reinforcing teaching for a client who is about to begin a prescription for an oral contraceptive. The nurse should tell the client that oral contraceptives work by doing which of the following? (Select all that apply.)

   _____ Thickening the cervical mucus to slow sperm passage

   _____ Inducing maturation of ovarian follicle

   _____ Increasing the development of the corpus luteum

   _____ Altering the endometrial lining to prevent implantation

   _____ Inhibiting ovulation

3. A nurse is caring for a male client who has a new prescription for testosterone cypionate (Depo-Testosterone) IM every 2 to 4 weeks for hypogonadism. The nurse should plan to monitor which of the following laboratory values?

   A. Serum creatinine

   B. Cholesterol levels

   C. BUN

   D. Serum potassium

4. A nurse is reinforcing teaching for a client who takes sildenafil (Viagra) several times weekly and has a new prescription for oral erythromycin (E-Mycin) to treat a respiratory tract infection. The nurse should instruct the client about an increased risk for which of the following findings due to an interaction between the two medications?

   A. Priapism

   B. Urinary frequency

   C. Weight gain

   D. Insomnia

5. A nurse is caring for a client who has a prescription for dutasteride (Avodart). Which of the following findings is an expected outcome for a client taking this medication?

   A. Increased blood pressure

   B. Increased testosterone levels

   C. Decreased prostate specific antigen (PSA)

   D. Decreased erectile dysfunction

APPLICATION EXERCISES ANSWER KEY

1. A nurse is reinforcing teaching for a female client who is beginning a prescription of conjugated estrogens (Premarin) for symptoms of menopause. For which of the following should the nurse plan to monitor the client?

    A. Lower leg pain and swelling

    B. Shortened stature

    C. Vulvar and vaginal atrophy

    D. Weight loss

    The client who takes estrogen is at an increased risk for cardiovascular events, including thrombophlebitis. The nurse should monitor the client for pain, swelling, and redness in the lower legs. Shortened stature may occur in a client who has osteoporosis, but estrogen therapy can help prevent the problem. Estrogen therapy can help prevent vulvar and vaginal atrophy in postmenopausal women. Weight loss is not an expected effect caused by estrogen therapy.

     NCLEX® Connection: Pharmacological Therapies, Adverse Effects/Contraindications/Side Effects/Interactions

2. A nurse is reinforcing teaching for a client who is about to begin a prescription for an oral contraceptive. The nurse should tell the client that oral contraceptives work by doing which of the following? (Select all that apply.)

    __X__   **Thickening the cervical mucus to slow sperm passage**

    _____   Inducing maturation of ovarian follicle

    _____   Increasing the development of the corpus luteum

    __X__   **Altering the endometrial lining to prevent implantation**

    __X__   **Inhibiting ovulation**

    Oral contraceptives thicken the cervical mucus (which causes a barrier to sperm), alter the endometrial lining to reduce the chance of fertilization, and stop conception by preventing ovulation. They do not induce maturation of ovarian follicles or increase the development of the corpus luteum.

     NCLEX® Connection: Pharmacological Therapies, Expected Actions/Outcomes

3. A nurse is caring for a male client with a new prescription for testosterone cypionate (Depo-Testosterone) IM every 2 to 4 weeks for hypogonadism. The nurse should plan to monitor which of the following laboratory values?

    A. Serum creatinine

    B. Cholesterol levels

    C. BUN

    D. Serum potassium

Androgens, such as testosterone cypionate, can elevate LDL levels and lower HDL levels, increasing the client's risk for atherosclerosis. Therefore, the nurse should plan to monitor cholesterol levels. It is not necessary to monitor serum creatinine, BUN, and serum potassium for the client taking androgens.

 NCLEX® Connection: Pharmacological Therapies, Adverse Effects/Contraindications/Side Effects/Interactions

4. A nurse is reinforcing teaching for a client who takes sildenafil (Viagra) several times weekly and has a new prescription for oral erythromycin (E-Mycin) to treat a respiratory tract infection. The nurse should instruct the client about an increased risk for which of the following findings due to an interaction between the two medications?

    A. Priapism

    B. Urinary frequency

    C. Weight gain

    D. Insomnia

Erythromycin, a strong inhibitor of CYP3A4, can greatly increase blood levels of sildenafil, increasing the client's risk for adverse effects, such as priapism. The medications do not interact to increase risk for infection, weight gain, or insomnia.

 NCLEX® Connection: Pharmacological Therapies, Adverse Effects/Contraindications/Side Effects/Interactions

5. A nurse is caring for a client who has a prescription for dutasteride (Avodart). Which of the following findings is an expected outcome for a client taking this medication?

    A. Increased blood pressure

    B. Increased testosterone levels

    C. Decreased prostate specific antigen (PSA)

    D. Decreased erectile dysfunction

Dutasteride is a 5-alpha reductase inhibitor, which is used to treat BPH (benign prostatic hypertrophy). Expected outcomes include a decrease in prostate size, decrease in PSA levels, and increased ability to urinate. The medication does not cause an increase in blood pressure or testosterone levels. Dutasteride can cause a decreased libido and does not decrease erectile dysfunction.

 NCLEX® Connection: Pharmacological Therapies, Expected Actions/Outcomes

UNIT 8: MEDICATIONS FOR JOINT AND BONE CONDITIONS

- Rheumatoid Arthritis

- Bone Disorders

NCLEX® CONNECTIONS

When reviewing the chapters in this section, keep in mind the relevant sections of the NCLEX® outline, in particular:

CLIENT NEEDS: PHARMACOLOGICAL THERAPIES

Relevant topics/tasks include:
- Adverse Effects/Contraindications/Side Effects/Interactions
  - Withhold medication dose if client experiences adverse effect to medication.
- Expected Actions/Outcomes
  - Reinforce education to client regarding medications.
- Pharmacological Pain Management
  - Identify client need for pain medication.

UNIT 8	MEDICATIONS FOR JOINT AND BONE CONDITIONS
Chapter 30	Rheumatoid Arthritis

 Overview

- Rheumatoid arthritis (RA) is a chronic disorder with autoimmune and inflammatory components. Pharmacological management provides symptomatic relief and some delay in progression of the disorder without resulting in cure. Use of disease-modifying antirheumatic drugs (DMARDs), glucocorticoids, and nonsteroidal anti-inflammatory drugs (NSAIDs) may be taken individually or in combination to manage this chronic disorder.

- The American College of Rheumatology (ACR) provides recommendations for management of rheumatoid arthritis. These guidelines can be found at http://www.rheumatology.org/

- Categories of medications in this section include disease-modifying antirheumatic drugs (DMARDs), glucocorticoids, immunosuppressants, and NSAIDs.

MEDICATION CLASSIFICATION: DISEASE-MODIFYING ANTIRHEUMATIC DRUGS (DMARDs)

- DMARDs I – Major Nonbiologic DMARDs

  - Cytotoxic medications: methotrexate (Rheumatrex), leflunomide (Arava)

  - Antimalarial agents: hydroxychloroquine (Plaquenil)

  - Antiinflammatory medication: sulfasalazine (Azulfidine)

  - Tetracycline antibiotic: minocycline (Minocin)

- DMARDs II – Major Biologic DMARDs

  - Etanercept (Enbrel)

  - Infliximab (Remicade)

  - Adalimumab (Humira)

  - Rituximab (Rituxan)

  - Abatacept (Orencia)

- DMARDs III – Minor Nonbiologic and Biologic DMARDs

  - Gold salts: aurothioglucose (Solganal)

  - Penicillamine (Cuprimine, Depen)

  - Cytotoxic medications: azathioprine (Imuran), cyclosporine (Sandimmune, Gengraf, Neoral)

- Glucocorticoids
  - Prednisone (Deltasone), prednisolone (Prelone)
- NSAIDs
  - Aspirin
  - Ibuprofen
  - Diclofenac (Voltaren)
  - Indomethacin (Indocin)
  - Meloxicam (Mobic)
  - Naproxen (Naprosyn)
  - Celecoxib (Celebrex)

Purpose

- Expected Pharmacological Action
  - DMARDs slow joint degeneration and progression of rheumatoid arthritis.
  - Glucocorticoids provide symptomatic relief of inflammation and pain.
  - NSAIDs provide rapid, symptomatic relief of inflammation and pain.
- Therapeutic Uses
  - Analgesia for pain, swelling, and joint stiffness
  - Maintenance of joint function
  - Slow/delay the worsening of the disease (DMARDs, glucocorticoids)
  - Short-term therapy until long-acting DMARDs take effect (NSAIDs, glucocorticoids)
  - Prevention of organ rejection in clients who have had an organ transplant (cytotoxic agents, glucocorticoids, immunosuppressants)
  - Management of inflammatory bowel disease (glucocorticoids, immunosuppressants, DMARDs)

Complications

SIDE/ADVERSE EFFECTS	NURSING INTERVENTIONS/CLIENT EDUCATION
Cytotoxic agents: methotrexate	
Increased risk of infection (fever and/or sore throat)	• Advise clients to notify the provider immediately if symptoms occur.
Hepatic fibrosis (anorexia, abdominal fullness, jaundice)	• Monitor liver function test. • Advise clients to notify the provider if symptoms occur.
Bone marrow suppression	• Obtain the client's baseline CBC and platelet counts. Repeat every 3 to 6 months.
Gastrointestinal (GI) ulceration (coffee-ground emesis or black, tarry stools)	• Advise clients to take the medication with food or a full glass of water. • Advise clients to monitor for signs of bleeding, to notify the provider, and to stop the medication if symptoms occur. • Advise clients to take H_2-receptor antagonists, such as ranitidine (Zantac), for prevention if prescribed.
Fetal death/congenital abnormalities	• Advise clients to avoid use during pregnancy. • Instruct clients to use adequate contraception during therapy.
Antimalarial agents: hydroxychloroquine	
Retinal damage (blindness)	• Advise clients to have a baseline eye examination and follow-up eye exams every 6 months with an ophthalmologist. • Advise clients to stop the medication and notify the provider if blurred vision occurs.
Sulfasalazine	
GI discomfort (nausea, vomiting, diarrhea, abdominal pain)	• Advise clients to use an enteric-coated preparation and divide dosage daily.
Skin reactions (pruritus, rash, urticaria)	• Advise clients to report skin reactions to the provider. May need to take antihistamine.
Hepatic dysfunction	• Monitor liver function tests.
Bone marrow suppression	• Monitor CBC and platelet counts.

SIDE/ADVERSE EFFECTS	NURSING INTERVENTIONS/CLIENT EDUCATION
Biologic response modifiers: etanercept, infliximab	
Subcutaneous injection-site irritation (redness, swelling, pain, itching)	• Monitor the client's injection site, and stop the medication if signs of irritation occur.
Risk of infection, especially TB (fever, sore throat, inflammation)	• Instruct clients to monitor for infection and notify the provider if symptoms occur. • Tell clients the provider may discontinue the medication. • Perform TB testing. Monitor closely for TB during treatment.
Severe skin reactions	• Instruct clients to monitor for adverse skin reactions and notify the provider if symptoms occur. The provider will discontinue the medication.
Heart failure (distended neck veins, crackles in lungs, dyspnea)	• Monitor for development or worsening of heart failure. Tell clients the provider will discontinue the medication.
Blood dyscrasias	• Monitor for signs of bleeding, bruising or fever. Medication should be discontinued.
Aurothioglucose	
Toxicity (severe pruritus, rashes, stomatitis)	• Stop medication. • Notify the provider if symptoms occur.
Renal toxicity, such as proteinuria	• Stop the medication. • Monitor I&O, BUN, creatinine, and UA.
Blood dyscrasias (thrombocytopenia, leukopenia, agranulocytosis, aplastic anemia)	• Monitor CBC, WBC, and platelet counts periodically. • Advise clients to observe for signs of bleeding and to notify the provider if these occur.
Hepatitis	• Monitor liver function tests.
GI discomfort (nausea, vomiting, abdominal pain)	• Observe for symptoms and notify the provider if they occur.
Penicillamine	
Bone marrow suppression	• Obtain the client's baseline CBC and platelet counts, and repeat every 3 to 6 months.
Toxicity (severe pruritus, rashes)	• Stop the medication. • Notify the provider if symptoms occur.

SIDE/ADVERSE EFFECTS	NURSING INTERVENTIONS/CLIENT EDUCATION
Cyclosporine	
Risk of infection (fever and/or sore throat)	• Advise clients to notify the provider immediately if symptoms occur.
Hepatotoxicity (jaundice)	• Monitor liver function and adjust dosage.
Nephrotoxicity	• Monitor BUN and serum creatinine. • Measure I&O.
Hirsutism	• Tell clients the provider may discontinue the medication which will reverse this side effect.
Glucocorticoids: prednisone	
Risk of infection (fever and/or sore throat)	• Advise clients to notify the provider immediately if symptoms occur.
Osteoporosis	• Advise clients to take calcium supplements, vitamin D, and/or bisphosphonates (etidronate [Didronel]).
Adrenal suppression	• Advise clients to observe for symptoms, and to notify the provider if symptoms occur. • Monitor clients receiving IV fluids (0.9% sodium chloride) and hydrocortisone IV doses. • Advise clients not to discontinue medication suddenly.
Fluid retention	• Monitor for signs of fluid excess, such as crackles, weight gain, and edema.
GI discomfort	• Advise clients to observe for symptoms and to notify the provider if symptoms occur. • Advise clients to use H_2-receptor antagonists if prescribed. • Advise client to report symptoms of GI bleeding.
Hyperglycemia	• Monitor blood glucose level. Clients who have diabetes mellitus may need to adjust hypoglycemic agent.
Hypokalemia	• Monitor serum potassium levels. • Advise clients to eat potassium-rich foods. • Administer potassium supplements.

 Contraindications/Precautions:

- Methotrexate

  o This medication is Pregnancy Risk Category X.

  o Methotrexate is contraindicated in clients who have psoriasis, renal or liver failure, alcoholism, or blood dyscrasias.

- o Use with caution in clients who have liver or kidney dysfunction, cancer and suppressed bone marrow function, peptic ulcer disease, ulcerative colitis, impaired nutritional status, or infections.

- o Use cautiously with children or older adult clients.

- Etanercept (Enbrel)

  - o Use caution in clients who have heart failure, CNS demyelinating disorders, such as multiple sclerosis, or blood dyscrasias.

- Cyclosporine is contraindicated in pregnancy, recent vaccination with live virus vaccines, and recent contact with or active infection of chickenpox or herpes zoster.

- Glucocorticoids are contraindicated in systemic fungal infections and live virus vaccines.

Interactions

MEDICATION/FOOD INTERACTIONS	NURSING INTERVENTIONS/CLIENT EDUCATION
Methotrexate	
Concurrent use may reduce digoxin level.	Monitor digoxin level. Monitor ECG.
NSAIDs, salicylates, and sulfonamides can cause methotrexate toxicity.	Monitor methotrexate levels.
Methotrexate can reduce levels of phenytoin (Dilantin).	Monitor phenytoin level.
Food can decrease absorption.	Advise clients to take on an empty stomach.
Alcohol use can increase risk of hepatotoxicity.	Advise clients to avoid alcohol.
Etanercept	
Concurrent use of etanercept with a live vaccine increases the risk of getting or transmitting infection.	Advise clients to avoid live vaccines.
Cyclosporine	
Concurrent use of phenytoin, phenobarbital, rifampin, carbamazepine, and trimethoprim-sulfamethoxazole decreases cyclosporine level, which can lead to organ rejection.	Monitor the client's cyclosporine levels and administer adjusted dosage as prescribed.
Concurrent use of ketoconazole, erythromycin, and amphotericin B can increase cyclosporine level, leading to toxicity.	Monitor cyclosporine dosage and administer adjusted dosage as prescribed.
Amphotericin B, aminoglycoside, and NSAIDs are nephrotoxic, and concurrent use with cyclosporine increases the risk for renal dysfunction.	Monitor BUN, serum creatinine, and I&O.
Consumption of grapefruit juice increases cyclosporine levels by 50%, which poses an increased risk of toxicity.	Advise clients to avoid drinking grapefruit juice.

MEDICATION/FOOD INTERACTIONS	NURSING INTERVENTIONS/CLIENT EDUCATION
Glucocorticoids	
Diuretics that promote potassium loss increase the risk of hypokalemia.	Monitor the client's potassium level and administer supplements as needed.
Because of the risk for hypokalemia, concurrent use of glucocorticoids with digoxin increases the risk of digoxin-induced dysrhythmias.	Monitor digoxin and potassium levels.
NSAIDs increase the risk of GI ulceration.	Advise clients to avoid use of NSAIDs. If GI distress occurs, instruct clients to notify the provider.
Glucocorticoids promote hyperglycemia, thereby counteracting the effects of hypoglycemic agents.	Monitor blood glucose levels. Instruct clients to notify provider of changes and expect a change in dosage.

Nursing Administration

- Advise clients that effects of DMARDs may take 3 to 6 weeks to experience, with full therapeutic effect taking several months.

- Administer etanercept by subcutaneous injection two times a week. Ensure solution is clear without particles present.

- Administer glucocorticoids as oral agents or as intra-articular injections. Use short-term therapy to control exacerbations of symptoms and also while waiting for the effects of DMARDs to develop.

- Cyclosporine

  o Monitor clients for hypersensitivity reactions. Stay with clients for 30 min after administration of cyclosporine.

  o Mix oral cyclosporine with milk or orange juice right before ingestion to increase palatability.

  o Instruct clients regarding the importance of lifelong therapy if used to prevent organ rejection.

Nursing Evaluation of Medication Effectiveness

- Depending on the therapeutic intent, effectiveness may be evidenced by:

  o Improvement of symptoms of rheumatoid arthritis (reduced swelling of joints, absence of joint stiffness, ability to maintain joint function, absence of pain)

  o Decrease in systemic complications, such as weight loss and fatigue

  o Prevention of organ rejection

APPLICATION EXERCISES

1. A nurse is to administer a regular intramuscular dose of aurothioglucose (Solganal) for a client who has rheumatoid arthritis. For which of the following should the nurse monitor and withhold the medication? (Select all that apply.)

    _____ Insomnia

    _____ Stomatitis

    _____ Visual changes

    _____ Bruising

    _____ Pruritus

2. A nurse is reinforcing teaching for a female client who has a new prescription for hydroxychloroquine (Plaquenil) for rheumatoid arthritis. The nurse evaluates that the client understands the teaching when she states, "While taking hydroxychloroquine I should

    A. go to the dentist more frequently."

    B. call my doctor if I develop blurred vision."

    C. have a Pap test twice a year."

    D. let my doctor know if my urine becomes darker."

3. A nurse is caring for a client who has rheumatoid arthritis and is being treated with a variety of medications. The nurse should monitor the client carefully for tuberculosis if the client is taking which of the following medications?

    A. Indomethacin (Indocin)

    B. Sulfasalazine (Azulfidine)

    C. Prednisone (Deltasone)

    D. Etanercept (Enbrel)

4. A nurse is caring for a client who has a prescription for cyclosporine (Sandimmune) to treat rheumatoid arthritis. Which of the following medications, if taken concurrently with cyclosporine, should the nurse anticipate causing a risk for cyclosporine toxicity?

    A. Phenytoin (Dilantin)

    B. Trimethoprim/sulfamethoxazole (Septra)

    C. Carbamazepine (Tegretol)

    D. Erythromycin (E-Mycin)

APPLICATION EXERCISES ANSWER KEY

1. A nurse is to administer a regular intramuscular dose of aurothioglucose (Solganal) for a client who has rheumatoid arthritis. For which of the following should the nurse monitor and withhold the medication? (Select all that apply.)

_____	Insomnia
__X__	**Stomatitis**
_____	Visual changes
__X__	**Bruising**
__X__	**Pruritus**

    The nurse should withhold the medication and notify the provider for stomatitis, bruising (possible thrombocytopenia), and pruritus. Insomnia and visual changes are not side effects of aurothioglucose therapy.

     NCLEX® Connection: Pharmacological Therapies, Adverse Effects/Contraindications/Side Effects/Interactions

2. A nurse is reinforcing teaching for a female client who has a new prescription for hydroxychloroquine (Plaquenil) for rheumatoid arthritis. The nurse evaluates that the client understands the teaching when she states, "While taking hydroxychloroquine I should

    A. go to the dentist more frequently."

    B. call my doctor if I develop blurred vision."

    C. have a Pap test twice a year."

    D. let my doctor know if my urine becomes darker."

    Toxicity to hydroxychloroquine can cause retinal damage. The client should report any blurred vision to her provider and should see the ophthalmologist before starting her prescription and every 6 months while taking hydroxychloroquine. There is no reason to see the dentist more frequently or have pap smears every 6 months while taking the medication. Darkening of the urine is not an adverse effect of hydroxychloroquine.

     NCLEX® Connection: Pharmacological Therapies, Adverse Effects/Contraindications/Side Effects/Interactions

3. A nurse is caring for a client who has rheumatoid arthritis and is being treated with a variety of medications. The nurse should monitor the client carefully for tuberculosis if the client is taking which of the following medications?

    A. Indomethacin (Indocin)

    B. Sulfasalazine (Azulfidine)

    C. Prednisone (Deltasone)

    D. Etanercept (Enbrel)

The development of severe, disseminated tuberculosis is a risk factor for a client taking etanercept, a DMARD used to decrease inflammation in rheumatoid arthritis. The other medications do not increase the client's risk for tuberculosis.

 NCLEX® Connection: Pharmacological Therapies, Adverse Effects/Contraindications/Side Effects/Interactions

4. A nurse is caring for a client who has a prescription for cyclosporine (Sandimmune) to treat rheumatoid arthritis. Which of the following medications, if taken concurrently with cyclosporine, should the nurse anticipate causing a risk for cyclosporine toxicity?

    A. Phenytoin (Dilantin)

    B. Trimethoprim/sulfamethoxazole (Septra)

    C. Carbamazepine (Tegretol)

    D. Erythromycin (E-Mycin)

Erythromycin can increase levels of cyclosporine and increase the risk for toxicity. Phenytoin, carbamazepine, and trimethoprim/sulfamethoxazole can decrease cyclosporine levels and not increase the risk of toxicity.

 NCLEX® Connection: Pharmacological Therapies, Adverse Effects/Contraindications/Side Effects/Interactions

UNIT 8	MEDICATIONS FOR JOINT AND BONE CONDITIONS
Chapter 31	Bone Disorders

 Overview

- Calcium is necessary for the proper functioning of bones, nerves, muscles, the heart, and blood coagulation.

- Give calcium as a supplement when dietary intake is insufficient. Uses for other medications that affect the bones include prevention and treatment of osteoporosis and prevention of fractures.

- Medication classifications include calcium supplements, selective estrogen receptor modulators, bisphosphonates, and calcitonin.

MEDICATION CLASSIFICATION: CALCIUM SUPPLEMENTS

- Select Prototype Medication – Calcium citrate (Citracal)

- Other Medications:

  ○ Calcium carbonate (Tums, Os-Cal)

  ○ Calcium acetate (PhosLo)

  ○ For IV administration:

    ▪ Calcium chloride

    ▪ Calcium gluconate

Purpose

- Expected Pharmacological Action

  ○ Maintenance of normal musculoskeletal, neurological, and cardiovascular function

- Therapeutic Uses

  ○ Use oral calcium supplements for clients who have hypocalcemia or deficiencies of the parathyroid hormone, vitamin D, or dietary calcium.

  ○ Use oral calcium supplements for adolescents, older adults, and women who are postmenopausal, pregnant, or breastfeeding.

  ○ Use intravenous calcium agents for clients who have critically low levels of calcium.

Complications

SIDE/ADVERSE EFFECTS	NURSING INTERVENTIONS/CLIENT EDUCATION
Hypercalcemia – Calcium level greater than 10.5 mg/dL • Findings include muscle weakness and hypotonia, polyuria, nocturia, polydipsia, constipation, nausea, vomiting, abdominal pain, lethargy, and depression. Cardiovascular changes may start with elevated blood pressure and tachycardia but may progress to bradycardia.	• Instruct clients to monitor for symptoms and report to the provider. • Monitor serum calcium levels to maintain between 9.0 to 10.5 mg/dL.

 ## Contraindications/Precautions

- Calcium supplements are contraindicated in clients who have hypercalcemia, bone tumors, and hyperparathyroidism.

- Use cautiously in clients who have kidney disease or a decrease in GI function.

Interactions

MEDICATION/FOOD INTERACTIONS	NURSING INTERVENTIONS/CLIENT EDUCATION
Concurrent use of glucocorticoids reduces absorption of calcium.	• Give medications at least 1 hr apart.
Concurrent use of calcium decreases absorption of tetracyclines and thyroid hormone.	• Ensure 1 hr between administration of tetracyclines and several hr between administration of thyroid hormone medications.
Concurrent use of thiazide diuretics increases risk of hypercalcemia.	• Check clients for hypercalcemia. • Avoid concurrent use.
Spinach, rhubarb, Swiss chard, beets, bran, and whole grains can decrease calcium absorption.	• Do not administer calcium with foods that decrease absorption. • Instruct clients to avoid consuming these foods at the same time as taking calcium.

Nursing Administration

- Instruct clients to take calcium supplements with 240 mL (8 oz) of water. Inform clients that taking calcium with meals or soon after will enhance absorption.

- Instruct clients to take a calcium supplement at least 1 hr apart from glucocorticoids, tetracyclines, and/or thyroid hormones.

- Advise clients that chewable tablets provide more consistent bioavailability.

- Instruct clients to follow provider prescription due to variations in calcium formulations.

Nursing Evaluation of Medication Effectiveness

- Depending on therapeutic intent, effectiveness may be evidenced by:

    o Serum calcium level within expected reference range: 9.0 to 10.5 mg/dL

MEDICATION CLASSIFICATION: SELECTIVE ESTROGEN RECEPTOR MODULATORS/ SERMS

- Select Prototype Medication – Raloxifene (Evista)

Purpose

- Expected Pharmacological Action

    o Works as endogenous estrogen in bone, lipid metabolism, and blood coagulation

    o Decreases bone resorption, which results in slowing down of bone loss and preservation of bone mineral density

    o Works as an antagonist to estrogen on breast and endometrial tissue

    o Can decrease plasma levels of cholesterol

- Therapeutic Uses

    o Prevents and treats postmenopausal osteoporosis

    o Protects against breast cancer for postmenopausal women at high risk

Complications

SIDE/ADVERSE EFFECTS	NURSING INTERVENTIONS/CLIENT EDUCATION
Increases the risk for pulmonary embolism and deep vein thrombosis (DVT)	• Instruct clients to stop taking medication at least 72 hr prior to scheduled surgery or if on bed rest and to resume when fully mobile. • Discourage long periods of sitting and inactivity, as in traveling.
Hot flashes	• Inform clients that the medication may exacerbate, rather than reduce, hot flashes.

 Contraindications/Precautions

- Raloxifene is Pregnancy Risk Category X.

- This medication is contraindicated in clients who have a history of venous thrombosis.

Interactions

- No significant interactions

Nursing Administration

- For maximum benefit of the medication, encourage clients to consume adequate amounts of calcium, such as from dairy products, and vitamin D, such as from egg yolks. Inadequate amounts of dietary calcium and vitamin D cause release of parathyroid hormone, which stimulates calcium release from the bone.

- Instruct clients that medication may be taken with or without food once a day.

- Monitor the client's bone density; clients should undergo a bone density scan every 12 to 18 months.

- Monitor the client's serum calcium. Expected reference range is 9 to 10.5 mg/dL.

- Monitor liver function tests. Raloxifene levels may be increased in clients with hepatic impairment.

- Encourage clients to perform weight-bearing exercises daily, such as walking 30 to 40 min each day.

Nursing Evaluation of Medication Effectiveness

- Depending on therapeutic intent, effectiveness may be evidenced by:

  o Increase in bone density

  o No spinal fractures

MEDICATION CLASSIFICATION: BISPHOSPHONATES

- Select Prototype Medications – Alendronate (Fosamax)

- Other Medications:

  o Ibandronate (Boniva)

  o Risedronate (Actonel)

  o Zoledronate (Reclast, Zometa) – For IV infusion

Purpose

- Expected Pharmacological Action

  o Bisphosphonates decrease the number and action of osteoclasts, which thereby inhibits bone resorption.

- Therapeutic Uses

  o Prevents and treats postmenopausal osteoporosis

  o Treats osteoporosis in men

  o Prevents and treats osteoporosis produced by long-term glucocorticoid use

  o Treats Paget's disease of the bone and hypercalcemia of malignancy

Complications

SIDE/ADVERSE EFFECTS	NURSING INTERVENTIONS/CLIENT EDUCATION
Esophagitis and other GI disturbances (nausea, diarrhea, constipation, and dyspepsia)	• Instruct clients to sit upright or ambulate for 30 min (60 min with ibandronate) after taking this medication orally. • Instruct client to take tablets with at least 240 mL (8 oz) of water and liquid formulation with at least 60 mL (2 oz) of water.
Musculoskeletal pain	• Advise clients to take mild analgesic. • Instruct clients to notify the provider if pain persists. Tell clients the provider may prescribe a different medication.
Visual disturbances, such as blurred vision and eye pain	• Instruct clients to watch for symptoms and report to the provider. Medication should be discontinued.
Bisphosphonate-related osteonecrosis of the jaw with IV infusion	• Avoid dental work during administration of medication.
Risk for hyperparathyroidism at higher dose used for Paget's disease	• Monitor the client's parathyroid hormone (PTH) levels. The provider may prescribe calcium supplements.

 Contraindications/Precautions

- Bisphosphonates are Pregnancy Risk Category C.

- These medications are contraindicated for women who are lactating.

- These medications are contraindicated in clients who have esophageal stricture or difficulty swallowing, esophageal disorders, serious renal impairment, and hypocalcemia.

- Use cautiously in clients who have upper GI disorders, infection, and liver impairment.

Interactions

MEDICATION/FOOD INTERACTIONS	NURSING INTERVENTIONS/CLIENT EDUCATION
Alendronate absorption decreases when taken with calcium supplements, antacids, orange juice, and caffeine.	• Instruct clients to wait 30 min (60 min with ibandronate) before eating or drinking anything after taking the medication.

Nursing Administration

- Instructions for clients should include:

  ○ Take the medication first thing in the morning after getting out of bed.

  ○ Take oral medication on an empty stomach, drinking at least 8 oz of water with tablets and at least 2 oz of water with liquid formulation.

  ○ Sit or ambulate for 30 min after taking the medication.

  ○ Wait 30 min (60 min with ibandronate) before eating or drinking after taking the medication.

  ○ Avoid chewing or sucking on the tablet.

  ○ Perform weight-bearing exercises daily, such as walking 30 to 40 min each day.

  ○ Notify the provider of difficulty swallowing, painful swallowing, and/or new or worsening heartburn.

  ○ If a dose is skipped, wait until the next day to take the next dose. Do not take the skipped dose.

  ○ For maximum benefit of the medication, consume adequate amounts of calcium and vitamin D.

- Take tablets once daily or once a week. Take liquid form once a week.

- Monitor the client's bone density; clients should have a bone density scan every 12 to 18 months.

- Monitor the client's serum calcium – Expected reference range 9 to 10.5 mg/dL.

Nursing Evaluation of Medication Effectiveness

- Depending on therapeutic intent, effectiveness may be evidenced by:

  ○ Increase in bone density

  ○ No fractures

MEDICATION CLASSIFICATION: CALCITONIN

- Select Prototype Medication – Calcitonin-salmon (Fortical, Miacalcin)

Purpose

- Expected Pharmacological Action
  - Decreases bone resorption by inhibiting the activity of osteoclasts in osteoporosis
  - Increases renal calcium excretion by inhibiting tubular resorption
- Therapeutic Uses
  - Postmenopausal osteoporosis and moderate to severe Paget's disease
  - Hypercalcemia caused by hyperparathyroidism and cancer

Complications

SIDE/ADVERSE EFFECTS	NURSING INTERVENTIONS/CLIENT EDUCATION
Nausea	• Advise clients that nausea is usually self-limiting.
With intranasal route, nasal dryness and irritation can occur	• Instruct clients to alternate nostrils daily. • Inspect nasal mucosa periodically for ulceration.

 Contraindications/Precautions

- This medication is Pregnancy Risk Category C.
- The medication is contraindicated in clients who have hypersensitivity to the medication and fish protein. Perform an allergy skin test prior to administration if the client is at risk.
- Use cautiously with women who are lactating, children, and clients diagnosed with kidney disease.

Interactions

- Concurrent use with lithium can decrease serum lithium levels. Monitor lithium levels closely.

Nursing Administration

- Administer calcitonin-salmon intranasally as a nasal spray. Rotate injection sites to prevent inflammation. It is also administered IM or subcutaneously.
- Instruct clients to keep the container in an upright position.
- Tell clients to alternate nostrils daily.

- Monitor for hypocalcemia by checking for Chvostek's or Trousseau's signs.

- Monitor the client's bone density scans periodically.

- Encourage clients to consume a diet high in calcium and vitamin D.

Nursing Evaluation of Medication Effectiveness

- Depending on therapeutic intent, effectiveness may be evidenced by:

    o Increase in bone density

    o Serum calcium level within expected reference range of 9 to 10.5 mg/dL

APPLICATION EXERCISES

1. A nurse is reinforcing teaching to a client who is taking raloxifene (Evista) to prevent postmenopausal osteoporosis. What information should the nurse provide to the client?

2. A client who has osteoporosis is started on alendronate (Fosamax). The nurse should instruct the client to do which of the following? (Select all that apply.)

   _____ Take the medication in the morning after arising and before eating.

   _____ Chew tablets to increase bioavailability.

   _____ Drink 8 oz of water with each tablet.

   _____ Take the medication with an antacid if heartburn occurs.

   _____ Avoid lying down after taking the medication.

3. A nurse is reinforcing teaching to a client who has been prescribed daily calcium supplements. What foods should the nurse teach the client to avoid at the time she takes her calcium tablets?

4. A nurse is caring for a client who has been prescribed calcitonin-salmon to treat osteoporosis. When evaluating the client's therapy, the nurse should recognize that which of the following serum calcium levels is within the expected range?

   A. 8.6 mg/dL

   B. 9.6 mg/dL

   C. 10.6 mg/dL

   D. 11.6 mg/dL

APPLICATION EXERCISES ANSWER KEY

1. A nurse is reinforcing teaching to a client who is taking raloxifene (Evista) to prevent postmenopausal osteoporosis. What information should the nurse provide to the client?

   The client who takes raloxifene is at risk for DVT, pulmonary embolism, and stroke. Tell the client to monitor for thromboembolism as evidenced by swelling or redness in calf, shortness of breath, or weakness. Also, tell the client to stop taking prior to surgery or immobility, such as bed rest.

    NCLEX® Connection: Pharmacological Therapies, Adverse Effects/Contraindications/Side Effects/Interactions

2. A client who has osteoporosis is started on alendronate (Fosamax). The nurse should instruct the client to do which of the following? (Select all that apply.)

__X__	**Take the medication in the morning after arising and before eating.**
_____	Chew tablets to increase bioavailability.
__X__	**Drink 8 oz of water with each tablet.**
_____	Take the medication with an antacid if heartburn occurs.
__X__	**Avoid lying down after taking the medication.**

   To prevent esophagitis, the client should take the medication first thing in the morning before eating, swallow the tablet with at least a full 8 oz of water, and avoid lying down after taking the medication. The client should not chew as this can cause esophagitis. To optimize absorption, the client should not ingest anything for 30 min after taking the medication.

    NCLEX® Connection: Pharmacological Therapies, Medication Administration

3. A nurse is reinforcing teaching to a client who has been prescribed daily calcium supplements. What foods should the nurse teach the client to avoid at the time she takes her calcium tablets?

   The client should avoid taking calcium at the same time as eating spinach, bran, whole-grain breads and cereals, Swiss chard, rhubarb, and beets. These foods decrease the absorption of calcium.

    NCLEX® Connection: Pharmacological Therapies, Medication Administration

4. A nurse is caring for a client who has been prescribed calcitonin-salmon to treat osteoporosis. When evaluating the client's therapy, the nurse should recognize that which of the following serum calcium levels is within the expected range?

    A. 8.6 mg/dL

    B. 9.6 mg/dL

    C. 10.6 mg/dL

    D. 11.6 mg/dL

    The expected reference range for serum calcium is 9.0 to 10.5 mg/dL. The other values represent either hypocalcemia or hypercalcemia.

 NCLEX® Connection: Pharmacological Therapies, Expected Actions/Outcomes

UNIT 9: MEDICATIONS FOR PAIN AND INFLAMMATION

- Nonopioid Analgesics

- Opioid Agonists and Antagonists

- Adjuvant Medications for Pain

- Miscellaneous Pain Medications

NCLEX® CONNECTIONS

When reviewing the chapters in this section, keep in mind the relevant sections of the NCLEX® outline, in particular:

CLIENT NEEDS: PHARMACOLOGICAL THERAPIES

Relevant topics/tasks include:
- Adverse Effects/Contraindications/Side Effects/Interactions
  - Monitor and document client side effects to medications.
- Medication Administration
  - Count narcotics/controlled substances.
- Pharmacological Pain Management
  - Monitor and document client response to pharmacological interventions.

UNIT 9	MEDICATIONS FOR PAIN AND INFLAMMATION
Chapter 32	Nonopioid Analgesics

 Overview

- Nonopioid analgesics may have anti-inflammatory, antipyretic, and analgesic action. These medications include nonsteroidal anti-inflammatory drugs and acetaminophen.

MEDICATION CLASSIFICATION: NONSTEROIDAL ANTI-INFLAMMATORY DRUGS

- 1st generation NSAIDs (COX-1 and COX-2 inhibitors):

  o Aspirin

  o Ibuprofen (Motrin, Advil)

  o Naproxen (Naprosyn)

  o Indomethacin (Indocin)

  o Diclofenac (Voltaren)

  o Ketorolac (Toradol)

  o Meloxicam (Mobic)

- 2nd generation NSAIDs (selective COX-2 Inhibitor):

  o Celecoxib (Celebrex)

Purpose

- Expected Pharmacological Action

  o Inhibition of cyclooxygenase – Inhibition of COX-1 can result in decreased platelet aggregation and kidney damage. Inhibition of COX-2 results in decreased inflammation, fever, and pain.

- Therapeutic Uses

  o Inflammation suppression

  o Analgesia for mild to moderate pain, such as with osteoarthritis and rheumatoid arthritis

  o Fever reduction

  o Dysmenorrhea

  o Inhibition of platelet aggregation, which protects against stroke and myocardial infarction (low-dose aspirin)

Complications

SIDE/ADVERSE EFFECTS	NURSING INTERVENTIONS/CLIENT EDUCATION
• Gastrointestinal (GI) discomfort (dyspepsia, abdominal pain, heartburn, nausea) • Damage to gastric mucosa may lead to GI bleeding and perforation, especially with long-term use (passage of black or dark-colored stools, severe abdominal pain).	• Advise clients to take medication with food or with a full glass of water or milk. • Advise clients to avoid alcohol. • Observe for signs of bleeding. • Administer a proton pump inhibitor, such as omeprazole (Prilosec), or an H_2 receptor antagonist, such as ranitidine (Zantac), to decrease the risk of ulcer formation or for treatment. • Use prophylaxis agents such as misoprostol (Cytotec).
• Renal dysfunction (decreased urine output, weight gain from fluid retention, increased BUN and serum creatinine levels)	• Use cautiously with older adults and clients who have heart failure. • Monitor I&O and kidney function.
• Increased risk of heart attack and stroke (nonaspirin NSAIDs)	• Use the smallest effective dose for clients with known cardiovascular disease.
• Salicylism may occur with aspirin (tinnitus, sweating, headache and dizziness, and respiratory alkalosis).	• Advise clients to notify the provider and to stop taking aspirin if symptoms occur.
• Reye syndrome is rare, but serious in childhood. This occurs when aspirin is used for fever reduction in children who have a viral illness, such as chickenpox or influenza.	• Advise clients to not give aspirin to a child who has a viral illness, such as chickenpox or influenza.

• Aspirin toxicity	• Manage aspirin toxicity as a medical emergency in the hospital.
	• Therapy includes:
	  o Cooling with tepid water
	  o Correction of dehydration and electrolyte imbalance with IV fluids
	  o Reversal of acidosis and promotion of salicylate excretion with bicarbonate
	  o Gastric lavage
	• Activated charcoal decreases absorption.
	• Use hemodialysis as last resort.

Contraindications/Precautions

- Contraindications for aspirin and other 1st generation NSAIDs include:

  o Pregnancy (Pregnancy Risk Category D)

  o Peptic ulcer disease

  o Bleeding disorders, such as hemophilia and vitamin K deficiency

  o Hypersensitivity to aspirin and other NSAIDs

  o Children with chickenpox or influenza (aspirin)

- Use NSAIDs cautiously in older adults, clients who smoke cigarettes, and in clients with *H. pylori* infection, hypovolemia, asthma, chronic urticaria, and/or a history of alcoholism.

- Celecoxib is contraindicated in clients with allergy to sulfonamides.

- Ketorolac is contraindicated in clients with advanced renal dysfunction. Use should be no longer than 5 days because of the risk for kidney damage.

- Use 2nd generation NSAIDs cautiously in clients who have known cardiovascular disease.

Interactions

MEDICATION/FOOD INTERACTIONS	NURSING INTERVENTIONS/CLIENT EDUCATION
Anticoagulants, such as heparin and warfarin, increase the risk of bleeding.	• Monitor the client's aPTT, PT, and INR. • Instruct clients to report signs of bleeding.
Glucocorticoids increase the risk of gastric bleeding.	• Advise clients to take antiulcer prophylaxis, such as misoprostol (Cytotec), to decrease the risk for gastric ulcer.
Alcohol increases the risk of bleeding.	• Advise clients to avoid consuming alcoholic beverages.
Ibuprofen decreases the antiplatelet effects of low-dose aspirin used to prevent MI.	• Advise clients not to take ibuprofen.
Ketorolac and concurrent use of other NSAIDs increase the risk of known side effects.	• Avoid concurrent use.
Concurrent use of ACE inhibitors, or angiotensin receptor blockers and NSAIDs, increases the risk of acute renal failure.	• Avoid concurrent use. May continue therapy with low-dose aspirin if indicated.

Nursing Administration

- Advise clients to stop aspirin and other NSAIDs 1 week before an elective surgery or expected date of childbirth (or to stop aspirin per the provider's instructions).

- Advise clients to take NSAIDs with food, milk, or a full glass of water to reduce gastric discomfort.

- Instruct clients not to chew or crush enteric-coated or sustained-release aspirin tablets.

- Advise clients to notify the provider if signs and symptoms of gastric discomfort or ulceration occur.

- Advise clients to notify the provider if symptoms of salicylism occur. The client should discontinue the medication until symptoms are resolved. Medication can be restarted at a lower dose.

- Use ketorolac for short-term treatment of moderate to severe pain such as that associated with postoperative recovery.

  o Concurrent use with opioids allows for lower dosages of opioids and thus minimizes adverse effects such as constipation and respiratory depression.

  o Ketorolac is usually first administered parenterally and then switched to oral doses. Use should not be longer than 5 days because of the risk for kidney damage.

Nursing Evaluation of Medication Effectiveness

- Depending on therapeutic intent, effectiveness may be evidenced by:

  o Reduction in inflammation

  o Reduction of fever

  o Relief from mild to moderate pain

MEDICATION CLASSIFICATION: ACETAMINOPHEN

- Select Prototype Medication – Acetaminophen (Tylenol)

Purpose

- Expected Pharmacological Action

  o Acetaminophen slows the production of prostaglandins in the central nervous system.

- Therapeutic Uses

  o Analgesic (relief of pain) effect

  o Antipyretic (reduction of fever) effects

Complications

SIDE/ADVERSE EFFECTS	NURSING INTERVENTIONS/CLIENT EDUCATION
Acute toxicity that results in liver damage with early symptoms of nausea, vomiting, diarrhea, sweating, and abdominal discomfort progressing to hepatic failure, coma, and death	• Advise clients to take acetaminophen as prescribed and not to exceed 4 g/day. • Administer the antidote, acetylcysteine (Mucomyst).

Contraindications/Precautions

- Use cautiously in clients who consume three or more alcoholic drinks per day and those taking warfarin (interferes with metabolism).

Interactions

MEDICATION/FOOD INTERACTIONS	NURSING INTERVENTIONS/CLIENT EDUCATION
• Alcohol increases the risk of liver damage.	• Advise clients about the potential risk of liver damage with consumption of alcohol.
• Acetaminophen slows the metabolism of warfarin (Coumadin), leading to increased levels of warfarin. This places clients at risk for bleeding (bruising, petechiae, hematuria).	• Instruct clients to observe for signs of bleeding (bruising, petechiae, hematuria). • Monitor PT and INR levels and adjust dosages of warfarin accordingly.

Nursing Administration

- Instruct clients to keep a running total of daily acetaminophen intake and follow recommended dosages as prescribed by the provider to prevent toxicity, not to exceed 4 g/day.

- In the event of an overdose, administer acetylcysteine (Mucomyst), the antidote for acetaminophen, to prevent liver damage. Administer via an oroduodenal tube or IV infusion to prevent emesis and subsequent aspiration.

Nursing Evaluation of Medication Effectiveness

- Depending on therapeutic intent, effectiveness may be evidenced by:

  ○ Relief of pain

  ○ Reduction of fever

APPLICATION EXERCISES

1. A nurse is caring for an older adult client who is taking large doses of aspirin four times daily for severe rheumatoid arthritis pain. For which of the following should the nurse monitor the client?

   A. Hepatotoxicity

   B. Renal impairment

   C. Reye's syndrome

   D. Ischemic stroke

2. A nurse is caring for a toddler who was just admitted for an acetaminophen overdose. Which of the following medications should the nurse anticipate being administered to this client?

   A. Acetylcysteine (Mucomyst)

   B. Pegfilgrastim (Neulasta)

   C. Misoprostol (Cytotec)

   D. Naltrexone (ReVia)

3. A nurse is caring for a postoperative client who is prescribed ketorolac (Toradol) for pain management. The nurse should recognize that which of the following is true regarding the administration of ketorolac?

   A. Ketorolac is prescribed postoperatively to lower the dosage of opioids needed.

   B. Clients who take ketorolac avoid the adverse reactions of NSAIDS.

   C. Ketorolac is available as a timed-release transdermal patch.

   D. Clients may be prescribed ketorolac for long-term relief of chronic pain, such as arthritis

4. A nurse is collecting data for a client who has arthritis and who hopes to obtain a prescription for celecoxib (Celebrex) from his provider to treat chronic joint pain. Which of the following allergies reported by the client is a contraindication to the use of celecoxib?

   A. Penicillin

   B. Sulfonamide

   C. Aspirin

   D. Shellfish

APPLICATION EXERCISES ANSWER KEY

1. A nurse is caring for an older adult client who is taking large doses of aspirin four times daily for severe rheumatoid arthritis pain. For which of the following should the nurse monitor the client?

    A. Hepatotoxicity

    B. Renal impairment

    C. Reye's syndrome

    D. Ischemic stroke

    Impaired renal function is an adverse effect which may be caused by aspirin due to its ability to inhibit prostaglandins needed by the kidney to function properly. The older adult client is at increased risk for this adverse effect, and if signs of impaired kidney function occur (increased BUN, decreased urine output), the nurse should inform the provider immediately. Hepatotoxicity is not an adverse effect of aspirin. Reye's syndrome is a rare adverse effect found only in children who have influenza or chickenpox, and take aspirin. Aspirin is protective for ischemic stroke; therefore, this is not an adverse effect.

     NCLEX® Connection: Pharmacological Therapies, Adverse Effects/Contraindications/Side Effects/Interactions

2. A nurse is caring for a toddler who was just admitted for an acetaminophen overdose. Which of the following medications should the nurse anticipate being administered to this client?

    A. Acetylcysteine (Mucomyst)

    B. Pegfilgrastim (Neulasta)

    C. Misoprostol (Cytotec)

    D. Naltrexone (ReVia)

    Acetylcysteine (Mucomyst) is the antidote for acetaminophen overdose. Use pegfilgrastim as a long-acting medication to increase the body's production of neutrophils. Use misoprostol, a prostaglandin hormone, to prevent the formation of gastric ulcers. Use naltrexone, an opioid antagonist, to prevent alcohol cravings.

     NCLEX® Connection: Pharmacological Therapies, Expected Actions/Outcomes

3. A nurse is caring for a postoperative client who is prescribed ketorolac (Toradol) for pain management. The nurse should recognize that which of the following is true regarding the administration of ketorolac?

   A. Ketorolac is prescribed postoperatively to lower the dosage of opioids needed.

   B. Clients who take ketorolac avoid the adverse reactions of NSAIDS.

   C. Ketorolac is available as a timed-release transdermal patch.

   D. Clients may be prescribed ketorolac for long-term relief of chronic pain, such as arthritis

   Ketorolac is prescribed for acute postoperative pain along with an opioid, such as morphine sulfate. Pain relief from ketorolac may decrease the amount of opioid required and thus decrease the risk for opioid adverse effects. Ketorolac has the same adverse effects as other NSAIDS, and should not be prescribed concurrently with other NSAIDS. Ketorolac is available in IM, IV, and oral preparations. Due to the risk for adverse effects, ketorolac is prescribed for no more than 5 days for moderate to severe pain.

    NCLEX® Connection: Pharmacological Therapies, Medication Administration

4. A nurse is collecting data for a client who has arthritis and who hopes to obtain a prescription for celecoxib (Celebrex) from his provider to treat chronic joint pain. Which of the following allergies reported by the client is a contraindication to the use of celecoxib?

   A. Penicillin

   B. Sulfonamide

   C. Aspirin

   D. Shellfish

   In clients allergic to sulfonamides, an allergic reaction may occur if the client takes celecoxib since the medication contains a molecule of sulfur. There is no contraindication to celecoxib use in clients allergic to penicillin, aspirin, or shellfish.

    NCLEX® Connection: Pharmacological Therapies, Adverse Effects/Contraindications/Side Effects/Interactions

UNIT 9   MEDICATIONS FOR PAIN AND INFLAMMATION

Chapter 33   Opioid Agonists and Antagonists

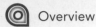 Overview

- Use opioid analgesics to treat moderate to severe pain. Most opioid analgesics reduce pain by attaching to a receptor in the central nervous system, altering perception and response to pain.

- Opioid classifications include agonists, agonist-antagonists, and antagonists.

- An agonist attaches to a receptor and produces a response.

- An agonist-antagonist binds to one receptor, causing a response, and binds to another receptor, which prevents a response.

- An antagonist attaches to a receptor site and prevents a response.

OPIOID AGONISTS

- Select Prototype Medication – Morphine

- Other Medications:

  ○   Fentanyl (Sublimaze, Duragesic)

  ○   Hydromorphone (Dilaudid)

  ○   Meperidine (Demerol)

  ○   Methadone (Dolophine)

  ○   Codeine, oxycodone (OxyContin)

Purpose

- Expected Pharmacological Action

  ○   Opioid agonists, such as morphine, codeine, meperidine, and other morphine-like medications (fentanyl), act on the mu receptors, and to a lesser degree on kappa receptors. Activation of mu receptors produces analgesia, respiratory depression, euphoria, and sedation, whereas kappa receptor activation produces analgesia, sedation, and decreased gastrointestinal (GI) motility.

- Therapeutic Uses
  - Relief of moderate to severe pain (postoperative, myocardial infarction, cancer)
  - Sedation
  - Reduction of bowel motility
  - Codeine – Cough suppression
- Route of administration:
  - Morphine – PO, rectal subcutaneous, IM, IV, epidural, and intrathecal
  - Other Medications:
    - Fentanyl – IV, IM, transmucosal and transdermal
    - Meperidine – Oral, subcutaneous IM, and IV
    - Codeine – Oral, subcutaneous, and IM
    - Methadone – Oral, subcutaneous IM, and IV
    - Oxycodone – Oral
    - Hydromorphone – Oral, subcutaneous, IM, IV

Complications

SIDE/ADVERSE EFFECTS	NURSING INTERVENTIONS/CLIENT EDUCATION
Respiratory depression	• Monitor the client's vital signs. • Stop opioids if the client's respiratory rate is less than 12/min, and then notify the provider. • Have naloxone (Narcan) and resuscitation equipment available. • Avoid the use of opioids with CNS depressant medications (barbiturates, benzodiazepines, consumption of alcohol).
Constipation	• Encourage increased fluid intake and physical activity. • Administer a stimulant laxative, such as bisacodyl (Dulcolax), or a stool softener, such as docusate sodium (Colace).
Orthostatic hypotension	• Advise clients to sit or lie down if symptoms of lightheadedness or dizziness occur. • Instruct clients to change positions slowly and to sit or lie down if symptoms occur. • Provide assistance with ambulation as needed.
Urinary hesitancy, retention	• Advise clients to void every 4 hr. • Monitor I&O. • Check the client's bladder for distention by palpating the lower abdomen area every 4 to 6 hr.

SIDE/ADVERSE EFFECTS	NURSING INTERVENTIONS/CLIENT EDUCATION
Seizures, neurotoxicity (delirium, agitation, myoclonus, hypoanalgesia)	• Encourage adequate fluid intake • Use lowest dose possible.
With meperidine – Accumulation of toxic metabolite (seizures, dysphoria, irritability, tremors)	• Minimize use, especially in older adult clients • Restrict use to less than 48 hr.
Cough suppression	• Advise clients to cough at regular intervals to prevent accumulation of secretions in the airway. • Auscultate the client's lungs for crackles, and instruct clients to increase intake of fluid to liquefy secretions.
Sedation	• Advise clients to avoid hazardous activities such as driving or operating heavy machinery.
Biliary colic	• Avoid giving morphine to clients who have a history of biliary colic. Use meperidine as an alternative.
Emesis	• Administer an antiemetic such as promethazine (Phenergan).
Opioid overdose triad of coma, respiratory depression, and pinpoint pupils	• Monitor the client's vital signs. • Assist with emergency care.

 Contraindications/Precautions

- Morphine is contraindicated after biliary tract surgery.

- Morphine is contraindicated for premature infants during and after delivery because of respiratory depressant effects.

- Meperidine is contraindicated for clients with renal failure because of the accumulation of normeperidine, which can result in seizures and neurotoxicity.

- Use cautiously with:

  ○ Clients who have asthma, emphysema, and/or head injuries; infants; and older adult clients (risk of respiratory depression)

  ○ Clients who are pregnant (risk of physical dependence of the fetus)

  ○ Clients who are extremely obese (greater risk for prolonged side effects because of the accumulation of medication that is metabolized at a slower rate)

  ○ Clients with inflammatory bowel disease (risk of megacolon or paralytic ileus)

  ○ Clients with an enlarged prostate (risk of acute urinary retention)

  ○ Clients with hepatic or renal disease

Interactions

MEDICATION/FOOD INTERACTIONS	NURSING INTERVENTIONS/CLIENT EDUCATION
CNS depressants (barbiturates, phenobarbital, benzodiazepines, alcohol) have additive CNS depression action.	• Warn clients about the use of these medications in conjunction with opioid agonists. • Advise clients to avoid consumption of alcohol.
Anticholinergic agents (atropine sulfate or scopolamine), antihistamines (diphenhydramine [Benadryl]), and tricyclic antidepressants (amitriptyline [Elavil]) have additive anticholinergic effects (constipation, urinary retention).	• Advise clients to increase fluids and dietary fiber to prevent constipation.
Monoamine oxidase inhibitors (MAOIs) may cause hyperpyrexic coma (excitation, seizures, and respiratory depression).	• Avoid the use of meperidine with MAOIs to prevent occurrence of this syndrome.
Antihypertensives have additive hypotensive effects.	• Inform clients of additive effects.

Nursing Administration

- Check the client's pain level on a regular basis. Document the client's response.

- Take the client's baseline vital signs. If the respiratory rate is less than 12/min, notify the provider and withhold the medication.

- Follow controlled substance procedures.

- Double check opioid doses with another nurse prior to administration.

- Have naloxone (Narcan) and resuscitation equipment available.

- Warn clients not to increase dosage without consulting the provider.

- For clients who have cancer, administer opioids on a fixed schedule around the clock. Administer supplemental doses as needed.

- Advise clients with physical dependence not to discontinue opioids abruptly. Reinforce to clients how to slowly taper dosage, usually over a period of 3 days.

- When switching clients from PCA to oral doses of opioids, make sure the client receives adequate PCA dosing until the onset of oral medication takes place.

- When starting clients on pain management therapy with a transdermal fentanyl patch, administer a short-acting opioid prior to onset of therapeutic effects of fentanyl, which typically takes several hours.

Nursing Evaluation of Medication Effectiveness

- Depending on the therapeutic intent, effectiveness may be evidenced by:

  o Relief of moderate to severe pain (postoperative pain, cancer pain, chest pain)

  o Cough suppression

  o Resolution of diarrhea

MEDICATION CLASSIFICATION: AGONIST-ANTAGONIST OPIOIDS

- Select Prototype Medication – Butorphanol (Stadol)

- Other Medications:

  o Nalbuphine hydrochloride (Nubain)

  o Buprenorphine hydrochloride (Buprenex)

Purpose

- Expected Pharmacological Action

  o These medications act as antagonists on mu receptors and agonists on kappa receptors.

  o Compared to pure opioid agonists, agonist-antagonists have:

    ▪ A low potential for abuse causing little euphoria. In fact, high doses can cause adverse effects (anxiety, restlessness, mental confusion).

    ▪ Less respiratory depression.

    ▪ Less analgesic effect.

- Therapeutic Uses

  o Relief of moderate to severe pain

  o Treatment of opioid dependence (buprenorphine)

  o Adjunct to balanced anesthesia

  o Relief of labor pain (butorphanol)

- Route of administration:

  o Butorphanol – IV, IM, intranasal

  o Nalbuphine – IV, IM, subcutaneous

  o Buprenorphine – IV, sublingual, epidural

Complications

SIDE/ADVERSE EFFECTS	NURSING INTERVENTIONS/CLIENT EDUCATION
Abstinence syndrome (cramping, hypertension, vomiting)	• Monitor clients closely when these medications are given to clients who are physically dependent on opioid agonists.
Sedation, respiratory depression	• Have naloxone (Narcan) and resuscitation equipment available. Monitor for respiratory depression.
Dizziness	• Advise clients to use caution in standing up and to avoid driving or using heavy machinery.
Increased intracranial pressure, headache	• Monitor for headache. Check level of consciousness.
Increased cardiac workload	• Do not use for angina or myocardial infarction.

 Contraindications/Precautions

- Use cautiously in clients who have a history of myocardial infarction, renal or liver disease, respiratory depression, or head injury, and clients who are physically dependent on opioids.

Interactions

MEDICATION/FOOD INTERACTIONS	NURSING INTERVENTIONS/CLIENT EDUCATION
CNS depressants and alcohol may cause additive effects.	• Use together cautiously. • Monitor respirations.
Opioid agonists may antagonize and reduce analgesic effects of the opioid.	• Do not use concurrently.

Nursing Administration

- Take the client's baseline vital signs. If the respiratory rate is less than 12/min, withhold the medication and notify the provider.

- Have naloxone and resuscitation equipment available.

- Check clients for opioid dependence prior to administration. Agonist-antagonists may trigger withdrawal symptoms.

- Warn clients not to increase dosage without consulting the provider.

- Advise clients to use caution when getting out of bed or standing. Clients should not operate heavy machinery or drive until CNS effects are known.

- Warn clients not to increase dosage without consulting the provider.

Nursing Evaluation of Medication Effectiveness

- Monitor for improvement of symptoms, such as relief of pain.

MEDICATION CLASSIFICATION: OPIOID ANTAGONISTS

- Select Prototype Medication – Naloxone (Narcan)

- Other Medications – Naltrexone (Re Via, Depade), nalmefene (Revex)

Purpose

- Expected Pharmacological Action

  o Opioid antagonists interfere with the action of opioids by competing for opioid receptors. Opioid antagonists have no effect in the absence of opioids.

- Therapeutic Uses

  o Treatment of opioid overdose

  o Reversal of effects of opioids, such as respiratory depression

  o Reversal of respiratory depression in an infant

- Route of administration:

  o Naloxone, nalmefene – IV, IM, subcutaneous

  o Naltrexone – Oral

Complications

SIDE/ADVERSE EFFECTS	NURSING INTERVENTIONS/CLIENT EDUCATION
Tachycardia and tachypnea	- Monitor the client's heart rhythm (risk of ventricular tachycardia) and respiratory function. - Have resuscitative equipment, including oxygen, on standby during administration.
Abstinence syndrome (cramping, hypertension, vomiting)	- Monitor clients closely when given to clients who are physically dependent on opioid agonists.
Pulmonary edema	- Monitor for pulmonary edema (rales). - Use with caution in clients with history of pulmonary edema.

 Contraindications/Precautions

- Opioid antagonists are Pregnancy Risk Category B.

- These medications are contraindicated in clients with opioid dependency.

Interactions

- None noted

Nursing Administration

- Naloxone is given parenterally due to rapid first-pass inactivation and should be administered IV, IM, or SC. Do not administer orally.

- Observe clients for withdrawal symptoms and/or abrupt onset of pain. Be prepared to address the client's need for analgesia (if given for postoperative opioid-related respiratory depression).

- Monitor respirations for up to 2 hr after use to identify reoccurrence of respiratory depression and the need for repeat dosage of naloxone.

Nursing Evaluation of Medication Effectiveness

- Reversal of respiratory depression (respirations are regular, client is without shortness of breath, respiratory rate is 16 to 20/min in adults and 40 to 60/min in newborns)

APPLICATION EXERCISES

1. A nurse is monitoring a client who received regular doses of meperidine (Demerol) for post-operative pain for 36 hr. For which of the following should the nurse monitor the client?

   A. Hypothermia

   B. Bradycardia

   C. Delirium

   D. Watery diarrhea

2. A nurse is caring for a client who has been receiving morphine for postoperative pain for the past few days. For which of the following should the nurse monitor the client? (Select all that apply.)

   _____ Dilated pupils

   _____ Urinary retention

   _____ Orthostatic hypotension

   _____ Constipation

   _____ Nausea

3. A nurse is caring for a client with severe pain whose prescription for morphine IV bolus has been changed to transdermal fentanyl (Duragesic). The nurse should understand which of the following information when administering a fentanyl transdermal patch?

   A. Apply a hot pack to the area containing the patch to enhance therapeutic effect.

   B. Administer a short-term opioid for pain for the first 24 hr after patch application.

   C. Have the client replace the patch daily.

   D. Remove the patch for immediate relief of the respiratory depression and do not give any further treatment.

4. A nurse is caring for a client who has back pain and has been prescribed nalbuphine (Nubain). The nurse should know that agonist-antagonist opioids, such as nalbuphine, differ from pure opioid agonists in that they

   A. have a greater risk for abuse due to an increase in euphoria.

   B. cause a higher incidence of respiratory depression.

   C. may not be reversed with an opioid antagonist.

   D. may cause abstinence syndrome in clients physically dependent to opioids.

APPLICATION EXERCISES ANSWER KEY

1. A nurse is monitoring a client who received regular doses of meperidine (Demerol) for post-operative pain for 36 hr. For which of the following should the nurse monitor the client?

    A. Hypothermia

    B. Bradycardia

    C. Delirium

    D. Watery diarrhea

    Repeated use of meperidine can result in accumulation of normeperidine, which can result in neurotoxicity and findings such as irritability, delirium, seizures, and eventually coma and death. Meperidine may be the opioid of choice in some situations, but should not be used for more than 48 hr. Toxicity is more likely in clients who have renal failure. Hypothermia, bradycardia, and watery diarrhea are not expected toxic effects seen in clients receiving meperidine.

 NCLEX® Connection: Pharmacological Therapies, Adverse Effects/Contraindications/ Side Effects/Interactions

2. A nurse is caring for a client who has been receiving morphine for postoperative pain for the past few days. For which of the following should the nurse monitor the client? (Select all that apply.)

    _____ Dilated pupils

    __X__ Urinary retention

    __X__ Orthostatic hypotension

    __X__ Constipation

    __X__ Nausea

    Besides the serious adverse effects of respiratory depression and sedation, a client receiving opioids may also experience urinary retention, orthostatic hypotension, constipation, and nausea/vomiting. Pinpoint pupils (miosis), rather than dilated pupils may occur.

 NCLEX® Connection: Pharmacological Therapies, Adverse Effects/Contraindications/ Side Effects/Interactions

3. A nurse is caring for a client with severe pain whose prescription for morphine IV bolus has been changed to transdermal fentanyl (Duragesic). The nurse should understand which of the following information when administering a fentanyl transdermal patch?

    A. Apply a hot pack to the area containing the patch to enhance therapeutic effect.

    B. Administer a short-term opioid for pain for the first 24 hr after patch application.

    C. Have the client replace the patch daily.

    D. Remove the patch for immediate relief of the respiratory depression and do not give any further treatment.

The full analgesic effect may take up to 24 hr to develop and the client may require short-term opioids during that period of time for breakthrough pain relief. Avoid hot packs, warm water, and a fever which may increase the release of fentanyl from the patch and thus increase the risk of toxicity. Have the client change the patch as prescribed, usually every 48 to 72 hr. Effects of opioid toxicity continue for several hours following transdermal patch removal. The nurse should monitor the client and anticipate that the client may require naloxone (Narcan) to reverse the opioid effects.

 NCLEX® Connection: Pharmacological Therapies, Medication Administration

4. A nurse is caring for a client who has back pain and has been prescribed nalbuphine (Nubain). The nurse should know that agonist-antagonist opioids, such as nalbuphine, differ from pure opioid agonists in that they

    A. have a greater risk for abuse due to an increase in euphoria.

    B. cause a higher incidence of respiratory depression.

    C. may not be reversed with an opioid antagonist.

    D. may cause abstinence syndrome in clients physically dependent to opioids.

Clients physically dependent on opioids may develop withdrawal symptoms with the use of an agonist-antagonist opioid. Symptoms include abdominal pain, fever, and irritability. Agonist-antagonist opioids produce less respiratory depression and have a lower potential for abuse due to less euphoria. They may be reversed or partially reversed with an opioid antagonist, such as naloxone.

 NCLEX® Connection: Pharmacological Therapies, Expected Actions/Outcomes

UNIT 9	MEDICATIONS FOR PAIN AND INFLAMMATION
Chapter 34	Adjuvant Medications for Pain

 Overview

- Use adjuvant medications for pain with a primary pain medication, usually an opioid agonist, to increase pain relief while reducing the dosage of the opioid agonist.

- Reduced dosage of the opioid results in reduced adverse reactions, such as respiratory depression, sedation, and constipation. Targeting pain stimulus using different types of medications often provides improved pain reduction.

- Categories of medications in this section include tricyclic antidepressants, anticonvulsants, CNS stimulants, antihistamines, glucocorticoids, bisphosphonates, and nonsteroidal anti-inflammatory drugs (NSAIDs).

MEDICATION CLASSIFICATION: ADJUVANT MEDICATIONS FOR PAIN

- Select Prototype Medication:

    o Tricyclic antidepressants: Amitriptyline (Elavil) – Oral/IM

    o Anticonvulsants: Carbamazepine (Tegretol), Gabapentin (Neurontin) – Oral

    o CNS stimulants: Methylphenidate (Ritalin) – Oral

    o Antihistamines: Hydroxyzine (Vistaril) – Oral/IM

    o Glucocorticoids: Dexamethasone (Decadron) – Oral, IV, IM

    o Bisphosphonates: Etidronate (Didronel) – Oral

    o NSAIDs: Ibuprofen (Motrin) – Oral

- Other Medications:

    o Tricyclic antidepressants: Imipramine (Tofranil) – Oral

    o Anticonvulsants: Phenytoin (Dilantin) – Oral, IV, IM

    o CNS stimulants: Dextroamphetamine (Dexedrine) – Oral

    o Glucocorticoids: Prednisone (Deltasone) – Oral

    o NSAIDs – Ketorolac (Toradol)

Purpose

- Expected Pharmacological Action

  o Adjuvant medications for pain complement the effects of opioids.

- Therapeutic Uses

  o NSAIDs treat inflammation.

  o Tricyclic antidepressants reduce neuropathic pain, such as cramping, aching, burning, darting, and lancinating pain.

  o Anticonvulsants relieve neuropathic pain.

  o CNS stimulants augment analgesia and decrease sedation.

  o Antihistamines promote analgesia in patients with anxiety.

  o Glucocorticoids decrease pain from intracranial pressure and spinal cord compression.

  o Bisphosphonates manage hypercalcemia and bone pain.

Complications

SIDE/ADVERSE EFFECTS	NURSING INTERVENTIONS/CLIENT EDUCATION
Tricyclic antidepressants: amitriptyline	
Orthostatic hypotension	• Advise clients to sit or lie down if symptoms of lightheadedness or dizziness occur and to change positions slowly. • Provide assistance with ambulation as needed. • Monitor the client's blood pressure while the client is lying down, sitting, and standing.
Sedation	• Advise clients to avoid hazardous activities, such as driving or operating heavy machinery.
Anticholinergic effects, (dry mouth, urinary hesitancy or retention, constipation, and blurred vision)	• Advise clients to increase fluid intake, sip fluids throughout the day, chew gum, or suck on hard candy. • Instruct clients to increase physical activity by engaging in a regular exercise routine. • Administer a stimulant laxative, such as bisacodyl (Dulcolax) to counteract decreased bowel motility, and a stool softener, such as docusate sodium (Colace), to prevent constipation. • Advise clients to void every 4 hr and to report urinary hesitancy or retention. • Advise clients to report blurred vision. • Monitor the client's I/O and check the client's bladder for distention by palpating the lower abdomen area every 4 to 6 hr.

SIDE/ADVERSE EFFECTS	NURSING INTERVENTIONS/CLIENT EDUCATION
Anticonvulsants: carbamazepine, gabapentin	
Bone marrow suppression (bruising, bleeding, fever, sore throat)	• Periodically monitor the client's complete blood count and platelets. • Advise clients to observe for signs and to notify the provider if they occur.
Gastrointestinal (GI) distress (nausea, vomiting, diarrhea)	• Advise clients to take the medication with food.
CNS stimulants: methylphenidate	
Weight loss	• Monitor the client's weight. Encourage good nutrition.
Insomnia	• Instruct clients to take the last dose of the day no later than 4 p.m.
Antihistamines: hydroxyzine	
Sedation	• Advise clients to avoid hazardous activities, such as driving or operating heavy machinery. Reduce dosage in older adult clients.
Dry mouth	• Advise clients to increase fluid intake, sip fluids throughout the day, chew gum, or suck on hard candy.
Glucocorticoids: dexamethasone	
Adrenal insufficiency (hypotension, dehydration, weakness, lethargy, vomiting, diarrhea associated with prolonged use)	• Advise clients to observe for symptoms and to notify the provider if symptoms occur.
Osteoporosis	• Advise clients to take calcium supplements, vitamin D, and/or bisphosphonate (alendronate [Fosamax]) as prescribed.
Hypokalemia	• Monitor the client's potassium levels and administer potassium supplements as needed.
Glucose intolerance	• Monitor the client's blood glucose levels.
Peptic ulcer disease	• Advise clients to take the medication with meals. • Encourage prophylactic use of an H_2 receptor-antagonist such as ranitidine (Zantac).
NSAIDs: ibuprofen	
Bone marrow suppression	• Periodically monitor the client's complete blood count and platelets. • Advise clients to observe for signs of easy bruising and bleeding, fever or sore throat, and to notify the provider if they occur.
GI distress (nausea, vomiting, diarrhea, or coffee-ground emesis; bloody, tarry stools; abdominal pain)	• Advise client to take with food or meals. • Monitor for GI bleed.

Contraindications/Precautions

MEDICATION	CONTRAINDICATIONS
Tricyclic antidepressants – Amitriptyline	• These medications are contraindicated in clients recovering from an MI and within 14 days of taking an MAOI. • Use caution with clients who have a seizure disorder, urinary retention, prostatic hypertrophy, angle-closure glaucoma, hyperthyroidism, and liver or kidney disease.
Anticonvulsants – Carbamazepine, gabapentin	• These medications are contraindicated in clients who have bone marrow suppression and within 14 days of taking a MAOI. • Use caution with clients who have a seizure disorder.
CNS stimulants – Methylphenidate	• Methylphenidate is contraindicated in clients with hyperthyroidism and hypertension and within 14 days of taking an MAOI. • Use caution with clients who have agitation or tics.
Antihistamines – Hydroxyzine	• Hydroxyzine is contraindicated in clients who are hypersensitive to this medication. • Use caution with older adults.
Glucocorticoids – Dexamethasone	• Dexamethasone is contraindicated in clients who have fungal infection. • Use caution with clients who have a seizure disorder, peptic ulcer disease, hypertension, hypothyroidism, diabetes mellitus, or liver disease.
Bisphosphonates – Etidronate	• Etidronate is contraindicated in clients who are hypersensitive to this medication. • Use caution with clients who have kidney disease.
NSAIDs – Ibuprofen	• Ibuprofen is contraindicated in clients who have a history of bronchospasms with aspirin or NSAIDs. • Use caution with clients who have peptic ulcers, hypertension, and liver or kidney disease.

Interactions

MEDICATION/FOOD INTERACTIONS	NURSING INTERVENTIONS/CLIENT EDUCATION
Tricyclic antidepressants: amitriptyline	
Barbiturates, CNS depressants, and alcohol may cause additive CNS depression.	• Do not use together.

MEDICATION/FOOD INTERACTIONS	NURSING INTERVENTIONS/CLIENT EDUCATION
Anticonvulsants: carbamazepine, gabapentin	
Carbamazepine causes a decrease in the effects of oral contraceptives and warfarin (Coumadin) because of the stimulation of hepatic drug-metabolizing enzymes.	• Advise clients to increase dose of oral contraceptives. • Monitor for therapeutic effects of warfarin with PT and INR. • Tell clients the provider may adjust the dosage.
Grapefruit juice inhibits metabolism, and thus increases carbamazepine levels.	• Advise clients to avoid intake of grapefruit juice.
Phenytoin and phenobarbital decrease the effects of carbamazepine.	• Avoid concurrent use.
CNS stimulants: methylphenidate	
Alkalizing medications may cause increase in reabsorption.	• Monitor for increase in amphetamine effects.
Acidifying medications may increase excretion of amphetamine.	• Monitor for decrease in amphetamine effects.
Hypoglycemic agents may decrease glucose level.	• Monitor blood glucose.
MAOIs may cause severe hypertension.	• Avoid concurrent use.
Caffeine may increase stimulant effect.	• Advise clients to avoid caffeine.
OTC medications with sympathomimetic action may lead to increased CNS stimulation.	• Instruct clients to avoid use of OTC medications.
Antihistamines: hydroxyzine	
Barbiturates, CNS depressants, and alcohol may cause additive CNS depression.	• Do not use together.
Glucocorticoids: dexamethasone	
Glucocorticoids promote hyperglycemia, thereby counteracting the effects of hypoglycemic agents.	• Tell clients the provider may increase the dosage of the hypoglycemic agents.
Concurrent use of salicylates and NSAIDs may increase the risk for GI bleed.	• Monitor for GI bleed. Use together cautiously.
Because of the risk for hypokalemia there is an increased risk of dysrhythmias caused by digoxin.	• Monitor serum potassium level and cardiac rhythm. • Administer potassium supplements.
Diuretics that promote potassium loss increase the risk for hypokalemia.	• Monitor serum potassium level. • Encourage clients to eat potassium-rich foods. • Administer potassium supplements.

MEDICATION/FOOD INTERACTIONS	NURSING INTERVENTIONS/CLIENT EDUCATION
NSAIDs: ibuprofen	
NSAIDs may reduce effectiveness of antihypertensives, furosemide, and thiazide diuretics.	• Monitor for medication effectiveness.
Aspirin and corticosteroids may increase GI effects.	• Do not use together.
NSAIDs may increase levels of oral anticoagulants and lithium.	• Monitor medication levels.

Nursing Administration

- Contribute to the client's pain management plan.

- Encourage clients who have cancer to voice fears and concerns about cancer, cancer pain, and pain treatment.

- Advise clients to take pain medications on a fixed schedule around the clock, and not as needed.

- Advise clients that physical dependence is not considered addiction.

Nursing Evaluation of Medication Effectiveness

- Depending on the therapeutic intent, effectiveness may be evidenced by:

  o Relief of depression, seizures, dysrhythmias, and other symptoms that aggravate the client's pain level

  o Decreased opioid side effects

  o Relief of neuropathic pain

  o Decreased cancer bone pain

(A) APPLICATION EXERCISES

1. A nurse is caring for a client who has severe pain and has been receiving hydroxyzine (Vistaril) along with each opioid injection. The client asks why she is receiving the medication. The nurse should recognize that use of adjuvant medications in conjunction with an opioid agonist is to accomplish which of the following?? (Select all that apply.)

    _____ Reduce the dosage of the opioid

    _____ Reduce the side effects of the opioid

    _____ Increase the analgesic effects

    _____ Increase CNS stimulation

    _____ Increase opioid tolerance

2. A nurse is caring for a hospitalized client who has cancer and has a variety of prescribed adjuvant medications which may be administered along with opioids for pain. When the client describes having "burning pain shooting down my leg," which of the following adjuvants should the nurse administer?

    A. Etidronate (Didronel)

    B. Gabapentin (Neurontin)

    C. Methylphenidate (Ritalin)

    D. Hydroxyzine (Vistaril)

3. A nurse is caring for a client who has cancer and is receiving opioids along with prednisone (Deltasone) daily for pain control. While the client is taking prednisone, the nurse should plan to monitor the client for which of the following findings?

    A. Hypoglycemia

    B. GI bleeding

    C. Weight loss

    D. Asthma

4. A nurse is reinforcing teaching for a client who has cancer pain and has a new prescription for methylphenidate (Ritalin). What instructions should the nurse give the client regarding administration of the medication?

APPLICATION EXERCISES ANSWER KEY

1. A nurse is caring for a client who has severe pain and has been receiving hydroxyzine (Vistaril) along with each opioid injection. The client asks why she is receiving the medication. The nurse should recognize that use of adjuvant medications in conjunction with an opioid agonist is to accomplish which of the following?? (Select all that apply.)

    <u> X </u>   **Reduce the dosage of the opioid**

    <u> X </u>   **Reduce the side effects of the opioid**

    <u> X </u>   **Increase the analgesic effects**

    <u>   </u>   Increase CNS stimulation

    <u>   </u>   Increase opioid tolerance

    Use of adjuvant medications for pain with an opioid is to increase pain relief while reducing the dosage of the opioid agonist. Reduced dosage of the opioid agonist results in reduced adverse reactions, such as respiratory depression, sedation, and constipation. Targeting pain stimulus using different types of medications often provides increased pain reduction. Adjuvant medications do not increase CNS stimulation or increase opioid tolerance.

     NCLEX® Connection: Pharmacological Therapies, Expected Actions/Outcomes

2. A nurse is caring for a hospitalized client who has cancer and has a variety of prescribed adjuvant medications which may be administered along with opioids for pain. When the client describes having "burning pain shooting down my leg," which of the following adjuvants should the nurse administer?

    A. Etidronate (Didronel)

    B. Gabapentin (Neurontin)

    C. Methylphenidate (Ritalin)

    D. Hydroxyzine (Vistaril)

    Anticonvulsant medications, such as gabapentin, treat neuropathic pain which stems from a nerve injury and may be described as sharp or burning. Use biphosphonates, such as etidronate, for hypercalcemia and bone pain. Use stimulants, such as methylphenidate, to augment analgesia and decrease sedation. Use antihistamines, such as hydroxyzine, to relieve nausea and anxiety and promote sleep.

     NCLEX® Connection: Pharmacological Therapies, Pharmacological Pain Management

3. A nurse is caring for a client who has cancer and is receiving opioids along with prednisone (Deltasone) daily for pain control. While the client is taking prednisone, the nurse should plan to monitor the client for which of the following findings?

   A. Hypoglycemia

   B. GI bleeding

   C. Weight loss

   D. Asthma

   GI bleeding may occur when using prednisone over time because prednisone increases the risk of peptic ulcer formation. This is more likely to occur if the client takes NSAIDs, which also increase the risk of bleeding. The client taking prednisone is at risk for hyperglycemia, edema, and weight gain. Taking prednisone does not increase a client's risk of asthma.

 NCLEX® Connection: Pharmacological Therapies, Adverse Effects/Contraindications/Side Effects/Interactions

4. A nurse is reinforcing teaching for a client who has cancer pain and has a new prescription for methylphenidate (Ritalin). What instructions should the nurse give the client regarding administration of the medication?

   To prevent problems with insomnia, the client should take his last dose of the day by 4 p.m.

 NCLEX® Connection: Pharmacological Therapies, Medication Administration

| UNIT 9 | MEDICATIONS FOR PAIN AND INFLAMMATION |
| Chapter 35 | Miscellaneous Pain Medications |

Overview

- Pain is subjective and may indicate tissue injury or impending tissue injury.

- Pain may result from the release of chemical mediators, inflammation, or pressure.

- Elevated levels of uric acid, which may accumulate and cause localized inflammation in synovial areas, may result in gout. Antigout medications act either by reducing inflammation or decreasing serum uric acid levels.

- Inflammation and vasodilation of cerebral blood vessels may result in migraine headaches. Use medications to stop an oncoming migraine or to prevent a migraine from occurring.

- Local anesthetics block motor and sensory neurons to a specific area. They may be given topically, injected directly into an area, or given regionally, epidurally, or into the subarachnoid (spinal) space.

MEDICATION CLASSIFICATION: ANTIGOUT MEDICATION

MEDICATIONS	EXPECTED PHARMACOLOGICAL ACTION	THERAPEUTIC USES
Anti-inflammatory agents		
• Select Prototype Medication – Colchicine • Other Medications: ○ NSAIDs – Indomethacin (Indocin), naproxen (Naprosyn), diclofenac (Voltaren)	• These medications decrease inflammation. • Colchicine is only effective for inflammation of gout.	• Abort an acute gout attack if given in response to precursor symptoms • Treatment of acute attacks • Decrease in incidence of acute attacks for clients with chronic gout
○ Glucocorticoids – Prednisone (Deltasone)		• Acute gout for clients who are unable to take or unresponsive to NSAIDs.
Agents for hyperuricemia		
• Select Prototype Medication – Allopurinol (Zyloprim) • Other Medications – Febuxostat (Uloric), probenecid	• Allopurinol inhibits uric acid production. • Probenecid inhibits uric acid reabsorption by renal tubules.	• Hyperuricemia due to chronic gout or secondary to cancer chemotherapy

Route of Administration

- Colchicine – Oral, IV (IV rarely used)

- Allopurinol – Oral, IV

Complications

SIDE/ADVERSE EFFECTS	NURSING INTERVENTIONS/CLIENT EDUCATION
Colchicine	
Mild gastrointestinal (GI) distress which may progress to GI toxicity (abdominal pain, diarrhea, nausea, vomiting)	• Advise clients to take oral medications with food. • Provide antidiarrheal agents as prescribed. • Instruct clients to stop colchicine if symptoms are severe.
Thrombocytopenia, suppressed bone marrow	• Advise clients to notify the provider of bleeding, bruising or sore throat.
Hepatic necrosis	• Monitor liver enzymes.
Allopurinol	
Hypersensitivity reaction, fever, and rash	• Severe reaction may require hemodialysis or glucocorticoids.
Renal injury	• Alkalinize the urine and encourage intake of 2 to 3 L of fluids/day. Monitor I&O, BUN, and serum creatinine.
Hepatitis	• Monitor liver enzymes.
GI distress (nausea and vomiting)	• Give with food.

 Contraindications/Precautions

- Colchicine:

  o Avoid use during pregnancy (Pregnancy Risk Category C with oral use; Category D with IV use).

  o Use cautiously in older adults, clients who are debilitated, and clients who have renal, cardiac, and gastrointestinal dysfunction.

- Allopurinol:

  o Allopurinol is Pregnancy Risk Category C.

  o This medication is contraindicated in clients who have medication hypersensitivity or idiopathic hemochromatosis.

Interactions

MEDICATION/FOOD INTERACTIONS	NURSING INTERVENTIONS/CLIENT EDUCATION
Colchicine	
Salicylates may lessen the effectiveness of probenecid and may precipitate gout.	• Advise clients not to use salicylates during colchicine/probenecid therapy.
Loop diuretics may lessen the effectiveness of colchicine.	• Do not use together.
Alcohol use may lessen the effectiveness of colchicine.	• Do not use together.
Allopurinol	
Allopurinol slows the metabolism of warfarin (Coumadin) within the liver, which places clients at risk for bleeding (bruising, petechiae, hematuria).	• Instruct clients to observe for signs of bleeding and to report to the provider. • Monitor the client's PT and INR levels and administer adjusted dosage.

Nursing Administration

- Monitor CBC and uric acid levels.

- Instruct clients to take the oral form with meals.

- Advise clients to report sore throat, fever, or bleeding.

- Advise clients to avoid aspirin.

- Monitor BUN, serum creatinine, and urine output.

- If a rash develops, advise clients to stop the medication and report the occurrence to the provider.

- Instruct clients to concurrently take preventive measures, such as avoiding alcohol and foods high in purine (red meat, scallops, cream sauces). Encourage clients to consume an adequate intake of water, exercise regularly, and maintain an appropriate body weight.

Nursing Evaluation of Medication Effectiveness

- Depending on the therapeutic intent, effectiveness may be evidenced by:

  ○ Improvement of pain caused by a gout attack (decrease in joint swelling, redness, uric acid levels)

  ○ Decrease in number of gout attacks

  ○ Decrease in uric acid levels

MEDICATION CLASSIFICATION: MIGRAINE MEDICATIONS

- Select Prototype Medications:

  o Ergot alkaloids – Ergotamine (Ergostat)

  o Serotonin receptor agonists (Triptans) – Sumatriptan (Imitrex)

  o Beta-blockers – Propranolol (Inderal)

  o Anticonvulsants – Divalproex (Depakote ER)

  o Tricyclic antidepressants – Mitriptyline (Elavil)

  o Calcium channel blockers – Verapamil (Calan)

  o Estrogens – Estrogen gel and estrogen patches (Alora, Climara, Estraderm) for menstrual migraine

Purpose

- Expected Pharmacological Action

  o Migraine medications prevent the inflammation and dilation of the intracranial blood vessels, thereby relieving migraine pain.

- Therapeutic Uses

  ■ Stop acute migraine attacks

  ■ Prevent migraine attacks

- Route of Administration

  o Ergotamine – Oral, sublingual, rectal

  o Sumatriptan – Oral, subcutaneous, intranasal

  o Propranolol, divalproex, verapamil – Oral

  o Amitriptyline – Oral, IM

Complications

SIDE/ADVERSE EFFECTS	NURSING INTERVENTIONS/CLIENT EDUCATION
Ergot alkaloids: ergotamine	
GI discomfort (nausea and vomiting)	• Administer metoclopramide (Reglan).
Ergotism (muscle pain; paresthesias in fingers and toes; cold, pale extremities)	• Advise clients to stop taking the medication, and immediately seek medical attention.
Physical dependence	• Advise clients not to exceed the prescribed dose. • Inform clients regarding symptoms of withdrawal (headache, nausea, vomiting, restlessness). • Instruct clients to notify the provider if symptoms occur.
Fetal abortion	• Instruct clients to use adequate contraception during therapy.
Serotonin receptor antagonists (Triptans): sumatriptan	
Chest pressure (heavy arms or chest tightness)	• Warn clients about symptoms, and reassure clients that symptoms are self-limiting and not dangerous. • Advise clients to notify the provider for continuous or severe chest pain.
Coronary artery vasospasm/angina	• Do not administer to a client who has, or is at risk for, coronary artery disease (CAD).
Dizziness or vertigo	• Advise client to avoid driving or operating machinery until medication effects are known.
Beta-blockers: propranolol	
Extreme tiredness, fatigue, depression, and asthma exacerbation	• Advise clients to observe for symptoms and notify the provider if they occur.
Bradycardia, hypotension	• Monitor heart rate and blood pressure. Instruct clients to take apical pulse prior to dosage. Notify the provider of significant change.
Anticonvulsants: divalproex	
Neural tube defects	• Instruct clients to use adequate contraception during therapy.
Liver toxicity	• Monitor liver enzymes. Notify the provider of lethargy or fever.
Pancreatitis (abdominal pain, nausea, vomiting, and anorexia)	• Instruct clients to report symptoms. • Tell clients the provider will discontinue the medication.

SIDE/ADVERSE EFFECTS	NURSING INTERVENTIONS/CLIENT EDUCATION
Tricyclic antidepressants: amitriptyline	
Anticholinergic effects (dry mouth, constipation, urinary hesitancy or retention, blurred vision, tachycardia)	• Advise clients to: ○ Increase fiber and fluid intake. ○ Increase physical activity by engaging in regular exercise. ○ Administer stimulant laxatives, such as bisacodyl (Dulcolax), to counteract reduced bowel motility, or stool softeners, such as docusate sodium (Colace), to prevent constipation. ○ Void every 4 hr and report urinary retention. ○ Report blurred vision.
Drowsiness or dizziness	• Advise clients to avoid driving or operating machinery until medication effects are known.
Calcium channel blockers: verapamil	
Orthostatic hypotension or bradycardia	• Advise clients to sit or lie down if symptoms of lightheadedness or dizziness occur and to change positions slowly. • Provide assistance with ambulation as needed. • Monitor heart rate.
Constipation	• Advise clients to increase fiber and fluid intake, and to exercise regularly.

 Contraindications/Precautions

- Ergotamine is contraindicated in clients with renal and/or liver dysfunction, sepsis, and CAD, as well for patients who are pregnant or who are taking triptans.

    ○ Pregnancy Risk Category X

- Triptans are contraindicated in clients with liver failure, ischemic heart disease, a history of myocardial infarction, or uncontrolled hypertension.

    ○ Pregnancy Risk Category C

- Do not administer a triptan within 24 hours of another triptan.

- Propranolol is contraindicated in clients with greater than first-degree heart block, bradycardia, bronchial asthma, cardiogenic shock, or heart failure.

    ○ Use with caution in clients taking other antihypertensives, liver or renal impairment, diabetes mellitus, or Wolff-Parkinson-White syndrome.

    ○ Pregnancy Risk Category C

- Divalproex sodium (Depakote) is contraindicated in clients with liver disease.

  o Pregnancy Risk Category D

- Amitriptyline (Elavil) is contraindicated in clients with recent MI or within 14 days of a MAO inhibitor. Use with caution in clients with seizure history, urinary retention, prostatic hypertrophy, angle-closure glaucoma, hyperthyroidism and others.

  o Pregnancy Risk Category C

- Verapamil is contraindicated in clients with greater than first-degree heart block, bradycardia, hypotension, left ventricle disease, atrial fibrillation or flutter, or heart failure.

  o Use with caution in clients who have liver or renal impairment or increased intracranial pressure.

  o Pregnancy Risk Category C

Interactions

MEDICATION/FOOD INTERACTIONS	NURSING INTERVENTIONS/CLIENT EDUCATION
Ergotamine	
Sumatriptan can lead to spastic reaction of the blood vessels.	• Avoid concurrent use of these medications.
Some HIV protease inhibitors, antifungal medications, and macrolide antibiotics may increase ergotamine levels, causing increased vasospasm.	• Do not use together.
Sumatriptan	
Concurrent use of MAOIs can lead to MAO toxicity.	• Do not give triptans within 2 weeks of stopping MAOIs.
Combining a triptan with an ergot alkaloid or another triptan can lead to spastic reaction of the blood vessels.	• Avoid concurrent use of these medications.
SSRIs may cause weakness and hyperreflexia.	• Monitor carefully.
Propranolol	
Verapamil (Calan) and diltiazem (Cardizem) have additive cardiosuppression effects.	• Monitor ECG, heart rate, and blood pressure.
Diuretics and antihypertensive medications have additive hypotensive effects.	• Monitor blood pressure.
Propranolol use can mask the hypoglycemic effect of insulin and prevent the breakdown of fat in response to hypoglycemia.	• Use with caution for clients with diabetes mellitus. Advise clients who have diabetes to monitor blood glucose.

MEDICATION/FOOD INTERACTIONS	NURSING INTERVENTIONS/CLIENT EDUCATION
Divalproex	
Aspirin, chlorpromazine, and cimetidine may cause divalproex sodium toxicity.	• Monitor medication levels.
Benzodiazepines may cause CNS depression.	• Do not use together.
Divalproex may increase levels of phenobarbital and phenytoin.	• Monitor medication levels.
Amitriptyline	
Barbiturates may cause increased CNS depression.	• Do not use together.
Cimetidine may increase amitriptyline levels.	• Monitor medication effects.
MAOIs may increase CNS excitation or cause seizures.	• Do not give amitriptyline within 2 weeks of stopping MAOIs.
Verapamil	
Carbamazepine and digoxin may increase medication levels.	• Monitor medication levels.
Atenolol, esmolol, propranolol, and timolol may potentiate medication effects.	• Monitor medication effects. • Adjust dosage.

Nursing Administration

- Advise clients who have migraines to avoid trigger factors (stress, alcohol, fatigue, and tyramine-containing foods, such as wine and aged cheese).

- Advise clients that lying down in a dark, quiet place may help ease symptoms.

- Advise clients to check apical pulse before dosage (propranolol).

- Advise clients to take dosage with food to reduce GI distress (Divalproex sodium, verapamil) and increase absorption (propranolol).

- Advise clients to protect skin from sun (amitriptyline) and avoid driving or operating machinery until medication effects are known (amitriptyline, verapamil).

- Advise clients to use caution in case of orthostatic hypotension (amitriptyline).

Nursing Evaluation of Medication Effectiveness

- Depending on the therapeutic intent, effectiveness may be evidenced by:

  o Reduction in intensity and frequency of migraine attacks

  o Prophylaxis against migraine attacks

  o Termination of migraine headaches

MEDICATION CLASSIFICATION: LOCAL ANESTHETICS

- Select Prototype Medications:

  o Amide type – Lidocaine (Xylocaine)

- Other Medications:

  o Ester type – Tetracaine (Pontocaine), procaine (Novocain)

  o Amide type – Eutectic mixture of 2.5% lidocaine/2.5% prilocaine (EMLA Cream)

Purpose

- Expected Pharmacological Action

  o These medications decrease pain by blocking conduction of pain impulses in a circumscribed area. Loss of consciousness does not occur.

- Therapeutic Uses

  o Parenteral administration includes:

    - Pain management for dental procedures, minor surgical procedures, labor and delivery, and diagnostic procedures

    - Regional anesthesia (spinal, epidural)

  o Topical administration includes:

    - Skin and mucous membrane disorders

    - Minor procedures, such as IV insertion, injection (pediatric), and wart removal

Complications

SIDE/ADVERSE EFFECTS	NURSING INTERVENTIONS/CLIENT EDUCATION
CNS excitation (seizures, followed by respiratory depression, leading to unconsciousness)	• Monitor for signs of seizure activity, sedation, change in mental status (decrease in level of consciousness). • Monitor the client's vital signs and respiratory status. • Have equipment ready for resuscitation.
Hypotension, cardiosuppression as evidenced by bradycardia, heart block, and cardiac arrest (common in spinal anesthesia because of sympathetic block)	• Monitor the client's vital signs and ECG. • If symptoms occur, assist with emergency management.
Allergic reactions (more likely with ester-type agents, such as procaine)	• Observe for symptoms of allergy to anesthetics, such as allergic dermatitis or anaphylaxis. • Treat with antihistamines or per agency protocol.

SIDE/ADVERSE EFFECTS	NURSING INTERVENTIONS/CLIENT EDUCATION
During labor and delivery, local anesthetics can result in fetal bradycardia and CNS depression.	• Monitor fetal heart rate (FHR) for bradycardia and decreased variability.
Spinal headache	• Monitor clients for signs of severe headache. • Advise client to remain flat in bed for 12 hr postprocedure.
Urinary retention (can occur with spinal anesthesia)	• Monitor the client's urinary output. • Notify the provider if clients have not voided within 8 hr.

 Contraindications/Precautions

- Local anesthetics are Pregnancy Risk Category B.

- These medications are contraindicated in clients with supraventricular dysrhythmias and/or heart block.

- Use cautiously in clients who have liver and kidney dysfunction, heart failure, and myasthenia gravis.

Interactions

MEDICATION/FOOD INTERACTIONS	NURSING INTERVENTIONS/CLIENT EDUCATION
Antihypertensive medications have additive hypotensive effects with parenteral administration of local anesthetics.	• Monitor heart rate and blood pressure.

Nursing Administration

- Advise clients to avoid hazardous activities when recovering from anesthesia.

- Maintain clients in a comfortable position during recovery.

- Injection of local anesthetic

  o Vasoconstrictors, such as epinephrine (adrenaline), are often used in combination of local anesthetics to prevent the spread of the local anesthetic. Containing the local anesthetic prolongs the anesthesia and decreases the chance of systemic toxicity.

  o Prepare injection site for local anesthetic.

  o Maintain IV access for administration of emergency medications if necessary.

  o Have equipment ready for resuscitation.

  o For regional block, protect the area of numbness from injury.

- Spinal or epidural nerve blocks

- Monitor during insertion for hypotension, anaphylaxis, seizure, and dura puncture.

- Monitor for respiratory depression and sedation.

- Monitor insertion site for hematoma and signs of an infection.

- Check level of sensory block. Evaluate leg strength prior to ambulating.

- Client Education

  - Advise clients to notify the provider for signs of infection, such as fever, swelling and redness, increase in pain or severe headache, sudden weakness to lower extremities, or decrease in bowel or bladder control.

  - Notify the provider for signs of systemic infection, such as a metallic taste, ringing in ears, perioral numbness, and seizures.

- Topical cream (EMLA):

  - Apply to intact skin 1 hr before routine procedures or superficial puncture and 2 hr before more extensive procedures or deep puncture. Cover with occlusive dressing.

  - Prior to the procedure, remove the dressing and clean the skin with aseptic solution.

  - Instruct clients to apply EMLA at home prior to coming to a health care facility for a procedure.

Nursing Evaluation of Medication Effectiveness

- Depending on the therapeutic intent, effectiveness may be evidenced by the following:

  - The client undergoes procedure without experiencing pain

  - The client reports a decrease in pain level.

APPLICATION EXERCISES

1. A nurse is providing teaching to a client who is to start colchicine (Colgout) for acute gouty arthritis. The nurse should advise the client to do which of the following? (Select all that apply.)

     _____ Decrease fluid intake.

     _____ Avoid alcohol use.

     _____ Take the medication on an empty stomach to increase absorption.

     _____ Notify the provider of bleeding, bruising, or sore throat.

     _____ Avoid aspirin or products containing salicylates.

2. A nurse is caring for a client who has severe pain in his right foot. Which of the following laboratory values tell the nurse that the client is having a flare-up of gout?

     A. Increased serum creatinine

     B. Decreased creatine kinase

     C. Decreased total protein

     D. Increased uric acid

3. A nurse is caring for a client who has migraine headaches and is planning to ask her provider for a prescription for ergotamine (Ergostat), which she heard is helpful for treating migraines. The nurse should be aware that ergotamine is contraindicated for clients who have which of the following conditions?

     A. Seizure disorders

     B. Angle closure glaucoma

     C. Coronary artery disease

     D. Peptic ulcer disease

4. A nurse is reinforcing teaching to a client with migraine headaches who has a new prescription for sumatriptan (Imitrex). The nurse should plan to monitor the client for which of the following?

     A. Nausea and vomiting

     B. Pressure in the chest

     C. Fever and sore throat

     D. Bleeding and bruising

5. A nurse is caring for a postoperative client who received spinal anesthesia. For which of the following adverse effects should the nurse monitor the client? (Select all that apply.)

     _____ Hypotension

     _____ Tachycardia

     _____ Sedation

     _____ Urinary retention

     _____ Headache

APPLICATION EXERCISES ANSWER KEY

1. A nurse is providing teaching to a client who is to start colchicine (Colgout) for acute gouty arthritis. The nurse should advise the client to do which of the following? (Select all that apply.)

    _____ Decrease fluid intake.

    __X__ **Avoid alcohol use.**

    _____ Take the medication on an empty stomach to increase absorption.

    __X__ **Notify the provider of sore throat, fever, or bruising.**

    __X__ **Avoid aspirin or products containing salicylates.**

    Colchicine is an anti-inflammatory agent limited to the treatment of gout. Instruct the client to take it with food to reduce GI symptoms, and to stop the medication for severe GI effects that may lead to hemorrhagic gastroenteritis. Instruct the client to increase fluid intake, avoid alcohol, and notify the provider of a sore throat, fever, or bruising. Instruct the client to avoid aspirin and salicylates.

     NCLEX® Connection: Pharmacological Therapies, Medication Administration

2. A nurse is caring for a client who has severe pain in his right foot. Which of the following laboratory values tell the nurse that the client is having a flare-up of gout?

    A. Increased serum creatinine

    B. Decreased creatine kinase

    C. Decreased total protein

    D. Increased uric acid

    Hyperuricemia is found in clients who are experiencing an episode of gout. Increased serum creatinine, decreased creatine kinase, and decreased total protein do not characterize gout.

     NCLEX® Connection: Physiological Adaptations, Basic Pathophysiology

3. A nurse is caring for a client who has migraine headaches and is planning to ask her provider for a prescription for ergotamine (Ergostat), which she heard is helpful for treating migraines. The nurse should be aware that ergotamine is contraindicated for clients who have which of the following conditions?

    A. Seizure disorders

    B. Angle closure glaucoma

    C. Coronary artery disease

    D. Peptic ulcer disease

    Ergotamine constricts dilated blood vessels in the brain and is contraindicated in clients with coronary artery disease, peripheral vascular disease, and renal or liver disease. It is also contraindicated in pregnancy because it may cause uterine contractions. Ergotamine is not contraindicated for clients with a seizure disorder, those who have angle closure glaucoma, or those with peptic ulcer disease.

     NCLEX® Connection: Pharmacological Therapies, Adverse Effects/Contraindications/Side Effects/Interactions

4. A nurse is reinforcing teaching to a client with migraine headaches who has a new prescription for sumatriptan (Imitrex). The nurse should plan to monitor the client for which of the following?

    A. Nausea and vomiting

    B. Pressure in the chest

    C. Fever and sore throat

    D. Bleeding and bruising

    The nurse should advise the client that pressure in the chest occurs frequently when taking sumatriptan and that this symptom is not related to heart disease. Clients who actually have coronary artery disease should not take sumatriptan. Nausea/vomiting, fever and sore throat (signs of infection), and bleeding/bruising, are not adverse effects of sumatriptan.

     NCLEX® Connection: Pharmacological Therapies, Adverse Effects/Contraindications/Side Effects/Interactions

5. A nurse is caring for a postoperative client who received spinal anesthesia. For which of the following adverse effects should the nurse monitor the client? (Select all that apply.)

__X__	**Hypotension**
_____	Tachycardia
_____	Sedation
__X__	**Urinary retention**
__X__	**Headache**

    The nurse should monitor the client for hypotension, urinary retention, and spinal headache. The nurse should notify the provider if the client has not voided within 8 hr after spinal anesthesia. Have the client lie supine for about 12 hr following surgery to prevent a spinal headache. Tachycardia and sedation are not adverse effects expected from spinal anesthesia.

     NCLEX® Connection: Pharmacological Therapies, Adverse Effects/Contraindications/Side Effects/Interactions

UNIT 10: MEDICATIONS AFFECTING THE ENDOCRINE SYSTEM

- Diabetes Mellitus

- Endocrine Disorders

NCLEX® CONNECTIONS

When reviewing the chapters in this section, keep in mind the relevant sections of the NCLEX® outline, in particular:

CLIENT NEEDS: PHARMACOLOGICAL THERAPIES

Relevant topics/tasks include:
- Adverse Effects/Contraindications/Side Effects/Interactions
  - Reinforce client teaching on possible effects of medications.
- Expected Actions/Outcomes
  - Reinforce education to client regarding medications.
- Medication Administration
  - Mix client medication from two vials as necessary.

UNIT 10   MEDICATIONS AFFECTING THE ENDOCRINE SYSTEM

Chapter 36   Diabetes Mellitus

 Overview

- Diabetes mellitus is a chronic illness that results from an absolute or relative deficiency of insulin.

   o   Various insulins are available to manage diabetes. These medications differ in their onset, peak, and duration.

   o   Oral hypoglycemic agents work in various ways to increase available insulin or modify carbohydrate metabolism.

   o   There are now newer injectable medications to supplement insulin or oral agents to manage blood glucose control.

MEDICATION CLASSIFICATION: INSULIN

- Select Prototype Medications

CLASSIFICATION	GENERIC (TRADE NAME)	ONSET	PEAK	DURATION
Rapid-acting	Insulin lispro (Humalog)	Less than 15 min	0.5 to 1 hr	3 to 4 hr
Short-acting	Regular insulin (Humulin R)	0.5 to 1 hr	2 to 3 hr	5 to 7 hr
Intermediate-acting	NPH insulin (Humulin N)	1 to 2 hr	4 to 12 hr	18 to 24 hr
Long-acting	Insulin glargine (Lantus)	1 hr	None	10.4 to 24 hr

- Other Medications

CLASSIFICATION	GENERIC (TRADE NAME)
Rapid-acting	• Insulin aspart (NovoLog) • Insulin glulisine (Apidra)
Short-acting	• Regular insulin (Novolin R)
Intermediate-acting	• Insulin detemir (Levemir)

- Premixed insulins

  - 70% NPH and 30% Regular (Humulin 70/30) – mixture of intermediate acting and short-acting insulin

  - 75% insulin lispro protamine and 25% insulin lispro (Humalog Mix 75/25) – mixture of intermediate acting and rapid-acting insulin

Purpose

- Expected Pharmacological Action

  - Promotes cellular uptake of glucose (decreases glucose levels)

  - Converts glucose into glycogen

  - Moves potassium into cells (along with glucose)

- Therapeutic Uses

  - Blood glucose control of diabetes mellitus (type 1, type 2, gestational) to prevent complications.

  - Clients who have type 2 diabetes mellitus may require insulin when:

    - Oral hypoglycemics, diet, and exercise are unable to control blood glucose levels

    - Severe renal or liver disease is present

    - Painful neuropathy is present

    - Undergoing surgery or diagnostic tests

    - Experiencing severe stress such as infection and trauma

    - Undergoing emergency treatment of diabetes ketoacidosis (DKA) and hyperosmolar hyperglycemic nonketotic syndrome (HHNS)

    - Requiring treatment of hyperkalemia

Complications

SIDE/ADVERSE EFFECTS	NURSING INTERVENTIONS/CLIENT EDUCATION
<ul><li>Risk for hypoglycemia (too much insulin)</li><li>If abrupt onset, client will experience sympathetic nervous system (SNS) symptoms (tachycardia, palpitations, diaphoresis, shakiness).</li><li>If gradual onset, client will experience parasympathetic nervous system (PNS) symptoms (headache, tremors, weakness).</li></ul>	<ul><li>Monitor clients for signs of hypoglycemia.</li><li>Administer glucose. For conscious clients, administer a snack of 15 g of carbohydrate (4 oz [120 mL] orange juice, 2 oz [60 mL] grape juice, 8 oz [240 mL] milk, glucose tablets per manufacturer's suggestion to equal 15 g).</li><li>If client is not fully conscious, do not risk aspiration. Administer SC/IM glucagon.</li><li>Encourage clients to wear a medical alert bracelet.</li></ul>
<ul><li>Lipohypertrophy</li></ul>	<ul><li>Instruct clients to systematically rotate injection sites and to allow 1 inch between injection sites.</li></ul>

Interactions

MEDICATION/FOOD INTERACTIONS	NURSING INTERVENTIONS/CLIENT EDUCATION
Sulfonylureas, meglitinides, beta blockers, and alcohol have additive hypoglycemic effects with concurrent use.	• Monitor the client's serum glucose levels for hypoglycemia (less than 50 mg/dL) and adjust insulin or oral hypoglycemic dosages accordingly.
Concurrent use of thiazide diuretics and glucocorticoids may raise blood glucose levels and thereby counteract the effects of insulin.	• Monitor the client's serum glucose levels for hyperglycemia and adjust insulin doses accordingly. Tell clients the provider may prescribe a higher insulin dose.
Beta blockers may mask SNS response to hypoglycemia (tachycardia, tremors), making it difficult for clients to identify hypoglycemia.	• Advise clients of the importance of monitoring blood glucose levels and not relying on SNS symptoms as an alert to developing hypoglycemia. • Instruct clients to maintain a regular eating schedule to ensure adequate glucose during times of hypoglycemic action.

Nursing Administration

- Adjust the client's insulin dosage to meet insulin needs.

  o Administer an increased dose in response to the client's increase in caloric intake, infection, stress, growth spurts, and in the second and third trimesters of pregnancy.

  o Administer a reduced dose in response to level of exercise or first trimester of pregnancy.

- Ensure adequate glucose is available at the time of onset of insulin and during all peak times.

- When mixing short-acting insulin with longer-acting insulin, draw the short-acting insulin up into the syringe first, then the longer-acting insulin. This prevents the possibility of accidentally injecting some of the longer-acting insulin into the shorter-acting insulin vial (this can pose a risk for unexpected insulin effects with subsequent uses of the vial).

- Gently rotate the vial of insulin suspensions between the palms to disperse the particles throughout the vial prior to withdrawing insulin.

- Do not administer short-acting insulins, insulin glargine or insulin detemir if they appear cloudy or discolored. These insulins are clear.

- Do not mix insulin glargine and insulin detemir in a syringe with any other insulin.

- Administer lispro, aspart, glulisine, and regular insulins by subcutaneous injection or continuous subcutaneous infusion. These insulins may also be administered by the IV route, but only regular insulin is used routinely.

- Administer NPH, insulin glargine, and insulin detemir by subcutaneous route.

- Instruct clients to administer SC insulin in one general area for consistent rates of absorption. Absorption rates from subcutaneous tissue increase from thigh to upper arm to abdomen.

- Use only insulin-specific syringes that correspond to the concentration of insulin being administered. Administer U-100 insulin with an U-100 syringe; administer U-500 insulin with an U-500 syringe.

- Select an appropriate needle length to ensure insulin is injected into subcutaneous tissue versus intradermal (too short) or intramuscular (too long).

- Encourage clients to enhance their diabetes medication therapy with a proper diet and consistent activity.

- Instruct clients in proper storage of insulin.

  o Store unopened vials of a single type of insulin in the refrigerator until their expiration date.

  o Store vials of premixed insulins for up to 3 months.

  o Keep insulins premixed in syringes for 1 to 2 weeks under refrigeration. Keep the syringes in a vertical position, with the needles pointing up. Prior to administration, resuspend the insulin by gently moving the syringe.

  o Store the vial that is in use at room temperature, avoiding proximity to sunlight and intense heat. Discard after 1 month.

MEDICATION CLASSIFICATION: ORAL HYPOGLYCEMICS

MEDICATIONS	EXPECTED PHARMACOLOGICAL ACTION

Sulfonylureas
• Select Prototype Medications:
  o 1st generation – tolbutamide (Orinase)
  o 2nd generation – glipizide (Glucotrol, Glucotrol XL)
• Other Medications:
  o 1st generation – chlorpropamide (Diabinese)
  o 2nd generation – glyburide (DiaBeta, Micronase) glimepiride (Amaryl)
	• Results in insulin release from the pancreas

Meglitinides • Select Prototype Medication – Repaglinide (Prandin) • Other Medication – Nateglinide (Starlix)	• Results in insulin release from the pancreas
Biguanides • Select Prototype Medication – Metformin (Glucophage)	• Reduces the production of glucose within the liver through suppression of gluconeogenesis • Increases muscles' glucose uptake and use
Thiazolidinediones (Glitazones) • Select Prototype Medication – Rosiglitazone (Avandia) • Other Medication – Pioglitazone (Actos)	• Increases cellular response to insulin by decreasing insulin resistance • Results in increased glucose uptake and decreased glucose production

MEDICATIONS	EXPECTED PHARMACOLOGICAL ACTION
Alpha glucosidase inhibitors • Select Prototype Medication – Acarbose (Precose) • Other Medications – Miglitol (Glyset)	• Slows carbohydrate absorption and digestion
Gliptins • Sitagliptin (Januvia)	• Augments naturally occurring incretin hormones, which promote release of insulin and decrease secretion of glucagon • Lowers fasting and postprandial blood glucose levels

- Therapeutic Uses

  o All classifications of oral hypoglycemic agents control blood glucose levels in clients who have type 2 diabetes mellitus and are used in conjunction with diet and exercise life-style changes.

  o Metformin is used to treat polycystic ovary syndrome (PCOS).

Complications

SIDE/ADVERSE EFFECTS	NURSING INTERVENTIONS/CLIENT EDUCATION
Glipizide and repaglinide	
• Hypoglycemia • If abrupt onset, the client will experience SNS symptoms such as tachycardia, palpitations, diaphoresis, and shakiness. • If gradual onset, the client will experience PNS symptoms such as headache, tremors, and weakness.	• Monitor clients for signs of hypoglycemia. • Instruct clients to self-administer a snack of 15 g of carbohydrate (4 oz [120 mL] orange juice, 2 oz [60 mL] grape juice, 8 oz [240 mL] milk, glucose tablets per manufacturer's suggestion to equal 15 g). • Instruct clients to notify the provider if there is a recurrent problem. • Treat severe hypoglycemia with IV glucose. • Encourage clients to wear a medical alert bracelet.
Metformin HCl	
Gastrointestinal (GI) effects (anorexia, nausea, vomiting – which frequently results in weight loss of 3 to 4 kg [6 to 8 lb])	• Monitor clients for severity of these effects. • Tell clients the provider may discontinue the medication.
Vitamin B$_{12}$ and folic acid deficiency caused by altered absorption	• Provide supplements as needed.
Lactic acidosis (hyperventilation, myalgia, sluggishness, somnolence) – 50% mortality rate	• Instruct clients to discontinue medication if these symptoms occur, and to inform the provider immediately. • Treat severe lactic acidosis with hemodialysis.

SIDE/ADVERSE EFFECTS	NURSING INTERVENTIONS/CLIENT EDUCATION
Rosiglitazone	
Fluid retention	• Monitor clients for edema, weight gain, and/or signs of heart failure.
Elevations in low density lipoproteins (LDL) cholesterol	• Monitor the client's cholesterol levels.
Hepatotoxicity (jaundice or dark urine).	• Perform baseline and periodic liver function tests. • Instruct clients to report any hepatotoxicity symptoms.
Acarbose	
Intestinal effects (abdominal distention and cramping, hyperactive bowel sounds, diarrhea, excessive gas)	• Monitor impact of these symptoms on clients. • Tell clients the provider may discontinue the medication.
Risk for anemia due to the decrease of iron absorption	• Monitor the client's hemoglobin and iron levels. • Discontinue the medication if necessary.
Hepatoxicity with long-term use	• Check the client's baseline liver function and perform periodic liver function tests. • Tell clients the provider may discontinue the medication. • Advise clients that liver function will return to normal after the medication is discontinued.
Sitagliptin – Generally well tolerated	

 Contraindications/Precautions

- Pregnancy Risk Category C – Glipizide, repaglinide, rosiglitazone

- Pregnancy Risk Category B – Metformin HCl (Glucophage), acarbose (Precose), sitagliptin (Januvia)

- These oral agents are generally avoided in pregnancy and lactation, but the provider may decide to prescribe them.

- Use cautiously in clients who have renal failure, hepatic dysfunction, or heart failure because of the risk of medication accumulation and resulting hypoglycemia. Severity of disease may indicate contraindication.

- Contraindicated in the treatment of diabetic ketoacidosis (DKA)

- Metformin HCl is contraindicated for clients who have severe infection, shock, and any hypoxic condition.

- Acarbose is contraindicated for clients who have gastrointestinal (GI) disorders, such as inflammatory disease, ulceration, or obstruction.

Interactions

MEDICATION/FOOD INTERACTIONS	NURSING INTERVENTIONS/CLIENT EDUCATION
Glipizide	
Use of alcohol can result in disulfiram-like reaction (intense nausea and vomiting, flushing, palpitations).	• Inform clients about the risk and encourage them to avoid alcohol.
Alcohol, NSAIDs, sulfonamide antibiotics, ranitidine (Zantac), and cimetidine (Tagamet) have additive hypoglycemia effect.	• Inform clients of the risk and encourage them to avoid alcohol. • Instruct clients to closely monitor blood glucose levels.
Beta-adrenergic blockers may mask SNS response to hypoglycemia (tachycardia, tremors, palpitations, diaphoresis), making it difficult for clients to identify hypoglycemia.	• Advise clients of the importance of monitoring blood glucose levels and not relying on SNS symptoms as an alert to developing hypoglycemia. • Instruct clients to maintain a regular eating schedule to ensure adequate glucose during times of hypoglycemic action.
Repaglinide and rosiglitazone	
Concurrent use of gemfibrozil (Lopid) results in inhibition of repaglinide metabolism, leading to an increased risk for hypoglycemia.	• Avoid concurrent use of repaglinide and gemfibrozil. • Monitor clients for signs of hypoglycemia with concurrent use.
Metformin	
Alcohol increases the risk of lactic acidosis with concurrent use.	• Inform clients of the risks and encourage them to avoid consuming alcohol.
Concurrent use of iodine-containing contrast for diagnostic tests may result in acute renal failure.	• Clients taking metformin should discontinue medication 24 to 48 hr prior to procedure. They may resume medication 48 hr after test if lab results indicate normal renal function.
Acarbose	
Concurrent use of acarbose with sulfonylureas or insulin increases the risk for hypoglycemia.	• Monitor clients for signs of hypoglycemia with concurrent use.
Concurrent use of metformin causes additive gastrointestinal effects and risk for hypoglycemia.	• If acarbose is combined with metformin, monitor clients carefully for gastrointestinal symptoms and hypoglycemia.
Sitagliptin – No significant interactions	

Nursing Administration

- Encourage clients to consistently exercise and to follow appropriate dietary guidelines.

- Encourage clients to maintain a log of blood glucose levels and to note patterns that impact glucose levels (increased dietary intake, infection).

- Request a referral to a registered dietician and/or diabetic nurse educator if indicated.

- Administer medications orally at appropriate times:

  o Glipizide – Instruct clients it's best taken 30 min prior to a meal.

  o Repaglinide – Instruct clients to eat within 30 min of taking a dose of the medication, three times a day.

  o Metformin – Instruct clients to take immediate-release tablets twice a day with breakfast and dinner and to take sustained-release tablets once a day with dinner.

  o Rosiglitazone – Instruct clients to take once or twice a day, with or without food.

  o Acarbose – Instruct clients to take with the first bite of food, three times a day. If a dose is missed, instruct clients to take the dose at the next meal but not to take two doses.

  o Sitagliptin – Instruct clients to take once a day with or without food

- Instruct clients that formulations may combine two medications.

- Instruct clients who are also taking insulin to monitor for signs of hypoglycemia.

MEDICATION CLASSIFICATION: AMYLIN MIMETICS

- Select prototype medication – Pramlintide (Symlin)

Purpose

- Expected Pharmacological Action

  o Pramlintide mimics the actions of the naturally occurring peptide hormone amylin, resulting in reduction of postprandial blood glucose levels from decreased gastric emptying time and inhibition of secretion of glucagon. There is also an increase in the sensation of satiety, which helps decrease caloric intake.

- Therapeutic Uses

  o Supplemental glucose control for clients who have type 1 or type 2 diabetes

  o Use in conjunction with insulin or an oral hypoglycemic agent, usually metformin or a sulfonylurea

Complications

SIDE/ADVERSE EFFECTS	NURSING INTERVENTIONS/CLIENT EDUCATION
Nausea	Instruct clients to report symptom to the provider. Tell clients the provider may decrease the dose.
Reaction at injection sites	Generally self-limiting

Contraindications/Precautions

- Pramlintide is Pregnancy Risk Category C.

- This medication is contraindicated for clients who have renal failure or are receiving dialysis.

- Use cautiously in clients who have thyroid disease, osteoporosis, or alcoholism.

Interactions

MEDICATION/FOOD INTERACTIONS	NURSING INTERVENTIONS/CLIENT EDUCATION
Insulin increases risk for hypoglycemia.	Concurrent use may require decrease in insulin dose, usually 50% of rapid- or short-acting insulin. Avoid use in clients unable to self-monitor blood glucose levels.
Concurrent use with medications that slow gastric emptying such as opioids, or medications that delay food absorption, such as acarbose, may further slow gastric emptying time.	Avoid concurrent use.
Oral medication absorption is delayed.	Administer oral medications 1 hr before or 2 hr after injection of pramlintide.

Nursing Administration

- Administer subcutaneously prior to meals, using the thigh or abdomen.

- Instruct clients to keep unopened vials in the refrigerator and not to freeze. Instruct clients to keep opened vials cool or at room temperature and to discard them after 28 days. Keep vials out of direct sunlight.

- Instruct clients not to mix medication with insulin in the same syringe.

MEDICATION CLASSIFICATION: INCRETIN MIMETICS

- Select Prototype Medication – Exenatide (Byetta)

Purpose

- Expected Pharmacological Action

  ○ Mimics the effects of naturally occurring glucagon-like peptide-1, and thereby promotes release of insulin, decreases secretion of glucagon, and slows gastric emptying. This results in lowered fasting and postprandial blood glucose levels.

- Therapeutic Uses

  ○ Supplemental glucose control for clients who have type 2 diabetes

  ○ May be used in conjunction with an oral hypoglycemic agent, usually metformin or a sulfonylurea

Complications

SIDE/ADVERSE EFFECTS	NURSING INTERVENTIONS/CLIENT EDUCATION
GI effects (nausea, vomiting and diarrhea)	Instruct clients to notify provider if symptoms are intolerable.
Pancreatitis (severe and intolerable abdominal pain)	Instruct clients to stop taking medication and to notify provider.

Contraindications/Precautions

- Pregnancy Risk Category C

- Contraindicated with clients who have renal failure, ulcerative colitis, Crohn's disease

- Use cautiously in older adult clients and clients who have renal impairment or thyroid disease.

Interactions

MEDICATION/FOOD INTERACTIONS	NURSING INTERVENTIONS/CLIENT EDUCATION
Oral medication absorption is delayed, especially oral contraceptives and antibiotics.	Administer oral medications 1 hr before or 2 hr after injection of exenatide.
Concurrent use of sulfonylurea increases risk of hypoglycemia.	Clients may require a lower dose of sulfonylurea. Instruct clients to monitor blood glucose levels.

Nursing Administration

- Instruct clients that this medication is supplied in prefilled injector pens.

- Administer subcutaneously in the thigh, abdomen, or upper arms.

- Give injection within 60 min before the morning and evening meal. Never administer after a meal.

- Instruct clients to keep the injection pen in the refrigerator and to discard after 30 days.

Nursing Evaluation of Medication Effectiveness

- Depending on therapeutic intent, effectiveness may be evidenced by:

  ○ Preprandial glucose levels of 90 to 130 mg/dL and postprandial levels of less than 180 mg/dL

  ○ HgbA1c less than 7%

MEDICATION CLASSIFICATION: HYPERGLYCEMIC AGENT

- Select Prototype Medication – Glucagon

Purpose

- Expected Pharmacological Action

  o Increases blood glucose levels by increasing the breakdown of glycogen into glucose, decreasing glycogen synthesis enhances the synthesis of glucose

- Therapeutic Uses

  o Emergency management of hypoglycemic reactions, such as insulin overdose in clients who do not have IV glucose available or clients who are unable to take oral glucose

  o Decrease in gastrointestinal motility in clients undergoing radiological procedures of the stomach and intestines

Complications

SIDE/ADVERSE EFFECTS	NURSING INTERVENTIONS/CLIENT EDUCATION
GI distress (nausea, vomiting)	Turn clients onto their left side following administration to reduce the risk of aspiration if emesis occurs.

 Contraindications/Precautions

- Glucagon is ineffective for hypoglycemia resulting from inadequate glycogen stores (starvation).

- This medication is Pregnancy Risk Category B.

- Use cautiously in clients who have cardiovascular disease.

Nursing Administration

- Administer glucagon SC, or IM immediately following reconstitution parameters.

- Provide food as soon as the client regains full consciousness and is able to swallow.

- Instruct clients to maintain access to a source of glucose and glucagon kit at all times.

Nursing Evaluation of Medication Effectiveness

- Depending on therapeutic intent, effectiveness may be evidenced by:

  o Elevation in blood glucose level to greater than 50 mg/dL

Ⓐ APPLICATION EXERCISES

1. Match each of the following types of insulin with the time of its onset:

    _____ NPH insulin (Humulin N)   A. Less than 15 min

    _____ Insulin glargine (Lantus)   B. 0.5 to 1 hr

    _____ Regular insulin (Humulin R)   C. 1 to 2 hr

    _____ Lispro insulin (Humalog)   D. 1 hr

2. A nurse is caring for a group of clients who need insulin injections. The nurse should recognize that he can mix which of the following insulins in the same syringe with another insulin? (Select all that apply.)

    _____ Insulin detemir (Levemir)

    _____ Insulin lispro (Humalog)

    _____ Insulin glargine (Lantus)

    _____ Insulin glulisine (Apidra)

    _____ Insulin aspart (Novolog)

3. A nurse is caring for a client who has type 2 diabetes mellitus and a prescription for rosiglitazone (Avandia). For which of the following findings should the nurse monitor the client?

    A. Edema

    B. Palpitations

    C. Seizures

    D. Urinary retention

4. A nurse is reinforcing teaching for a client newly diagnosed who has type 2 diabetes mellitus. Which of the following should the nurse include in the teaching? (Select all that apply.)

    _____ Check blood glucose levels less frequently when feeling ill.

    _____ Take an extra dose of the oral hypoglycemic agent the next day if a dose is missed.

    _____ Carry a fast-acting glucose source at all times.

    _____ Eat a snack prior to planned exercise.

    _____ Inspect feet surfaces daily.

5. A nurse is reinforcing teaching to a client who is prescribed pramlintide (Symlin) for type 1 diabetes. Which of the following should the nurse include in the teaching?

    A. Use subcutaneous tissue in the upper arms as an injection site.

    B. Expect a lower risk for hypoglycemia when using pramlintide with insulin.

    C. Take oral medications 1 hr before or 2 hr after pramlintide.

    D. Discard open vials of pramlintide after 3 months.

APPLICATION EXERCISES ANSWER KEY

1. Match each of the following types of insulin with the time of its onset:

__C__	NPH insulin (Humulin N)	A. Less than 15 min
__D__	Insulin glargine (Lantus)	B. 0.5 to 1 hr
__B__	Regular insulin (Humulin R)	C. 1 to 2 hr
__A__	Lispro insulin (Humalog)	D. 1 hr

     NCLEX® Connection: Pharmacological Therapies, Expected Actions/Outcomes

2. A nurse is caring for a group of clients who need insulin injections. The nurse should recognize that he can mix which of the following insulins in the same syringe with another insulin? (Select all that apply.)

    > _____ Insulin detemir (Levemir)
    > **__X__ Insulin lispro (Humalog)**
    > _____ Insulin glargine (Lantus)
    > **__X__ Insulin glulisine (Apidra)**
    > **__X__ Insulin aspart (Novolog)**

    Only four types of clear insulin may be mixed in the same syringe with another insulin (usually NPH insulin). These include insulin lispro, regular insulin, insulin glulisine, and insulin aspart. Do not mix insulin detemir and insulin glargine in a syringe with another insulin.

    NCLEX® Connection: Pharmacological Therapies, Medication Administration

3. A nurse is caring for a client who has type 2 diabetes mellitus and a prescription for rosiglitazone (Avandia). For which of the following findings should the nurse monitor the client?

    A. Edema
    B. Palpitations
    C. Seizures
    D. Urinary retention

    The client who takes rosiglitazone is at risk for edema and weight gain. The nurse should monitor the client who takes rosiglitazone and has mild heart failure carefully. Rosiglitazone is contraindicated for clients with severe heart failure. The client is not at risk for palpitations, seizures, or urinary retention while taking the medication.

     NCLEX® Connection: Pharmacological Therapies, Adverse Effects/Contraindications/Side Effects/Interactions.

4. A nurse is reinforcing teaching for a client newly diagnosed who has type 2 diabetes mellitus. Which of the following should the nurse include in the teaching? (Select all that apply.)

_____ Check blood glucose levels less frequently when feeling ill.

_____ Take an extra dose of the oral hypoglycemic agent the next day if a dose is missed.

__X__ **Carry a fast-acting glucose source at all times.**

__X__ **Eat a snack prior to planned exercise.**

__X__ **Inspect feet surfaces daily.**

A client who has diabetes should always carry a fast-acting glucose source to treat unexpected hypoglycemia. Active muscle cells can take in glucose without insulin, and therefore prior to exercising the client should eat a snack to ensure enough glucose is available to prevent hypoglycemia. A client who has diabetes should inspect his feet daily to monitor for skin breakdown and signs of infection. A client who has newly diagnosed diabetes should check blood glucose levels at least before meals and at bedtime, and more frequently when ill as acute illness can lead to hyperglycemia. The client should not take an extra dose of medication if a dose is missed.

 NCLEX® Connection: Pharmacological Therapies, Medication Administration

5. A nurse is reinforcing teaching to a client who is prescribed pramlintide (Symlin) for type 1 diabetes. Which of the following should the nurse include in the teaching?

A. Use subcutaneous tissue in the upper arms as an injection site.

B. Expect a lower risk for hypoglycemia when using pramlintide with insulin.

C. Take oral medications 1 hr before or 2 hr after pramlintide.

D. Discard open vials of pramlintide after 3 months.

Oral medication absorption is delayed by pramlintide and should be taken 1 hr before or 2 hr following pramlintide injections. Inject pramlintide into the thighs or abdomen. Hypoglycemia is not a risk when pramlintide is used alone, but when given with insulin, the client is at high risk for hypoglycemia. Refrigerate open vials of pramlintide should be refrigerated and discard after 28 days.

 NCLEX® Connection: Pharmacological Therapies, Medication Administration

UNIT 10	MEDICATIONS AFFECTING THE ENDOCRINE SYSTEM
Chapter 37	Endocrine Disorders

 Overview

- The endocrine system is made up of glands that secrete hormones, which act on specific receptor sites. Hormones target receptor sites to regulate response to stress, growth, metabolism, and homeostasis.

- An endocrine disorder usually involves the over-secretion or under-secretion of hormones or an altered response by the target area or receptor.

- Medications used to treat disorders of the thyroid, anterior and posterior pituitary, and adrenal glands are discussed in this chapter.

MEDICATION CLASSIFICATION: THYROID HORMONE

- Select Prototype Medication – Levothyroxine (Synthroid, Levothroid)

- Other Medications:

  o Liothyronine (Cytomel)

  o Liotrix (Thyrolar)

  o Thyroid (Thyroid USP)

Purpose

- Expected Pharmacological Action

  o Thyroid hormones are a synthetic form of thyroxine (T_4) that increase metabolic rate, protein synthesis, cardiac output, renal perfusion, oxygen use, body temperature, blood volume, and growth processes.

- Therapeutic Uses

  o Treat hypothyroidism (all ages, all forms).

  o Treat emergency myxedema coma (IV route).

- Route of administration – Oral, IV (myxedema coma)

Complications

SIDE/ADVERSE EFFECTS	NURSING INTERVENTIONS/CLIENT EDUCATION
Overmedication can result in signs of hyperthyroidism (anxiety, tachycardia, palpitations, altered appetite, abdominal cramping, heat intolerance, fever, diaphoresis, weight loss, menstrual irregularities)	• Instruct clients to report signs of overmedication to the provider.

 Contraindications/Precautions

- These medications are Pregnancy Risk Category A.

- Use cautiously in pregnancy and lactation.

- Use is contraindicated for clients who have thyrotoxicosis.

- Because of cardiac stimulant effects, use is contraindicated following a MI.

- Use cautiously in clients who have cardiovascular problems (hypertension, angina pectoris, ischemic heart disease) because of cardiac stimulant effects.

- Thyroid hormone replacement is not for use in the treatment of obesity.

Interactions

MEDICATION/FOOD INTERACTIONS	NURSING INTERVENTIONS/CLIENT EDUCATION
Binding agents (cholestyramine, antacids, iron and calcium supplements) and sucralfate (Carafate) reduce levothyroxine absorption with concurrent use.	• Allow at least 3 hr between medication administrations.
Many antiseizure and antidepressant medications, including carbamazepine (Tegretol), phenytoin (Dilantin), phenobarbital, and sertraline (Zoloft) can increase levothyroxine metabolism.	• Monitor clients for therapeutic effects of levothyroxine. The provider may increase the dose.
Levothyroxine can increase the anticoagulant effects of warfarin (Coumadin) by breaking down vitamin K.	• Monitor the client's INR. • Instruct clients to report signs of bleeding. • Tell clients the provider may decrease the dose of warfarin.

Nursing Administration

- Obtain the client's baseline vital signs, weight, and height, and monitor periodically throughout treatment.

- Monitor and report signs of cardiac excitability (angina, chest pain, palpitations, dysrhythmias).

- o Monitor the client's T_4 and TSH levels.

- o Instruct clients to take daily on an empty stomach (before breakfast daily).

- o Reinforce to clients the importance of lifelong replacement (even after improvement of symptoms). Advise clients not to discontinue or change the dose of the medication without checking with the provider.

Nursing Evaluation of Medication Effectiveness

- • Depending on therapeutic intent, evidence of effectiveness may include:

  - o Decreased TSH levels

  - o Normal T_4 levels

  - o Absence of hypothyroidism symptoms (depression, weight gain, bradycardia, anorexia, cold intolerance, dry skin, menorrhagia)

MEDICATION CLASSIFICATION: ANTITHYROID MEDICATIONS

- • Select Prototype Medication – Propylthiouracil (Propyl-Thyracil)

- • Other Medications – Methimazole (Tapazole)

Purpose

- • Expected Pharmacological Action

  - o Blocks the synthesis of thyroid hormones

  - o Prevents the oxidation of iodide

  - o Blocks conversion of T_4 into T_3

- • Therapeutic Uses

  - o Treatment of Graves' disease

  - o Produce an euthyroid state prior to thyroid removal surgery

  - o As an adjunct to irradiation of the thyroid gland

  - o Emergency treatment of thyrotoxicosis

- • Route of administration – Oral

Complications

SIDE/ADVERSE EFFECTS	NURSING INTERVENTIONS/CLIENT EDUCATION
Overmedication can result in signs of hypothyroidism (drowsiness, depression, weight gain, edema, bradycardia, anorexia, cold intolerance, dry skin, menorrhagia)	• Instruct clients to report signs of overmedication to the provider. • Tell clients the provider may reduce the dose or prescribe a temporary thyroid replacement.
Agranulocytosis (sore throat, fever)	• Monitor clients for early signs of agranulocytosis and instruct clients to report them promptly to provider. • Monitor the client's blood counts at baseline and periodically. • If agranulocytosis occurs, stop treatment and monitor the client for reversal of agranulocytosis. • Administer Neupogen to treat agranulocytosis if prescribed.

 Contraindications/Precautions

- Use is contraindicated in pregnancy (Pregnancy Risk Category D) and during lactation because of the risk of neonatal hypothyroidism.

- Use cautiously in clients who have bone marrow depression and/or immunosuppression.

Interactions

MEDICATION/FOOD INTERACTIONS	NURSING INTERVENTIONS/CLIENT EDUCATION
Concurrent use of antithyroid medications and anticoagulants may increase anticoagulation.	• Monitor the client's PT, INR, and activated partial thromboplastin time (aPTT), and administer adjusted dosages of anticoagulants accordingly.
Concurrent use of antithyroid medications and digoxin (Lanoxin) may increase glycoside level.	• Monitor digoxin level and administer reduced digoxin dose as prescribed.

Nursing Administration

- Advise clients that therapeutic effects may take 1 to 2 weeks to be evident. Propylthiouracil does not destroy the thyroid hormone that is present, but rather prevents continued synthesis of thyroid hormone.

- Monitor the client's vital signs, weight, and I&O at baseline and periodically.

- Instruct clients to take medication at consistent times each day and with meals to maintain a consistent therapeutic level and decrease gastric distress.

- Instruct clients not to discontinue the medication abruptly (risk of thyroid crisis due to stress response).

- Monitor clients for signs of hyperthyroidism (indicating inadequate medication).

- Expect to administer a beta-adrenergic antagonist, such as propranolol (Inderal), to decrease tremors and tachycardia.

- Monitor for symptoms of hypothyroidism (indicating overmedication), such as drowsiness, depression, weight gain, edema, bradycardia, anorexia, cold intolerance and dry skin.

- Monitor CBC for leukopenia or thrombocytopenia.

Nursing Evaluation of Medication Effectiveness

- Depending on therapeutic intent, evidence of effectiveness may include:

  o Weight gain

  o Normal vital signs

  o Decreased T_4 levels

  o Absence of signs of hyperthyroidism (anxiety, tachycardia, palpitations, increased appetite, abdominal cramping, heat intolerance, fever, diaphoresis, weight loss, menstrual irregularities)

MEDICATION CLASSIFICATION: ANTITHYROID MEDICATIONS

- Select Prototype Medication – Radioactive iodine (^{131}I)

Purpose

- Expected Pharmacological Action

  o Radioactive iodine is absorbed by the thyroid and destroys some of the thyroid producing cells. At high doses, thyroid-radioactive iodine destroys thyroid cells.

- Therapeutic Uses

  o At high doses

    ▪ Hyperthyroidism

    ▪ Thyroid cancer

  o At low doses

    ▪ Thyroid function studies (visualization of the degree of iodine uptake by the thyroid gland is helpful in the diagnosis of thyroid disorders)

- Route of administration – Oral

Complications

SIDE/ADVERSE EFFECTS	NURSING INTERVENTIONS/CLIENT EDUCATION
Radiation sickness (hematemesis, epistaxis, intense nausea, vomiting)	• Monitor clients for symptoms of radiation sickness. • Stop treatment and notify the provider.
Bone marrow depression	• Monitor clients for anemia, leukopenia, and thrombocytopenia.
Hypothyroidism (intolerance to cold, edema, bradycardia, increase in weight, depression)	• Instruct clients to report signs of hypothyroidism to the provider.

 Contraindications/Precautions

- Because of irradiating effects, use is contraindicated in pregnancy (Pregnancy Risk Category X), clients of childbearing age/intent, and during lactation.

Interactions

MEDICATION/FOOD INTERACTIONS	NURSING INTERVENTIONS/CLIENT EDUCATION
Concurrent use of other antithyroid medications reduces uptake of radioactive iodine.	• Instruct clients to discontinue use of other antithyroid medications for a week prior to therapy.

Nursing Administration

- Instruct clients regarding radioactivity precautions.

  o Void frequently to avoid irradiation of gonads.

  o Limit contact with others to 30 min/day per person.

  o Increase fluid intake, usually 2 to 3 L/day.

  o Dispose of body wastes per protocol.

  o Avoid coughing and expectoration (source of radioactive iodine).

MEDICATION CLASSIFICATION: ANTITHYROID MEDICATIONS

- Select Prototype Medication – Strong iodine solution (Lugol's Solution) – nonradioactive iodine

- Other Medications:

  o Sodium iodide

  o Potassium iodide

Purpose

- Expected Pharmacological Action

  o Thyroid-nonradioactive iodine creates high levels of iodide that will reduce iodine uptake (by the thyroid gland), inhibit thyroid hormone production, and block the release of thyroid hormones into the bloodstream.

- Therapeutic Uses

  o Induce euthyroid state and reduction of thyroid gland size prior to thyroid removal surgery.

  o Use thyroid-nonradioactive iodine for the emergency treatment of thyrotoxicosis.

- Route of administration – Oral

Complications

SIDE/ADVERSE EFFECTS	NURSING INTERVENTIONS/CLIENT EDUCATION
Iodism symptoms due to corrosive property (metallic taste, stomatitis, sore teeth and gums, gastric distress, small bowel lesions)	• Instruct clients to drink through a straw to prevent tooth discoloration. • Instruct clients to take the medication with meals to reduce gastrointestinal (GI) distress.

 ## Contraindications/Precautions

  o Use in pregnancy is contraindicated (Pregnancy Risk Category D).

Interactions

MEDICATION/FOOD INTERACTIONS	NURSING INTERVENTIONS/CLIENT EDUCATION
Concurrent intake of foods high in iodine (iodized salt, seafood) increases risk for iodism (brassy taste in mouth, burning sensation in mouth, sore teeth).	• Monitor clients for signs of iodism. • Instruct clients regarding foods high in iodine.

Nursing Administration

- Obtain the client's baseline vital signs, weight, and I&O, and monitor periodically.

- Instruct clients to dilute strong iodine solution (Lugol's Solution) with juice to improve taste.

- Instruct clients to take at the same time each day to maintain therapeutic levels.

- Encourage clients to increase fluid intake, unless contraindicated.

Nursing Evaluation of Medication Effectiveness

- Depending on therapeutic intent, effectiveness may be evidenced by the following:

    o Weight gain

    o Normal vital signs

    o Decreased T_4 levels

    o Reduction in size of thyroid gland

    o Clients will be able to get adequate sleep, achieve and maintain appropriate weight, maintain blood pressure and heart rate within expected reference range, and be free of complications of hyperthyroidism.

MEDICATION CLASSIFICATION: ANTERIOR PITUITARY HORMONES/ GROWTH HORMONES

- Select Prototype Medication – Somatropin (Genotropin, Nutropin)

- Other Medication – Somatrem (Protropin)

Purpose

- Expected Pharmacological Action

    o Anterior pituitary hormones/growth hormones stimulate overall growth and the production of protein, and decrease the use of glucose.

- Therapeutic Uses

    o Anterior pituitary hormones/growth hormones are used to treat growth hormone deficiencies (pediatric and adult growth hormone deficiencies, Turner's syndrome, Prader-Willi syndrome).

- Routes of administration – IM or subcutaneous

Complications

SIDE/ADVERSE EFFECTS	NURSING INTERVENTIONS/CLIENT EDUCATION
Hyperglycemia (polyphagia, polydipsia, polyuria)	• Observe clients for signs of hyperglycemia.
Hypothyroidism	• Monitor thyroid function.

 Contraindications/Precautions

- These medications are Pregnancy Risk Category C.

- Use is contraindicated in clients who are severely obese or have severe respiratory impairment (sleep apnea) because of higher risk of fatality.

- Use cautiously in clients who have diabetes because of the risk of hyperglycemia.

Interactions

MEDICATION/FOOD INTERACTIONS	NURSING INTERVENTIONS/CLIENT EDUCATION
Concurrent use of glucocorticoids can counteract growth-promoting effects.	• Avoid concurrent use.

Nursing Administration

- Obtain the client's baseline height and weight.

- Monitor growth patterns during medication administration, usually monthly.

- Reconstitute medication per directions. Rotate gently, and do not shake, prior to administration.

- Instruct clients that therapy will be discontinued prior to epiphyseal closure.

Nursing Evaluation of Medication Effectiveness

- Depending on therapeutic intent, effectiveness may be evidenced by the following:

  o Client increases height.

MEDICATION CLASSIFICATION: POSTERIOR PITUITARY HORMONES/ ANTIDIURETIC HORMONES

- Select Prototype Medication – Vasopressin

- Other Medication – Desmopressin (DDAVP, Stimate)

Purpose

- Expected Pharmacological Action

  o Posterior pituitary hormones/antidiuretic hormones promote reabsorption of water within the kidneys.

  o Posterior pituitary hormones/antidiuretic hormones cause vasoconstriction because of the contraction of vascular smooth muscle (Vasopressin).

- Therapeutic Uses

  o Treat diabetes insipidus.

  o Use during cardiac arrest (Vasopressin).

- Route of Administration

  o Vasopressin – Intranasal, subcutaneous, IM, IV

  o Desmopressin – Oral, intranasal, subcutaneous, IV

Complications

SIDE/ADVERSE EFFECTS	NURSING INTERVENTIONS/CLIENT EDUCATION
Water intoxication	• Monitor clients for signs of overhydration (drowsiness, lethargy, pounding headache). • In general, clients should be instructed to reduce fluid intake during therapy.
Myocardial ischemia from vasoconstriction.	• Monitor ECG and blood pressure. Advise clients to notify the provider of chest pain or tightness, and diaphoresis.

 Contraindications/Precautions

- Use of vasopressin is contraindicated in clients who have coronary artery disease (risk for angina, MI) or with decreased peripheral circulation (risk for gangrene) and in clients who have chronic nephritis.

Interactions

MEDICATION/FOOD INTERACTIONS	NURSING INTERVENTIONS/CLIENT EDUCATION
Carbamazepine (Tegretol) and tricyclic antidepressants may increase the antidiuretic action.	• Use cautiously together.

Nursing Administration

- Monitor vital signs, central venous pressure, I&O, specific gravity, and laboratory studies (serum electrolytes, BUN, serum creatinine, urine specific gravity, osmolality).

- Monitor blood pressure and heart rate.

- Monitor for headache, confusion, or other signs of water intoxication.

- Monitor clients receiving IV therapy of vasopressin, due to risk of extravasation at IV site, which can lead to gangrene.

Nursing Evaluation of Medication Effectiveness

- Depending on therapeutic intent, evidence of effectiveness may include:

  ○ A reduction in the large volumes of urine output associated with diabetes insipidus to expected levels of urine output

  ○ Cardiac arrest survival

MEDICATION CLASSIFICATION: ADRENAL HORMONE REPLACEMENT

- Select Prototype Medication – Hydrocortisone (Hydrocortone, Solu-Cortef))

- Other Medications:

    o Prednisone (Deltasone), dexamethasone (Decadron)

    o Mineral corticoids – Fludrocortisone acetate (Florinef)

Purpose

- Expected Pharmacological Action

    o Mimic effect of natural hormones

- Therapeutic Uses

    o Acute and chronic replacement therapy for adrenocortical insufficiency (Addison's disease)

    o Nonendocrine disorders include cancer, inflammation, and allergic reactions.

- Route of administration – Oral, IV

Complications

SIDE/ADVERSE EFFECTS	NURSING INTERVENTIONS/CLIENT EDUCATION
Glucocorticoids: hydrocortisone	
Osteoporosis	• Advise clients to take calcium supplements, vitamin D, and/or bisphosphonate (Etidronate).
Adrenal suppression (hyperpigmentation, weakness and fatigue, nausea and vomiting, orthostatic hypotension, dehydration, hyponatremia, hyperkalemia, hypoglycemia, hypercalcemia)	• Advise clients to observe for symptoms, and to notify the provider if symptoms occur. • Instruct clients how to taper dosage slowly. • Instruct clients to notify provider at times of stress for increase in dosage.
Peptic ulcer, GI discomfort (coffee-ground emesis, bloody or tarry stools, abdominal pain)	• Advise clients to observe for signs and symptoms, and to notify the provider if symptoms occur. • Administer prophylactic H_2 receptor antagonists.
Infection (fever, sore throat)	• Advise clients to avoid contact with people who have a communicable disease. Monitor for signs of infection.
Mineralocorticoid: fludrocortisone acetate	
Retention of sodium and water, which may lead to hypertension, edema, heart failure and hypokalemia (muscle weakness, irregular heart rate)	• Monitor weight, blood pressure, and serum potassium. Monitor breath sounds and urine output.

Contraindications/Precautions

- Pregnancy Risk Category

  o Hydrocortisone is not rated.

  o Mineralocorticoid – Fludrocortisone acetate is Pregnancy Risk Category C.

- Use is contraindicated in clients who have a systemic fungal infection.

- Use with caution in clients who have a recent MI, gastric ulcer, hypertension, kidney disorder, osteoporosis, diabetes mellitus, hypothyroidism, myasthenia gravis and seizure disorder.

Interactions

MEDICATION/FOOD INTERACTIONS	NURSING INTERVENTIONS/CLIENT EDUCATION
NSAIDs or alcohol use may cause increased gastric distress or bleed.	Use together with caution.
Concurrent use with oral anticoagulants may increase or decrease anticoagulation.	Monitor coagulations studies and medication levels.
Concurrent use with potassium depleting agents may cause increased potassium loss.	Monitor serum potassium and ECG.
Concurrent use with vaccines and toxoids may reduce the antibody response.	Avoid concurrent use.
Fludrocortisone acetate	
Barbiturates and phenytoin may reduce effects of fludrocortisone acetate.	Monitor for reduced medication effects.

Nursing Administration

- Monitor weight, blood pressure, and serum electrolytes.

- Give with food to reduce gastric distress.

- Advise clients to observe for signs and symptoms of peptic ulcer (coffee-ground emesis, bloody or tarry stools, abdominal pain) and to notify the provider if symptoms occur.

- Instruct clients not to stop the medication suddenly. Reinforce how to taper dosage slowly.

Nursing Evaluation of Medication Effectiveness

- Depending on therapeutic intent, evidence of effectiveness may include:

  o Relief of symptoms of adrenocortical deficiency, such as weakness, hypoglycemia, hyperkalemia, and fatigue, with minimal adverse effects

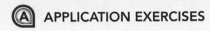 **APPLICATION EXERCISES**

1. A nurse is caring for a client who is taking levothyroxine (Synthroid). For which of the following should the nurse monitor to identify levothyroxine toxicity?

    A. Hair loss

    B. Lethargy

    C. Weight loss

    D. Cold intolerance

2. A nurse is reinforcing teaching for a client with hyperthyroidism who has a new prescription for propranolol (Inderal). The nurse should teach the client that propranolol should perform which of the following actions?

    A. Increase blood flow to the thyroid gland

    B. Prevent thyroid hormone synthesis

    C. Suppress tachycardia

    D. Promote conversion of T_4 to T_3

3. A nurse is reinforcing teaching for a client who is prescribed strong iodide solution (Lugol's solution) prior to thyroid surgery. For which of the following adverse effects should the nurse monitor the client?

    A. Blurred vision

    B. Metallic taste

    C. Absence seizures

    D. Frontal headache

4. A nurse is caring for a client who is prescribed somatropin (Genotropin) to stimulate growth. The nurse should plan to monitor the client's laboratory values for which of the following?

    A. Anemia

    B. Hyperglycemia

    C. Decreased urine specific gravity

    D. Increased urine amylase

5. A nurse is caring for a client who is prescribed vasopressin (Pitressin) for diabetes insipidus. For which of the following adverse effects should the nurse monitor the client? (Select all that apply.)

    _____ Headache

    _____ Drowsiness

    _____ Chest pain

    _____ Urinary hesitation

    _____ Bone pain

6. A client taking hydrocortisone for adrenocortical insufficiency (Addison's disease) is admitted to the hospital for a total hip arthroplasty. Which of the following actions is the highest priority?

   A. Administration of supplemental doses of hydrocortisone

   B. Instruction on coughing and deep breathing

   C. Insertion of an indwelling urinary catheter

   D. Requesting a referral for physical therapy

APPLICATION EXERCISES ANSWER KEY

1. A nurse is caring for a client who is taking levothyroxine (Synthroid). For which of the following should the nurse monitor to identify levothyroxine toxicity?

   A. Hair loss

   B. Lethargy

   C. Weight loss

   D. Cold intolerance

   Overmedication with levothyroxine may result in toxicity. Findings of toxicity include weight loss despite increased appetite, insomnia, nervousness, and palpitations. Hair loss, lethargy, and cold intolerance are findings seen in the client who have hypothyroidism.

 NCLEX® Connection: Pharmacological Therapies, Adverse Effects/Contraindications/Side Effects/Interactions

2. A nurse is reinforcing teaching for a client with hyperthyroidism who has a new prescription for propranolol (Inderal). The nurse should teach the client that propranolol should perform which of the following actions?

   A. Increase blood flow to the thyroid gland

   B. Prevent thyroid hormone synthesis

   C. Suppress tachycardia

   D. Promote conversion of T_4 to T_3

   Propranolol is a beta-adrenergic antagonist that suppresses tachycardia, a common finding in hyperthyroidism. Propranolol lowers blood pressure, but does not increase blood flow to the thyroid gland. Propranolol does not have any effects on thyroid hormone synthesis.

 NCLEX® Connection: Pharmacological Therapies, Expected Actions/Outcomes

3. A nurse is reinforcing teaching for a client who is prescribed strong iodide solution (Lugol's solution) prior to thyroid surgery. For which of the following adverse effects should the nurse monitor the client?

   A. Blurred vision

   B. Metallic taste

   C. Absence seizures

   D. Frontal headache

   Metallic taste and burning sensations in the mouth are signs of iodism (mild toxicity to strong iodide solution). The nurse should notify the provider if these findings occur. Severe toxicity is manifested by GI distress and bleeding. Blurred vision, absence seizures, and frontal headache are not signs of an adverse reaction to strong iodide solution.

 NCLEX® Connection: Pharmacological Therapies, Adverse Effects/Contraindications/Side Effects/Interactions

4. A nurse is caring for a client who is prescribed somatropin (Genotropin) to stimulate growth. The nurse should plan to monitor the client's laboratory values for which of the following?

   A. Anemia

   B. Hyperglycemia

   C. Decreased urine specific gravity

   D. Increased urine amylase

   Somatropin may increase blood glucose levels and the nurse should monitor the client for hyperglycemia. There is no indication to monitor laboratory values for anemia, decreased urine specific gravity, or increased urine amylase.

 NCLEX® Connection: Pharmacological Therapies, Adverse Effects/Contraindications/Side Effects/Interactions

5. A nurse is caring for a client who is prescribed vasopressin (Pitressin) for diabetes insipidus. For which of the following adverse effects should the nurse monitor the client? (Select all that apply.)

X	**Headache**
X	**Drowsiness**
X	**Chest pain**
_____	Urinary hesitation
_____	Bone pain

   Headache and drowsiness, progressing to seizures, and coma are signs of water intoxication, which may occur if fluid intake is not restricted after therapy begins. Vasopressin causes vasoconstriction, and chest pain is another adverse effect for which the nurse should monitor. Urinary hesitation and bone pain are not expected adverse reactions to vasopressin.

 NCLEX® Connection: Pharmacological Therapies, Adverse Effects/Contraindications/Side Effects/Interactions

6. A client taking hydrocortisone for adrenocortical insufficiency (Addison's disease) is admitted to the hospital for a total hip arthroplasty. Which of the following actions is the highest priority?

   A. Administration of supplemental doses of hydrocortisone

   B. Instruction on coughing and deep breathing

   C. Insertion of an indwelling urinary catheter

   D. Requesting a referral for physical therapy

   The greatest risk to a client with Addison's disease who is taking a glucocorticoid and undergoing surgery is adrenal crisis. To prevent adrenal crisis, the client should receive supplemental doses during times of increased stress, such as infection or surgery. Instruction on coughing and deep breathing, insertion of an indwelling urinary catheter, and a referral for physical therapy are important but not the highest priority.

 NCLEX® Connection: Pharmacological Therapies, Expected Actions/Outcomes

UNIT 11: MEDICATIONS AFFECTING THE IMMUNE SYSTEM AND FOR INFECTIOUS DISEASES

- Immunizations
- Principles of Antimicrobial Therapy
- Antibiotics Affecting the Bacterial Cell Wall
- Antibiotics Affecting Protein Synthesis
- Urinary Tract Infections
- Mycobacterial, Fungal, and Parasitic Infections
- Viral Infections, HIV, and AIDS

NCLEX® CONNECTIONS

When reviewing the chapters in this section, keep in mind the relevant sections of the NCLEX® outline, in particular:

CLIENT NEEDS: PHARMACOLOGICAL THERAPIES

Relevant topics/tasks include:
- Dosage Calculation
  - Use clinical decision making when calculating doses.
- Expected Actions/Outcomes
  - Evaluate client response to medication.
- Pharmacological Pain Management
  - Monitor client non-verbal signs of pain/discomfort.

UNIT 11	MEDICATIONS AFFECTING THE IMMUNE SYSTEM AND FOR INFECTIOUS DISEASES

Chapter 38   Immunizations

 Overview

- Administration of a vaccine causes production of antibodies that prevent illness from a specific microbe.

- Active natural immunity develops when the body produces antibodies in response to exposure to a live pathogen. Active artificial immunity develops when an immunization is given and the body produces antibodies in response to exposure to a killed or attenuated virus.

- Passive natural immunity occurs when antibodies are passed from the mother to the newborn/infant through the placenta and then breastfeeding. Passive artificial immunity is temporary, and occurs after antibodies in the form of immune globulins are administered to an individual who requires immediate protection against a disease after exposure has occurred.

- Immunizations may be made from killed viruses or live, attenuated, or weakened viruses.

MEDICATION CLASSIFICATION: VACCINATIONS

 Childhood Vaccinations (See www.cdc.gov for updates.)

- o Diphtheria and tetanus toxoids and acellular pertussis vaccine (DTaP) – Give doses at 2, 4, 6, 15 to 18 months, and at 4 to 6 years.

- o Tetanus, diphtheria toxoids, and pertussis vaccine (Tdap) – Give one dose at 11 to 12 years.

- o Tetanus diphtheria (Td) booster – Give one dose every 10 years following DTaP.

- o Haemophilus influenza Type B (Hib) – Give doses at 2, 4, 6, and at 12 to 15 months.

- o Rotavirus oral vaccine

  - Two formulations are available.

    - □ RotaTeq requires three doses beginning at age 6 weeks, with subsequent doses 4 to 10 weeks apart. Complete RotaTeq vaccination before age 32 weeks. Do not initiate immunization for infants 15 weeks or older.

    - □ Rotarix requires two doses beginning at age 6 weeks with the next dose 4 weeks later.

  - Complete all doses by age 8 months.

o   Inactivated poliovirus vaccine (IPV) – Give doses at 2, 4, and 6 to 18 months, and at 4 to 6 years.

o   Measles, mumps, and rubella vaccine (MMR) – Doses at 12 to 15 months, and at 4 to 6 years

o   Varicella vaccine – Give one dose at 12 to 15 months, and 4 to 6 years, or 2 doses administered 4 weeks apart if administered after age 13.

o   Pneumococcal conjugate vaccine (PCV) – Give doses at 2, 4, 6, and 12 to 15 months.

o   Hepatitis A vaccine – Give two doses 6 months apart after age 12 months.

o   Hepatitis B vaccine – Give within 12 hr after birth with additional doses at age 1 to 2 months and 6 to 18 months.

o   Seasonal Influenza vaccine

    ▪   Annually, beginning at age 6 months, give trivalent inactivated influenza vaccine (TIV).

    ▪   Starting at age 2, use the live attenuated influenza vaccine (LAIV).

    ▪   October through November is the ideal time, but December is acceptable.

o   Meningococcal vaccine (MCV4) – Give one dose at age 11 to 12 years (earlier if specific risk factors are present).

o   Human papillomavirus (HPV2 or HPV4) – Give three doses over a 6-month interval for girls at 9 to 12 years of age. HPV4 may be given to boys starting at age 9.

•   Adult Vaccinations – For adults 18 years of age and older (See www.cdc.gov for updates.)

o   Td booster – Give at least one dose of Tdap, and then Td every 10 years.

o   MMR vaccine – Give one or two doses at ages 19 to 49.

o   Varicella vaccine – Give two doses to adults who do not have evidence of previous infection. A second dose should be given for adults who had only one previous dose.

o   Pneumococcal polysaccharide vaccine (PPSV) – Vaccinate adults who are immunocompromised, who have a chronic disease, who smoke cigarettes, who are of Alaskan native and certain American Indian populations, or who live in a long-term care facility. Follow CDC guidelines for revaccination. If a client is not previously vaccinated or has no evidence of disease then give one dose at age 65.

o   Hepatitis A vaccine – Give two doses for high-risk individuals.

o   Hepatitis B vaccine – Give three doses for high-risk individuals.

o   Seasonal Influenza vaccine

    ▪   One dose annually is recommended for all adults over age 50; health care providers including those who care for young children; individuals with chronic medical conditions such as cerebral palsy, asthma, and diabetes; individuals who are immunocompromised; and individuals living in long-term care settings.

    ▪   Note that LAIV, given as a nasal spray, is only indicated for adults under age 50 who are not pregnant or immunocompromised.

- MCV4 – Students entering college and living in college dormitories if not previously immunized. Meningococcal polysaccharide vaccine (MPSV4) is recommended for adults greater than 56 years of age. Revaccination may be recommended after 5 years for adults at high risk for infection.

- HPV2 or HPV4 – Three doses are recommended for females up to age 26 who were not vaccinated as children. HPV4 may be given to males up to age 26.

- Herpes zoster vaccine – This is recommended for all adults over age 60 years.

Purpose

- Expected Pharmacological Action

    o Immunizations produce antibodies that provide active immunity. Immunizations may take months to have an effect but confer long-lasting protection against infectious diseases.

- Therapeutic Uses

    o Eradication of infectious diseases (polio, smallpox)

    o Prevention of childhood and adult infectious diseases and their complications (measles, diphtheria, mumps, rubella, tetanus, *H. influenza*)

Complications, Contraindications, and Precautions

- Anaphylactic reaction to a vaccine is a contraindication for further doses of that vaccine.

- Anaphylactic reaction to a vaccine is a contraindication to use of other vaccines containing that substance.

- Moderate or severe illnesses with or without fever may be considered precautions or contraindications and must be evaluated on a case-by-case basis. The common cold and other minor illnesses are not contraindications.

Contraindications to vaccinations require the provider to analyze data and weigh the risks that come with vaccinating or not vaccinating.

- Immunocompromised individuals, as defined by the CDC, are those individuals with hematologic or solid tumors, congenital immunodeficiency, or on long-term immunosuppressive therapy, including corticosteroids, and are at special risk from live vaccines.

IMMUNIZATIONS	SIDE EFFECTS	CONTRAINDICATIONS/PRECAUTIONS
DTaP	<ul><li>Local reaction at injection site</li><li>Fever and irritability</li><li>Crying that cannot be consoled, lasting up to 3 hours</li><li>Seizures</li><li>Rare – Acute encephalopathy</li></ul>	<ul><li>An occurrence of encephalopathy</li><li>7 days after the administration of the DTaP immunization</li><li>An occurrence of seizures within 3 days of the vaccination</li><li>A history of uncontrollable crying or temperature of 105° F (40.5° C) or higher that occurred within 48 hr of vaccination.</li></ul>
Haemophilus influenza type b conjugate vaccine	<ul><li>Mild local reactions, low grade fever</li><li>Rarely fever, (temperature greater than 38.5° C [101.3° F]), vomiting, crying may occur</li></ul>	<ul><li>Children less than 6 weeks of age</li></ul>
Rotavirus vaccine		<ul><li>Infants with diarrhea and vomiting</li><li>Use caution with infants who are immunocompromised (with HIV infection or from medication administration).</li></ul>
IPV	<ul><li>Local reaction at injection site</li><li>Allergic reaction is possible in children allergic to streptomycin, neomycin, or bacitracin, as these medications are contained in the vaccine in small amounts.</li><li>Rare – Vaccine-associated paralytic poliomyelitis</li></ul>	<ul><li>Allergy to neomycin, streptomycin, polymyxin B</li><li>Pregnancy</li></ul>
MMR	<ul><li>Local reactions such as rash; fever; swollen glands in cheeks, neck and under the jaw</li><li>Possibility of joint pain lasting for days to weeks.</li><li>Risk for anaphylaxis and thrombocytopenia</li></ul>	<ul><li>Pregnancy</li><li>Allergy to gelatin and neomycin</li><li>Clients who are immunocompromised (with HIV infection or from medication administration)</li><li>Recent transfusion with blood products</li><li>History of thrombocytopenia</li></ul>

IMMUNIZATIONS	SIDE EFFECTS	CONTRAINDICATIONS/PRECAUTIONS
Varicella vaccine	• Varicella-like rash, local or generalized, such as vesicles on the body	• Pregnancy • Pregnant women should avoid close proximity to children recently vaccinated. • Cancers of the blood and lymphatic system • Allergy to gelatin and neomycin • Clients who are immunocompromised (with HIV infection or from medication administration)
PCV	• Mild local reactions, fever, and no serious adverse effects	• Pregnancy

Hepatitis A and B vaccines	• Local reaction at injection site, mild fever
	• Anaphylaxis
		• Hep A:
		  ○ Pregnancy may be a contraindication
		• Hep B:
		  ○ Allergy to baker's yeast

Seasonal influenza vaccine	• Inactivated – Mild local reaction, and fever • Live attenuated – Headache, cough, fever • Rare – Risk for Guillain-Barré syndrome manifested by ascending paralysis, beginning with weakness of lower extremities, and progressing to difficulty breathing	• LAIV, administered as nasal spray, is contraindicated for adults over 50 years and children under 2 years, for adults and children who are immunocompromised or who have a chronic disease. • History of Guillain-Barré syndrome
MCV4	• Mild local reaction • Rare – Risk of allergic response	• History of Guillain Barré syndrome
HPV2 or HPB4 vaccine	• Mild local reaction and fever • Fainting has occurred shortly after receiving vaccination • Rare – Risk for Guillain-Barré syndrome	• Pregnancy • Hypersensitivity to yeast
Herpes Zoster	• None	• Clients who are immunocompromised (with HIV infection or from medication administration)

Medication/Food Interactions

• None significant

Nursing Administration

- For infants and children:

  - Obtain parental consent for children.

  - Note the date, route, and site of vaccination on the child's immunization record at the time of immunization.

  - Give intramuscular vaccinations in the vastus lateralis muscle in infants and young children and into the deltoid muscle for older children and adolescents.

  - Give subcutaneous injections in the outer aspect of the upper arm or anterolateral thigh.

  - Use appropriate size of needle for route, site, age, and amount of medication.

  - Use strategies to minimize discomfort.

  - Provide for distraction.

  - Do not allow children to delay the procedure.

  - Encourage the parent to use comforting measures such as cuddling and pacifiers during the procedure, and measures such as application of cool compresses to injection site or gentle movement of the involved extremity after the procedure.

  - Provide praise afterward.

  - Apply a colorful bandage if appropriate.

  - Instruct parents to avoid administration of aspirin to children to treat fever or local reaction because of the risk of the development of Reye's syndrome.

  - Instruct parents to premedicate infants and children with nonopioid analgesic/antipyretic prior to immunizations and for the following 24 hr. Use acetaminophen for infants 2 to 6 months. Parents may administer ibuprofen starting at 6 months.

  - Instruct parents to apply topical anesthetic prior to the injection.

- For adults:

  - Give subcutaneous vaccinations in the outer aspect of the upper arm or anterolateral thigh.

  - Give intramuscular vaccinations into the deltoid muscle.

- For clients of all ages:

  - Have emergency medications and equipment on standby in case clients experience an allergic response such as anaphylaxis.

  - Follow storage and reconstitution directions. If reconstituted, use within 30 min.

  - Provide written vaccine information sheets and review the content with parents or clients.

- ○ Instruct parents and clients to observe for complications and to notify the provider if side effects occur.

- ○ Document administration of vaccines including date, route, and site of vaccination; type, manufacturer, lot number and expiration of vaccine; and name, address, and signature.

Nursing Evaluation of Medication Effectiveness

- Depending on therapeutic intent, effectiveness may be evidenced by:

- ○ Improvement of local reaction to vaccination with absence of pain, fever, and swelling at the site of injection

- ○ Development of immunity

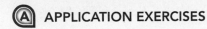 **APPLICATION EXERCISES**

1. A nurse is caring for a group of clients who came to the clinic for a seasonal influenza vaccination. Which of the following clients can receive the vaccine via nasal spray rather than an injection?

    A. A 1-year-old child with no health problems

    B. A 17-year-old client who has a hypersensitivity to penicillin

    C. A 25-year-old client who is pregnant

    D. A 52-year-old client who takes a multivitamin supplement

2. Which immunization should be administered to infants less than 8 months of age? Why are these young infants given this immunization?

3. A nurse is reinforcing teaching for the parents of a 12-month-old child who just received her first measles, mumps, and rubella (MMR) vaccine. For which of the following reactions should the nurse teach the parents?

    A. Fainting

    B. Inconsolable crying

    C. Ascending paralysis of the extremities

    D. Bruising on multiple areas of the body

4. A nurse is preparing to administer scheduled immunizations to a 2-month-old infant. Which of the following instructions should the nurse give the parent before discharge?

    A. Treat discomfort with liquid ibuprofen for the first 24 hr following the vaccinations.

    B. Apply warm compresses to injection site for comfort.

    C. Call the provider if the injection site becomes slightly reddened.

    D. Gently move the involved extremity to decrease discomfort.

APPLICATION EXERCISES ANSWER KEY

1. A nurse is caring for a group of clients who came to the clinic for a seasonal influenza vaccination. Which of the following clients can receive the vaccine via nasal spray rather than an injection?

    A. A 1-year-old child with no health problems

    B. A 17-year-old client who has a hypersensitivity to penicillin

    C. A 25-year-old client who is pregnant

    D. A 52-year-old client who takes a multivitamin supplement

    The adolescent can receive the immunization for influenza with the live vaccine (nasal spray). A hypersensitivity to eggs, not penicillin, is a contraindication for any influenza vaccination. The 1-year-old client and the 52-year-old client are not within the acceptable age range to receive the live vaccine via nasal spray, but both could receive the inactivated vaccine by IM injection. Women who are pregnant should not receive any live vaccine, but can receive the inactivated vaccine by IM injection.

     NCLEX® Connection: Pharmacological Therapies, Adverse Effects/Contraindications/Side Effects/Interactions

2. Which immunization should be administered to infants less than 8 months of age? Why are these young infants given this immunization?

    The rotavirus vaccine is administered to infants less than 8 months in age because the rotavirus causes severe gastroenteritis in very young clients.

     NCLEX® Connection: Pharmacological Therapies, Adverse Effects/Contraindications/Side Effects/Interactions

3. A nurse is reinforcing teaching for the parents of a 12-month-old child who just received her first measles, mumps, and rubella (MMR) vaccine. For which of the following reactions should the nurse teach the parents?

    A. Fainting

    B. Inconsolable crying

    C. Ascending paralysis of the extremities

    D. Bruising on multiple areas of the body

    Bruising can be a sign of thrombocytopenia, which should be reported to the provider following an MMR vaccination. Fainting is an adverse reaction that may occur following the human papilloma virus vaccination. Inconsolable crying is a reaction that may occur following a DTaP vaccination. Ascending paralysis of the extremities may be a sign of Guillain-Barré syndrome, an adverse reaction that may occur following the seasonal influenza vaccine.

     NCLEX® Connection: Pharmacological Therapies, Adverse Effects/Contraindications/Side Effects/Interactions

4. A nurse is preparing to administer scheduled immunizations to a 2-month-old infant. Which of the following instructions should the nurse give the parent before discharge?

   A. Treat discomfort with liquid ibuprofen for the first 24 hr following the vaccinations.

   B. Apply warm compresses to injection site for comfort.

   C. Call the provider if the injection site becomes slightly reddened.

   D. Gently move the involved extremity to decrease discomfort.

   The nurse should instruct the parent to gently move the extremity to help decrease discomfort, use acetaminophen for mild pain, use cool rather than warm compresses, and expect slight redness at the injection site. The nurse should instruct the parent to use acetaminophen until the infant is 6 months at which time ibuprofen is an appropriate analgesic.

 NCLEX® Connection: Pharmacological Therapies, Medication Administration

UNIT 11	MEDICATIONS AFFECTING THE IMMUNE SYSTEM AND FOR INFECTIOUS DISEASES

Chapter 39   Principles of Antimicrobial Therapy

 Overview

- Antimicrobial therapy (often termed "antibiotic therapy") is the use of medications to treat infections caused by bacteria, viruses, and fungi.

- Antimicrobials must use selective toxicity to kill or otherwise control microbes without destroying host cells. Methods of actions include:

  ○ Destroying the cell wall, which is present in bacteria but not in mammals.

  ○ Preventing viral replication through reduction of enzymes needed by the virus to reproduce.

- New antimicrobials must be continually created due to changes in DNA of micro-organisms, called conjugation, which produces resistance to multiple existing drugs.

- Suprainfection is a type of resistance caused when normal flora are killed by use of an antibiotic, thus favoring the emergence of a new infection that is difficult to eliminate.

- Selection of antimicrobial medications is based on multiple factors.

Selection of Antimicrobials

- Identification of the causative agent:

  ○ Gram stain – Examine an aspirate of body fluid under the microscope, where micro-organisms may be identified directly.

  ○ Culture of the fluid – Apply the aspirate to culture medium and allow colonies of the micro-organism to grow over several days. A culture may be preferable to gram stain in cases where positive identification cannot be made by the first method.

- Sensitivity of the micro-organism to the antimicrobial

  ○ Disk diffusion test (also called Kirby-Bauer test) is most common.

  ○ Broth dilution method is a quantitative method that helps determine the necessary amount of antibiotic for a specific infection.

- Host Factors
  - Immune System of Clients
    - In clients with an intact immune system, the antibiotic works with host defense systems to suppress organisms. Antibiotics that are not bactericidal may be used.
    - Clients who are immunocompromised need strong bactericidal antibiotics.
  - Site of the Infection
    - Certain sites are difficult for antimicrobials to reach.
      - Infections in cerebral spinal fluid, where the antimicrobial agent must cross the blood-brain barrier (meningitis)
      - Bacterial infiltration within the heart (endocarditis)
      - Purulent abscesses anywhere within the body, due to poor blood supply (Drainage through surgery increases the effect of antimicrobials.)
  - Age of Clients
    - Infants are at increased danger of antibiotic toxicity because of undeveloped renal and liver function.

    - Older adult clients may also develop toxicity because of reduction in drug metabolism and excretion.
  - Pregnancy

    - Antibiotics may harm the developing fetus.
  - Breastfeeding
    - Antimicrobials are generally avoided in breastfeeding mothers because of possible danger to the nursing infant.
  - Presence of a previous allergic reaction, especially with penicillin (Clients should not receive penicillin after an allergic reaction, narrowing the antibiotic choice for those clients.)
- Combination Therapy
  - Combining more than one antimicrobial may cause additive effects. Indications include:
    - Severe infections
    - Infections caused by more than one micro-organism
    - Infections, such as tuberculosis, where combination therapy actually prevents bacterial resistance from developing
    - Where use of combinations can decrease chance of toxicity by reducing necessary dosage
    - Where use of multiple antibiotics produces more effective treatment than use of only one

- o Combining antimicrobials can sometimes cause adverse effects, such as:

  - Increased resistance to antimicrobials

  - Increased cost of therapy

  - More adverse or toxic reactions

  - Antagonistic effects among the various antibiotics

Prophylactic Use

- Indications for prophylactic use include prevention of:

  - o Infections for clients undergoing surgery of the gastrointestinal tract, cardiac or vascular surgery, orthopedic surgery, or some gynecologic surgeries

  - o Influenza in susceptible individuals with amantadine (Symmetrel)

  - o Sexually transmitted diseases following sexual exposure

- Limit prophylactic use of antimicrobials to individuals with:

  - o Prosthetic heart valves, undergoing dental or other procedures because of the danger of bacterial endocarditis

  - o Recurring urinary tract infection

Ⓢ Nursing Interventions

- Perform hand hygiene before and after each client contact to prevent the spread of infection.

- Recognize invasive procedures that increase the chance of infection, such as urinary or other catheters.

- Encourage health measures to prevent infections:

  - o Maintaining up-to-date immunization status

  - o Hand hygiene

- Teach clients to take the full course of antibiotics prescribed to prevent medication resistance and recurrence of infection.

- Use infection control procedures to prevent transmission of resistant micro-organisms such as aseptic technique and appropriate transmission precautions.

- Evaluate effectiveness of treatment:

  - o Check post-treatment culture to determine if it is negative for bacteria.

  - o Monitor clients for clinical improvement, such as improved breath sounds.

APPLICATION EXERCISES

1. A nurse is caring for a school-age child who has been diagnosed with viral bronchitis. The mother tells the nurse, "I'm upset that the doctor didn't order an antibiotic for my child. I think I'll start giving her the left-over antibiotics from her last ear infection." What should concern the nurse in this situation?

2. A nurse is caring for a client who has a suspected bacterial infection in her urine. Which of the following prescribed laboratory tests will identify which micro-organism is responsible for the infection?

    A. Gram stain

    B. Culture

    C. Sensitivity

    D. Specific gravity

3. A nurse is caring for a group of clients. The nurse understands that prophylactic use of antibiotics is indicated for which of the following clients? (Select all that apply.)

    _____ An older adult client who has recovered from several episodes of severe pneumonia.

    _____ An adult client who is undergoing total hip replacement surgery today.

    _____ A young adult client who was exposed to gonorrhea last night.

    _____ A school-age child who will be having his tonsils and adenoids removed tomorrow.

    _____ A toddler who just completed treatment for the most recent of multiple ear infections.

APPLICATION EXERCISES ANSWER KEY

1. A nurse is caring for a school-age child who has been diagnosed with viral bronchitis. The mother tells the nurse, "I'm upset that the doctor didn't order an antibiotic for my child. I think I'll start giving her the left-over antibiotics from her last ear infection." What should concern the nurse in this situation?

The mother is promoting resistance toward antibiotics in her child by not giving the full dose of previously prescribed antibiotics, and by giving antimicrobials meant for a bacterial infection to the child for a viral infection, although these medications will be of no use for viral bronchitis. This indicates the mother needs reinforcing about the proper use of antibiotics.

 NCLEX® Connection: Pharmacological Therapies, Medication Administration

2. A nurse is caring for a client who has a suspected bacterial infection in her urine. Which of the following prescribed laboratory tests will identify which micro-organism is responsible for the infection?

   A. Gram stain

   B. Culture

   C. Sensitivity

   D. Specific gravity

A culture allows micro-organisms to reproduce over several days in order to positively identify them. A gram stain simply identifies the presence of micro-organisms through direct visualization under a microscope. A test for sensitivity tells which antibiotic will be effective in treating a specific infection. A test for specific gravity of urine does not indicate the presence of micro-organisms, rather, it tells the concentration of urine compared to water.

 NCLEX® Connection: Pharmacological Therapies, Expected Actions/Outcomes

3. A nurse is caring for a group of clients. The nurse understands that prophylactic use of antibiotics is indicated for which of the following clients? (Select all that apply.)

   _____ An older adult client who has recovered from several episodes of severe pneumonia.

   __X__ **An adult client who is undergoing total hip replacement surgery today.**

   __X__ **A young adult client who was exposed to gonorrhea last night.**

   _____ A school-age child who will be having his tonsils and adenoids removed tomorrow.

   _____ A toddler who just completed treatment for the most recent of multiple ear infections.

Prophylactic use of antibiotics is indicated for clients who undergo orthopedic, cardiac, peripheral vascular, gastrointestinal, and some gynecologic surgeries. It is also indicated for those who have been exposed to a sexually transmitted disease. Prophylactic use of antibiotics is not indicated for the other clients.

 NCLEX® Connection: Pharmacological Therapies, Expected Actions/Outcomes

UNIT 11	MEDICATIONS AFFECTING THE IMMUNE SYSTEM AND FOR INFECTIOUS DISEASES
Chapter 40	Antibiotics Affecting the Bacterial Cell Wall

 Overview

- Antibiotics that affect the cell wall are generally bactericidal. Bactericidal drugs are directly lethal to bacteria at clinically achievable concentrations. This group of antibiotics includes penicillins, cephalosporins, carbapenems, and monobactams.

MEDICATION CLASSIFICATION: PENICILLINS

- Select Prototype Medication – Penicillin G (Bicillin LA)

- Other Medications:

  o Broad-spectrum

  o Ampicillin (Principen)

  o Ampicillin/sulbactam (Unasyn) – Penicillin combined with beta-lactamase inhibitor

    ▪ Amoxicillin/clavulanate (Augmentin) – Penicillin combined with beta-lactamase inhibitor

  o Antistaphylococcal

    ▪ Nafcillin (Unipen)

    ▪ Methicillin

  o Antipseudomonas

    ▪ Carbenicillin (Geocillin)

    ▪ Ticarcillin/clavulanate (Timentin) – Penicillin combined with beta-lactamase inhibitor

    ▪ Piperacillin tazobactam (Zosyn)

Purpose

- Expected Pharmacological Action

  o Penicillins destroy bacteria by weakening the bacterial cell wall.

- Therapeutic Uses

  o Penicillins are the medication of choice for gram-positive cocci such as *Streptococcus pneumoniae* (pneumonia and meningitis), *Streptococcus viridans* (infectious endocarditis), and *Streptococcus pyogenes* (pharyngitis).

  o Penicillins are the medication of choice for meningitis caused by gram–negative cocci *Neisseria meningitides*.

  o Penicillins are the medication of choice for syphilis caused by *spirochete Treponema pallidum*.

  o Extended-spectrum penicillin (carbenicillin, piperacillin) is effective against organisms such as *Pseudomonas aeruginosa*, *Enterobacter species*, *Proteus*, *Bacteroides fragilis*, and *Klebsiella*.

  o Prophylaxis of bacterial endocarditis in at-risk clients prior to dental and other procedures.

Complications

SIDE/ADVERSE EFFECTS	NURSING INTERVENTIONS/CLIENT EDUCATION
• Allergies/Anaphylaxis	• Interview clients for prior allergy. • Advise clients to wear a medication alert bracelet. • Observe clients for 30 min following administration of parenteral penicillin.
• Renal impairment	• Monitor the client's kidney function. • Monitor the client's I&O.
• Hyperkalemia/dysrhythmias are possible with high doses of penicillin, penicillin G. • Hypernatremia may occur with IV carbenicillin and ticarcillin.	• Monitor the client's cardiac status and serum electrolyte levels. • Exercise caution with patients who follow a sodium-restricted diet.

 Contraindications/Precautions

- Penicillins are contraindicated for clients who have a severe history of allergies to cephalosporins.

 • Use cautiously in clients who have, or are at risk for, kidney dysfunction (clients who are acutely ill, older adults, or young children).

- Clients who are allergic to one penicillin should be considered cross allergic to other penicillins and at risk for a cross allergy to cephalosporin.

Interactions

MEDICATION/FOOD INTERACTIONS	NURSING INTERVENTIONS/CLIENT EDUCATION
Probenecid (Probalan) delays excretion of penicillin.	• Administer probenecid during penicillin therapy to prolong antibacterial action.

Nursing Administration

- o Instruct clients that penicillin V, amoxicillin, and amoxicillin-clavulanate may be taken with meals. All others should be taken with a full glass of water 1 hr before or 2 hr after meals.

- o Instruct clients to report any signs of an allergic response such as skin rash, itching, and/or hives.

- o Administer IM injections cautiously to avoid injection into a nerve or an artery.

- o Advise clients to complete the entire course of therapy regardless of presence of symptoms.

- o Encourage clients who have penicillin allergy to wear a medication alert bracelet.

MEDICATION CLASSIFICATION: CEPHALOSPORINS

- • Select Prototype Medication – Cephalexin (Keflex) – 1st generation

- • Other Medications:

  - o 1st generation – Cephradine (Anspor, Velosef)

  - o 2nd generation – Cefaclor (Ceclor), cefotetan (Cefotan)

  - o 3rd generation – Ceftriaxone (Rocephin), cefotaxime (Claforan), cefoperazone (Cefobid)

  - o 4th generation – Cefepime (Maxipime)

Purpose

- • Expected Pharmacological Action

  - o Cephalosporins are beta-lactam antibiotics, similar to penicillins that destroy bacterial cell walls, causing destruction of micro-organisms.

  - o Cephalosporins are bactericidal medications with a high therapeutic index.

  - o Cephalosporins are grouped into four generations. Each generation of cephalosporins is:

    - ■ More likely to reach cerebrospinal fluid

    - ■ Less likely to be destroyed by beta-lactamase

    - ■ More effective against gram-negative organisms and anaerobes

- Therapeutic Uses
  - Treat urinary tract infections, postoperative infections, pelvic infections, and meningitis.

Complications

SIDE/ADVERSE EFFECTS	NURSING INTERVENTIONS/CLIENT EDUCATION
- Hypersensitivity reactions or anaphylaxis (urticaria, rash, hypotension, and/or dyspnea) - Possible cross-sensitivity to penicillin	- If signs of allergy appear, stop cephalosporin immediately, and notify the provider. - Assist with emergency management of anaphylaxis (respiratory support and IV epinephrine). - Question clients carefully regarding past history of allergy to a penicillin or other cephalosporin, and notify the provider if present.
- Bleeding tendencies with use of cefotetan	- Cefotetan should be avoided in clients who have bleeding disorders and those taking anticoagulants/thrombolytic agents. - Observe clients for signs of bleeding. If bleeding develops, drug should be withdrawn. - Monitor clients for PT and bleeding time. Abnormal levels may require discontinuation of medication. - Administer parenteral vitamin K if indicated.
- Pain with IM injection	- Administer IM injection deep in large muscle mass.
- Antibiotic-associated pseudomembranous colitis	- Observe clients for diarrhea and notify the provider. - Tell clients the provider will discontinue the medication.

 Contraindications/Precautions

- Cephalosporins should not be given to clients who have a history of severe allergic reactions to penicillins.

- Use cautiously in clients who have renal impairment or bleeding tendencies.

Interactions

MEDICATION/FOOD INTERACTIONS	NURSING INTERVENTIONS/CLIENT EDUCATION
Disulfiram reaction (intolerance to alcohol) occurs with combined use of cefotetan and alcohol.	• Instruct clients not to consume alcohol while taking cefotetan.
Probenecid delays renal excretion of some cephalosporins.	• Administer probenecid during cephalosporin therapy to prolong antibacterial action.

Nursing Administration

- Instruct clients to complete the prescribed course of therapy, even though symptoms may resolve before the full course of antimicrobial treatment is completed.

- Advise clients to take oral cephalosporins with food.

- Instruct clients to store oral cephalosporin suspensions in a refrigerator.

MEDICATION CLASSIFICATION: CARBAPENEMS

- Select Prototype Medication – Imipenem (Primaxin)

Purpose

- Expected Pharmacological Action

  o Carbapenems are beta-lactam antibiotics that destroy bacterial cell walls, causing destruction of micro-organisms.

- Therapeutic Uses

  o Broad antimicrobial spectrum is effective against serious infections such as pneumonia, peritonitis, and urinary tract infections caused by gram-positive cocci, gram-negative cocci and bacilli, and anaerobic bacteria.

  o Resistance develops when imipenem is used alone to treat *Pseudomonas aeruginosa*. Use in combination with antipseudomonal medications to treat this micro-organism.

Complications

SIDE/ADVERSE EFFECTS	NURSING INTERVENTIONS/CLIENT EDUCATION
• Allergy/hypersensitivity (rash, pruritus) • Possible cross-sensitivity to penicillin or cephalosporins	• Monitor clients for signs of allergic reactions and report to the provider if present. • Question clients carefully regarding past history of allergy to a penicillin or other cephalosporin and notify provider if present.

SIDE/ADVERSE EFFECTS	NURSING INTERVENTIONS/CLIENT EDUCATION
• Gastrointestinal (GI) symptoms (nausea, vomiting, diarrhea)	• Observe clients for symptoms and notify the provider if present. • Monitor the client's I&O.
• Suprainfection (colitis [diarrhea], oral thrush, vaginal yeast infection)	• Monitor clients for signs and notify the provider if present.

 Contraindications/Precautions

- Use cautiously in clients who have renal impairment.

Nursing Administration

- Instruct clients to complete the prescribed course of antimicrobial therapy, even though symptoms may resolve before completing the full course.

MEDICATION CLASSIFICATION: MONOBACTAMS

- Select Prototype Medications:

    o Vancomycin (Vancocin)

    o Aztreonam (Azactam)

    o Fosfomycin (Monurol)

Purpose

- Expected Pharmacological Action

    o Monobactams are beta-lactam antibiotics that destroy bacterial cell walls, causing destruction of micro-organisms.

- Therapeutic Uses

    o Serious infections caused by methicillin resistant *Staphylococcus aureus* or *Staphylococcus epidermidis*

    o Antibiotic-associated pseudomembranous colitis caused by *Clostridium difficile*

Complications

SIDE/ADVERSE EFFECTS	NURSING INTERVENTIONS/CLIENT EDUCATION
Ototoxicity	• Check clients for signs of hearing loss. • Instruct clients to notify the provider if changes in hearing acuity develop. • Monitor vancomycin levels.
Infusion reactions (rashes, flushing, tachycardia, and hypotension)	• Monitor clients receiving IV infusions.
Thrombophlebitis	• Monitor the infusion site for redness, swelling, and inflammation.

Interactions

MEDICATION/FOOD INTERACTIONS	NURSING INTERVENTIONS/CLIENT EDUCATION
• Increased risk for ototoxicity with concurrent use with another medication that also produces ototoxicity (loop diuretics).	• Check for hearing loss.

 Contraindications/Precautions

- Use cautiously in clients who have renal impairment.

Nursing Administration

- Vancomycin peak blood levels should be collected 1 to 2 hr after completion of IV infusion.

Nursing Evaluation of Medication Effectiveness

- Depending on therapeutic intent, effectiveness may be evidenced by:

  o Reduction of signs and symptoms such as fever, pain, inflammation, and adventitious breath sounds

  o Resolution of infection

(A) APPLICATION EXERCISES

1. A nurse is caring for a group of clients in an outpatient facility who may require antibiotics for bacterial infections. For which of the following antibiotic prescriptions should the nurse be sure to collect data regarding previous penicillin allergies? (Select all that apply.)

    _____ Imipenem (Primaxin)

    _____ Vancomycin (Vancocin)

    _____ Cephalexin (Keflex)

    _____ Cefepime (Maxipime)

    _____ Teicoplanin (Targocid)

2. A nurse is caring for a client in an urgent care clinic who has pneumonia. The client is prescribed ampicillin (Principen). Two days later the client calls the clinic and reports to the nurse that she is experiencing an itchy rash. Which of the following actions should the nurse take first?

    A. Collect data about previous allergic reactions.

    B. Ask the client to describe her symptoms.

    C. Tell the client not to take the next dose of antibiotic.

    D. Have the client come to the clinic to see her provider.

3. A nurse is caring for a client who is receiving vancomycin (Vancocin) for a severe infection. For which of the following should the nurse monitor the client in order to collect data about a possible adverse reaction to vancomycin?

    A. Visual acuity

    B. Hearing ability

    C. Presence of ataxia

    D. Deep tendon reflexes

4. A nurse is reinforcing teaching for a client who has a urinary tract infection and a new prescription for imipenem (Primaxin). Which of the following adverse reactions should the nurse instruct the client to watch for?

    A. Oral thrush

    B. Chest pain

    C. Rapid pulse

    D. Peripheral neuropathy

APPLICATION EXERCISES ANSWER KEY

1. A nurse is caring for a group of clients in an outpatient facility who may require antibiotics for bacterial infections. For which of the following antibiotic prescriptions should the nurse be sure to collect data regarding previous penicillin allergies? (Select all that apply.)

    X   **Imipenem (Primaxin)**

    _____   Vancomycin (Vancocin)

    X   **Cephalexin (Keflex)**

    X   **Cefepime (Maxipime)**

    _____   Teicoplanin (Targocid)

    Clients who are allergic to penicillin may have a cross sensitivity to the carbapenem and cephalosporin antibiotics. Ask clients who are prescribed these medications about previous allergic reactions to the antibiotic prescribed, and any penicillin antibiotic. Vancomycin and teicoplanin do have cross sensitivity to penicillin and may be prescribed for clients with a penicillin allergy.

     NCLEX® Connection: Pharmacological Therapies, Adverse Effects/Contraindications/Side Effects/Interactions

2. A nurse is caring for a client in an urgent care clinic who has pneumonia. The client is prescribed ampicillin (Principen). Two days later the client calls the clinic and reports to the nurse that she is experiencing an itchy rash. Which of the following actions should the nurse take first?

    A. Collect data about previous allergic reactions.

    B. Ask the client to describe her symptoms.

    C. Tell the client not to take the next dose of antibiotic.

    D. Have the client come to the clinic to see her provider.

    The greatest risk to the client is anaphylaxis and therefore the nurse should first ask the client to fully describe her symptoms in order to evaluate whether she may need to call 911 to obtain emergency care. Findings that require immediate treatment include signs of anaphylaxis (laryngeal edema, severe hypotension, bronchoconstriction). If emergency care is not required, the nurse should collect data about previous allergic reactions, tell the client not to take the next dose of antibiotic, and have the client come to the clinic to see her provider.

     NCLEX® Connection: Pharmacological Therapies: Adverse Effects/Contraindications/Side Effects/Interactions

3. A nurse is caring for a client who is receiving vancomycin (Vancocin) for a severe infection. For which of the following should the nurse monitor the client in order to collect data about a possible adverse reaction to vancomycin?

   A. Visual acuity

   B. Hearing ability

   C. Presence of ataxia

   D. Deep tendon reflexes

   Vancomycin may cause ototoxicity and the nurse should monitor the client's hearing ability for changes during therapy with vancomycin. Visual acuity, gait (for presence of ataxia), and deep tendon reflexes do not require monitoring while the client is taking the medication.

 NCLEX® Connection: Pharmacological Therapies, Adverse Effects/Contraindications/Side Effects/Interactions

4. A nurse is reinforcing teaching for a client who has a urinary tract infection and a new prescription for imipenem (Primaxin). Which of the following adverse reactions should the nurse instruct the client to watch for?

   A. Oral thrush

   B. Chest pain

   C. Rapid pulse

   D. Peripheral neuropathy

   Imipenem may cause suprainfection, which may be manifested by oral thrush, colitis with diarrhea, or other yeast infections. Chest pain, rapid pulse, and peripheral neuropathy are not adverse reactions to imipenem.

 NCLEX® Connection: Pharmacological Therapies, Adverse Effects/Contraindications/Side Effects/Interactions

UNIT 11	MEDICATIONS AFFECTING THE IMMUNE SYSTEM AND FOR INFECTIOUS DISEASES

Chapter 41   Antibiotics Affecting Protein Synthesis

 Overview

- Antibiotics affecting protein synthesis may be bacteriostatic, such as tetracyclines and macrolides, or bactericidal, such as aminoglycosides.

- Uses include treatment of infections of the respiratory, gastrointestinal, urinary and reproductive tract and infections caused by rickettsia.

MEDICATION CLASSIFICATION: TETRACYCLINES

- Select Prototype Medication – Tetracycline (Sumycin)

- Other Medications – Doxycycline (Vibramycin), minocycline (Minocin)

Purpose

- Expected Pharmacological Action

  o Tetracyclines are broad-spectrum antibiotics that inhibit micro-organism growth by preventing protein synthesis.

- Therapeutic Uses

  o Topical and oral treatment for severe acne vulgaris and topically for periodontal disease

  o Rickettsial infections, such as typhus fever or Rocky Mountain spotted fever

  o Infections of the urethra or cervix caused by *Chlamydia trachomatis*

  o Brucellosis

  o Pneumonia caused by *Mycoplasma pneumonia*

  o Lyme disease

  o Anthrax

  o Gastrointestinal (GI) infections caused by *Helicobacter pylori*

Complications

SIDE/ADVERSE EFFECTS	NURSING INTERVENTIONS/CLIENT EDUCATION
Gastrointestinal (GI) discomfort (cramping, nausea, vomiting, diarrhea, and esophageal ulceration)	• Monitor clients for nausea, vomiting, and diarrhea. • Monitor the client's I&O. • Advise clients that doxycycline and minocycline may be taken with meals. • Instruct clients to avoid taking at bedtime to reduce esophageal ulceration.
Yellow/brown tooth discoloration and/or hypoplasia of tooth enamel	• Contraindicated for children less than 8 years of age.
Hepatotoxicity (lethargy, jaundice)	• Avoid administration of high IV doses.
Photosensitivity (exaggerated sunburn)	• Advise clients to take precautions when out in the sun such as wearing protective clothing and using sunscreen.
Suprainfection of the bowel – antibiotic-associated pseudomembranous colitis (diarrhea, yeast infections of the mouth, pharynx, vagina, and bowels)	• Instruct clients to observe for symptoms of diarrhea and notify the provider.
Dizziness, lightheadedness, with minocycline	• Instruct clients to notify the provider, who will discontinue the medication.

 Contraindications/Precautions

- Use of tetracycline during pregnancy after the fourth month is contraindicated in children less than 8 yr of age.

- Use cautiously in clients who have liver and renal disease. Doxycycline and minocycline may be used in clients who have renal disease.

Interactions

MEDICATION/FOOD INTERACTIONS	NURSING INTERVENTIONS/CLIENT EDUCATION
Interaction with milk products, calcium or iron supplements, laxatives containing magnesium such as magnesium hydroxide (Milk of Magnesia), and antacids causes formation of nonabsorbable chelates.	• Advise clients to take tetracycline on an empty stomach, generally 1 hr before or 2 hr after meals, with a full glass of water. • Instruct clients to take medication 2 hr before or 2 hr after consuming food and supplements containing calcium and magnesium.
Tetracycline decreases the efficacy of oral contraceptives.	• Advise clients to use an alternative form of birth control.

Nursing Administration

- Instruct clients to complete the prescribed course of antimicrobial therapy, even though symptoms may resolve before completing the full course.

Nursing Evaluation of Medication Effectiveness

- Depending on therapeutic intent, effectiveness may be evidenced by:

    o Improvement of infection symptoms, such as clear breath sounds

    o Resolution of yeast infections of the mouth, vagina, and bowels

    o Resolution of acne vulgaris facial lesions

MEDICATION CLASSIFICATION: MACROLIDES

- Select Prototype Medication – Erythromycin (E-Mycin)

- Other medication – Azithromycin (Zithromax)

Purpose

- Expected Pharmacological Action

    o Erythromycin slows the growth of micro-organisms by inhibiting protein synthesis.

- Therapeutic Uses

    o Treat infections in clients who have a penicillin allergy, such as for prophylaxis against rheumatic fever and bacterial endocarditis.

    o Treat Legionnaires' disease, whooping cough (pertussis), and acute diphtheria (eliminates the carrier state of diphtheria).

    o Treat chlamydia infections (urethritis and cervicitis; pneumonia caused by *Mycoplasma pneumoniae*; respiratory tract infections caused by *Streptococcus pneumoniae*, and group A *Streptococcus pyogenes*).

Complications

SIDE/ADVERSE EFFECTS	NURSING INTERVENTIONS/CLIENT EDUCATION
GI discomfort (nausea, vomiting, epigastric pain)	• Tell clients to observe for GI symptoms and to notify the provider. • Instruct clients to administer erythromycin with meals if GI upset occurs.
Hepatotoxicity (abdominal pain, lethargy, jaundice)	• Instruct clients to notify the provider, who will discontinue the medication.
Prolonged QT interval causing dysrhythmias and possible sudden cardiac death	• Avoid use in clients who have prolonged QT intervals and those taking antidysrhythmics. • Avoid concurrent use with medications that affect hepatic drug metabolizing enzymes.

Contraindications/Precautions

- Erythromycin should be avoided in clients who have pre-existing liver disease.

Interactions

MEDICATION/FOOD INTERACTIONS	NURSING INTERVENTIONS/CLIENT EDUCATION
Erythromycin inhibits metabolism of antihistamines, theophylline (Theo-24), carbamazepine (Tegretol), and warfarin (Coumadin), which can lead to toxicity of these medications.	• To minimize toxicity, avoid concurrent use.
Verapamil (Calan), and diltiazem (Cardizem), HIV protease inhibitors, antifungal azole medications, and nefazodone inhibit erythromycin metabolism.	• Avoid concurrent use.

Nursing Administration

- Administer oral preparation on an empty stomach (1 hr before meals or 2 hr after) with a full glass of water, unless GI upset occurs.

- Intravenous route for erythromycin is rarely used.

- Instruct clients to complete the prescribed course of antimicrobial therapy, even though symptoms may resolve before completing the full course.

Nursing Evaluation of Medication Effectiveness

- Depending on therapeutic intent, effectiveness may be evidenced by:

  o Improvement of infection symptoms (clear lung sounds; improvement of sore throat, cough, urinary tract symptoms; and resolution of bacterial endocarditis with negative blood cultures).

MEDICATION CLASSIFICATION: AMINOGLYCOSIDES

- Select Prototype Medication – Gentamicin (Garamycin) (IM, IV)

- Other Medications:

  o Amikacin (Amikin) (IM, IV)

  o Tobramycin sulfate (Nebcin) (IM, IV)

  o Streptomycin (IM, IV)

  o Neomycin (Mycifradin) (oral, topical)

Purpose

- Expected Pharmacological Action

  o Aminoglycosides are bactericidal antibiotics that destroy micro-organisms by disrupting protein synthesis.

- Therapeutic Uses

  o Use parenteral aminoglycosides to treat aerobic gram-negative bacilli, such as *Escherichia coli, Klebsiella pneumoniae, Proteus mirabilis,* and *Pseudomonas aeruginosa.*

  o Use oral neomycin prior to surgery of the GI tract to suppress normal flora.

  o Use topical neomycin for eye, ear, and skin infections.

Complications

SIDE/ADVERSE EFFECTS	NURSING INTERVENTIONS/CLIENT EDUCATION
Ototoxicity – Cochlear damage (hearing loss) and vestibular damage (loss of balance)	• Monitor clients for symptoms of tinnitus (ringing in the ears), headache, hearing loss, nausea, dizziness, and vertigo. • Instruct clients to notify the provider, who will discontinue the medication.
Nephrotoxicity related to high total cumulative dose resulting in acute tubular necrosis (proteinuria, casts in the urine, dilute urine, elevated BUN, creatinine levels)	• Monitor I&O, BUN, and serum creatinine levels. • Instruct clients to report a significant decrease in the amount of urine output.
Intensified neuromuscular blockade resulting in respiratory depression	• Closely monitor use in clients who have myasthenia gravis, clients taking skeletal muscle relaxants, and clients receiving general anesthetics.
Hypersensitivity (rash, pruritus, paresthesia of hands and feet, and urticaria)	• Monitor clients for allergic symptoms.
Streptomycin	
Neurologic disorder (peripheral neuritis, optic nerve dysfunction, tingling/numbness of the hands and feet)	• Instruct clients to promptly report any symptoms to the provider.

 Contraindications/Precautions

- Use cautiously with clients who have renal impairment, pre-existing hearing loss or myasthenia gravis.

- Use cautiously with clients taking ethacrynic acid (increases risk for ototoxicity), amphotericin B, cephalosporins, vancomycin (increases risk for nephrotoxicity), and neuromuscular blocking agents such as tubocurarine.

- Clients who have renal impairment should receive reduced doses of aminoglycosides.

Interactions

MEDICATION/FOOD INTERACTIONS	NURSING INTERVENTIONS/CLIENT EDUCATION
Concurrent use with other ototoxic medications (such as loop diuretics), the risk for ototoxicity greatly increases.	• Check frequently for hearing loss with concurrent medication use.

Nursing Administration

- Monitor parenteral aminoglycoside levels based on dosing schedules.

    o Once-a-day dosing – Only measure trough level. Take trough level 1 hr prior to the next dose.

    o Divided doses:

        ▪ Peak – 30 min after administration of aminoglycoside intramuscularly or 30 min after an IV infusion has finished

        ▪ Trough – Right before the next dose

Nursing Evaluation of Medication Effectiveness

- Depending on therapeutic intent, effectiveness may be evidenced by:

    o Improvement of infection symptoms (clear lung sounds, improvement of urinary tract symptoms, wound healing)

APPLICATION EXERCISES

1. A nurse is reinforcing teaching to a client prescribed tetracycline (Sumycin) to treat a gastrointestinal infection. Which of the following statements by the client indicates a need for further teaching?

    A. "I will be sure to wear long sleeves when out in the sun."

    B. "I will take the medication with a full glass of milk."

    C. "I will finish all the medicine even if I am feeling better."

    D. "I will take the medication first thing in the morning."

2. A nurse is caring for a client who will receive gentamicin (Garamycin) intermittent IV bolus at noon. The infusion will take 30 min. When should the nurse plan to have a peak level of gentamicin drawn by the laboratory?

    A. 12:30 p.m.

    B. 1:00 p.m.

    C. 2:30 p.m.

    D. 3:00 p.m.

3. A nurse is caring for a client with a prescription for erythromycin (E-Mycin) to treat a urethral infection. The client also takes daily prescriptions for furosemide (Lasix) and warfarin (Coumadin). For which of the following manifestations of a drug interaction should the nurse monitor the client?

    A. Bradycardia

    B. Urinary retention

    C. Bleeding

    D. Hypernatremia

4. A nurse is caring for a client who receives amikacin (Amikin) by intermittent IV bolus for a severe infection. Which of the following laboratory values should the nurse recognize as an adverse effect of amikacin?

    A. Elevated serum creatinine

    B. Elevated triglycerides

    C. Decreased serum potassium

    D. Decreased hematocrit

APPLICATION EXERCISES ANSWER KEY

1. A nurse is reinforcing teaching to a client prescribed tetracycline (Sumycin) to treat a gastrointestinal infection. Which of the following statements by the client indicates a need for further teaching?

    A. "I will be sure to wear long sleeves when out in the sun."

    B. "I will take the medication with a full glass of milk."

    C. "I will finish all the medicine even if I am feeling better."

    D. "I will take the medication first thing in the morning."

    Tetracycline can form a nonabsorbable chelate when taken with dairy products and should be taken with water. The client should wear long sleeves to protect against sun exposure. The client may feel better before the entire prescription is complete, but should finish the entire dose to ensure eradication of the infection. Taking the medication in the morning will reduce esophageal ulceration, which can occur if the medication is taken just before lying down at night.

 NCLEX® Connection: Pharmacological Therapies, Medication Administration

2. A nurse is caring for a client who will receive gentamicin (Garamycin) intermittent IV bolus at noon. The infusion will take 30 min. When should the nurse plan to have a peak level of gentamicin drawn by the laboratory?

    A. 12:30 p.m.

    B. 1:00 p.m.

    C. 2:30 p.m.

    D. 3:00 p.m.

    Draw the peak level of gentamicin 30 min following the completion of the IV infusion. None of the other times are correct since the infusion should be done by 12:30 p.m. if it starts at noon.

 NCLEX® Connection: Pharmacological Therapies, Medication Administration

3. A nurse is caring for a client with a prescription for erythromycin (E-Mycin) to treat a urethral infection. The client also takes daily prescriptions for furosemide (Lasix) and warfarin (Coumadin). For which of the following manifestations of a drug interaction should the nurse monitor the client?

    A. Bradycardia

    B. Urinary retention

    C. Bleeding

    D. Hypernatremia

    The nurse should monitor the client for bleeding because erythromycin interacts with warfarin to increase warfarin levels in the body. Erythromycin does not interact with furosemide. Bradycardia, urinary retention, and hypernatremia are not expected manifestations of an interaction with erythromycin and either medication.

NCLEX® Connection: Pharmacological Therapies, Adverse Effects/Contraindications/Side Effects/Interactions

4. A nurse is caring for a client who receives amikacin (Amikin) by intermittent IV bolus for a severe infection. Which of the following laboratory values should the nurse recognize as an adverse effect of amikacin?

    A. Elevated serum creatinine

    B. Elevated triglycerides

    C. Decreased serum potassium

    D. Decreased hematocrit

    Aminoglycosides, such as amikacin, can cause reversible renal injury. The nurse should monitor for increased serum creatinine and BUN, which would indicate renal damage. Elevated triglycerides, decreased serum potassium, or decreased hematocrit are not adverse effects of amikacin.

NCLEX® Connection: Pharmacological Therapies, Adverse Effects/Contraindications/Side Effects/Interactions

UNIT 11	MEDICATIONS AFFECTING THE IMMUNE SYSTEM AND FOR INFECTIOUS DISEASES
Chapter 42	Urinary Tract Infections

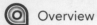 Overview

- Use sulfonamides, trimethoprim, and urinary antiseptics to treat urinary tract infections.

- Use these medications to treat active infections and for prophylaxis of recurrent infections for susceptible individuals.

- Regimens with these medications may be single-dose, a short-course of 3 days, or 7 to 14 days.

MEDICATION CLASSIFICATION: TRIMETHOPRIM AND SULFONAMIDES

- Select Prototype Medications:

  o Trimethoprim-sulfamethoxazole [TMP-SMZ] (Bactrim)

  o Co-trimoxazole (Cotrim, Septra)

Purpose

- Expected Pharmacological Action

  o Sulfonamides and trimethoprim inhibit bacterial growth by preventing the synthesis of folic acid. Folic acid is essential for the production of DNA, RNA, and proteins.

- Therapeutic Uses

  o Urinary tract infections from *E. coli, Klebsiella, Proteus, Pseudomonas,* and *Candida* species.

  o Other infections include otitis media, chronic bronchitis, shigellosis, and pneumonia caused by *Pneumocystis carinii.*

Complications

SIDE/ADVERSE EFFECTS	NURSING INTERVENTIONS/CLIENT EDUCATION

Hypersensitivity including Stevens-Johnson syndrome	• Do not administer TMP-SMZ to clients who have allergies to:
	   o Sulfonamides (sulfa)
	   o Thiazide diuretics [hydrochlorothiazide (HCTZ)]
	   o Sulfonylurea-type oral hypoglycemics [glipizide (Glucotrol)]
	   o Loop diuretics [furosemide (Lasix)]
	• Stop TMP-SMZ at the first indication of hypersensitivity, such as rash.

Blood dyscrasias (hemolytic anemia, agranulocytosis, aplastic anemia)	• Monitor the client's baseline and periodic CBC levels to detect any hematologic disorders. • Observe for any bleeding episodes, sore throat, or pallor. • If the above symptoms occur, instruct clients to notify the provider.
Crystalluria	• Maintain adequate oral fluid intake. • Instruct clients to consume 2 to 3 L/day of fluid a day from food and beverage sources.
Kernicterus (jaundice, increased bilirubin levels)	• Avoid administering TMP-SMZ to women who are pregnant, breastfeeding mothers, and infants younger than 2 months.
Photosensitivity	• Instruct clients to avoid prolonged exposure to sunlight, use sunscreen, and wear appropriate protective clothing.

 Contraindications/Precautions

- TMP-SMZ is contraindicated in clients who have folate deficiency manifested as megaloblastic anemia.

- TMP-SMZ is contraindicated in clients who have allergies to thiazide and loop diuretics and sulfonylurea-type oral hypoglycemic agents.

- Avoid use in pregnancy and lactation (risk of kernicterus).

- Use cautiously in clients who have renal dysfunction. Reduce dosage of TMP-SMZ by 50%.

- Do not use if creatinine clearance is less than 15 mL/min.

Interactions

MEDICATION/FOOD INTERACTIONS	NURSING INTERVENTIONS/CLIENT EDUCATION
Sulfonamides can increase the effects of warfarin (Coumadin), phenytoin (Dilantin), sulfonylurea oral hypoglycemics, and tolbutamide (Orinase) by inhibiting hepatic metabolism.	• Administer reduced dosages as prescribed during TMP-SMZ therapy.

Nursing Administration

- Instruct clients to take TMP-SMZ on an empty stomach with a full glass of water.

- Encourage clients to maintain adequate fluid intake throughout the day (2 to 3 L/day)

- Instruct clients to complete the prescribed course of antimicrobial therapy, even though symptoms may resolve before completing the full course.

Nursing Evaluation of Medication Effectiveness

- Depending on therapeutic intent, effectiveness may be evidenced by:

  o Improvement of infection symptoms, such as improvement of urinary tract symptoms (decreased frequency, burning, and pain during urination) and negative urine cultures

MEDICATION CLASSIFICATION: URINARY TRACT ANTISEPTICS

- Select Prototype Medication – Nitrofurantoin (Macrodantin)

- Other Medications – Methenamine (Mandelamine), nalidixic acid (NegGram)

Purpose

- Expected Pharmacological Action

  o These medications are active against the common urinary tract pathogens.

- Therapeutic Uses

  o Second-choice drugs for acute urinary tract infections

  o Prophylaxis for recurrent lower urinary tract infections

Complications

SIDE/ADVERSE EFFECTS	NURSING INTERVENTIONS/CLIENT EDUCATION
Gastrointestinal discomfort (anorexia, nausea, vomiting, diarrhea)	• Instruct clients to administer nitrofurantoin with milk or meals.
Hypersensitivity reactions with severe pulmonary manifestations (dyspnea, cough, malaise)	• Advise clients to stop the medication and call the provider if this occurs. • Pulmonary manifestations should subside within several days after nitrofurantoin is discontinued.
Blood dyscrasias (agranulocytosis, leukopenia, thrombocytopenia)	• Obtain baseline CBC and perform periodic blood tests. • Advise clients to monitor for signs of bleeding. • Instruct clients to notify the provider if symptoms occur.
Peripheral neuropathy (numbness, tingling of the hands and feet, muscle weakness)	• Instruct clients to notify the provider immediately if these symptoms occur.
Headache, drowsiness, dizziness	• Instruct clients to notify the provider if these symptoms occur.

 Contraindications/Precautions

- Nitrofurantoin is contraindicated in clients who have renal dysfunction and creatinine clearance less than 40 mL/min.

    o Impaired renal function will increase the risk of medication toxicity because of inability to excrete nitrofurantoin.

- Nitrofurantoin is contraindicated for pregnant women near term, and for infants under the age of 1 month.

Nursing Administration

- Inform clients that urine may have a brownish discoloration.

- Administer with milk or food if GI symptoms occur.

- Instruct clients to complete the prescribed course of antimicrobial therapy, even though symptoms may resolve before completing the full course.

Nursing Evaluation of Medication Effectiveness

- Depending on therapeutic intent, effectiveness may be evidenced by:

    o Improvement of infection symptoms, such as improvement of urinary tract symptoms (decreased frequency, burning, pain during urination) and negative urine cultures

    o Resolution of diarrhea, nausea, and vomiting

MEDICATION CLASSIFICATION: FLUOROQUINOLONES

- Select Prototype Medication – Ciprofloxacin (Cipro)

- Other Medications – Ofloxacin (Floxin), lomefloxacin (Maxaquin)

Purpose

- Expected Pharmacological Action

  o Fluoroquinolones are bactericidal as a result of inhibition of the enzyme necessary for DNA replication.

- Therapeutic Uses

  o Use to treat a wide variety of micro-organisms such as aerobic gram-negative bacteria, gram-positive bacteria, *Klebsiella*, and *Escherichia coli*.

  o Alternative to parenteral antibiotics for clients with severe infections

  o Urinary, respiratory, and gastrointestinal tract infections; infections of bones, joints, skin, and soft tissues

  o Medication of choice for prevention of anthrax in clients who have inhaled anthrax spore

Complications

SIDE/ADVERSE EFFECTS	NURSING INTERVENTIONS/CLIENT EDUCATION
Gastrointestinal discomfort (nausea, vomiting, diarrhea)	• Suggest clients take with food.
Achilles tendon rupture (pain, swelling, redness at Achilles tendon site)	• Instruct clients to observe for signs and symptoms, and to notify the provider. • The provider will discontinue the medication. • Clients should not exercise until inflammation subsides.
Suprainfection (thrush, vaginal yeast infection)	• Instruct clients to observe for signs and symptoms of yeast infection (cottage cheese/curd-like lesions on the mouth and genital area) and to notify the provider.
Phototoxicity (burning skin, erythema, blisters)	• Advise clients to wear sunscreen and protective clothing. • Advise clients to stop taking medication if symptoms occur and to notify the provider.

 Contraindications/Precautions

- Ciprofloxacin should not be administered to children younger than 18 years of age (due to risk of Achilles tendon rupture), unless the child is being treated for *Escherichia coli* infections of urinary tract or inhalational anthrax.

Interactions

MEDICATION/FOOD INTERACTIONS	NURSING INTERVENTIONS/CLIENT EDUCATION
Cationic compounds (aluminum-magnesium antacids, iron salts, sucralfate, milk and dairy products) decrease absorption of ciprofloxacin.	• Instruct clients to administer these compounds and foods 6 hr before or 2 hr after ciprofloxacin.
Plasma levels of theophylline (Theolair) can be increased with concurrent use of ciprofloxacin.	• Monitor levels and adjust dosage accordingly.
Plasma levels of warfarin (Coumadin) can be increased with concurrent use of ciprofloxacin.	• Monitor prothrombin time and INR, and adjust the dosage of warfarin accordingly.

Nursing Administration

- Administer ciprofloxacin orally.

- Monitor clients receiving ciprofloxacin by intermittent IV bolus.

- Administer decreased doses of ciprofloxacin in clients who have renal dysfunction.

- For inhalation anthrax infection, administer ciprofloxacin every 12 hr for 60 days.

- Instruct clients to complete the prescribed course of antimicrobial therapy, even though symptoms may resolve before completing the full course.

Nursing Evaluation of Medication Effectiveness

- Depending on therapeutic intent, effectiveness may be evidenced by:

  o Improvement of infection symptoms, such as improvement of urinary tract symptoms (decreased frequency, burning, pain during urination), negative urine cultures

  o No evidence of suprainfection such as absence of cottage cheese or curd-like lesions in the mouth and genital areas

APPLICATION EXERCISES

1. A nurse is caring for a group of clients who each have urinary tract infections. The nurse should know that trimethoprim-sulfamethoxazole is contraindicated in clients who have had a hypersensitivity reaction to which of the following medications?

    A. Digoxin (Lanoxin)

    B. Chlorothiazide (Diuril)

    C. Ranitidine (Zantac)

    D. Rosiglitazone (Avandia)

2. A nurse is reinforcing teaching for a client with a prescription for trimethoprim-sulfamethoxazole (Bactrim). Which of the following precautions should the nurse reinforce to the client in order to minimize an adverse effect of the medication?

    A. Avoid prolonged sun exposure.

    B. Sip water or suck hard candy frequently.

    C. Stop taking the medication if ringing in the ears occurs.

    D. Increase the amount of fiber and liquids in the diet.

3. A nurse is reinforcing teaching for a client who is prescribed nitrofurantoin (Macrodantin) for a urinary tract infection. Which of the following points should the nurse include in the instructions? (Select all that apply.)

    _____ The medication may cause the urine to be extremely pale yellow in color.

    _____ Cough and dyspnea are signs of a hypersensitivity reaction to nitrofurantoin.

    _____ Nitrofurantoin should be taken 1 hr before or 2 hr after a meal.

    _____ Notify the provider if nosebleeds or bruising easily occur.

    _____ Report numbness or tingling of hands or feet as soon as possible.

4. A nurse is reinforcing teaching to an adult client about her prescription for ciprofloxacin (Cipro). Which of the following adverse reactions should the nurse tell the client to watch for? (Select all that apply.)

    _____ Jaundice

    _____ Vaginal yeast infection

    _____ Irregular pulse rate

    _____ Urinary hesitancy

    _____ Achilles tendon pain

APPLICATION EXERCISES ANSWER KEY

1. A nurse is caring for a group of clients who each have urinary tract infections. The nurse should know that trimethoprim-sulfamethoxazole is contraindicated in clients who have had a hypersensitivity reaction to which of the following medications?

    A. Digoxin (Lanoxin)

    B. Chlorothiazide (Diuril)

    C. Ranitidine (Zantac)

    D. Rosiglitazone (Avandia)

    Trimethoprim-sulfamethoxazole is contraindicated in clients who have a history of hypersensitivity reactions to other sulfonamide medications and medications that are chemically related. These include thiazide diuretics (such as chlorothiazide), loop diuretics, and sulfonylurea-type oral hypoglycemics. Digoxin, ranitidine, and rosiglitazone are not chemically related to the sulfonamides, and are not contraindicated.

     NCLEX® Connection: Pharmacological Therapies, Adverse Effects/Contraindications/Side Effects/Interactions

2. A nurse is reinforcing teaching for a client with a prescription for trimethoprim-sulfamethoxazole (Bactrim). Which of the following precautions should the nurse reinforce to the client in order to minimize an adverse effect of the medication?

    A. Avoid prolonged sun exposure.

    B. Sip water or suck hard candy frequently.

    C. Stop taking the medication if ringing in the ears occurs.

    D. Increase the amount of fiber and liquids in the diet.

    Photosensitivity is a common adverse effect for clients taking trimethoprim-sulfamethoxazole. The nurse should instruct the client to wear protective clothing, sunscreen, and to avoid prolonged sun exposure. Sipping water and sucking hard candy is an intervention for dry mouth, which is not an adverse effect of the medication. Ringing in the ears (tinnitus) is not an adverse effect of the medication. Increasing the amount of fiber and liquids in the diet help to prevent constipation, which is not an adverse effect of the medication.

     NCLEX® Connection: Pharmacological Therapies, Adverse Effects/Contraindications/Side Effects/Interactions

3. A nurse is reinforcing teaching for a client who is prescribed nitrofurantoin (Macrodantin) for a urinary tract infection. Which of the following points should the nurse include in the instructions? (Select all that apply.)

    _____ The medication may cause the urine to be extremely pale yellow in color.

    __X__ **Cough and dyspnea are signs of a hypersensitivity reaction to nitrofurantoin.**

    _____ Nitrofurantoin should be taken 1 hr before or 2 hr after a meal.

    __X__ **Notify the provider if nosebleeds or bruising easily occur.**

    __X__ **Report numbness or tingling of hands or feet as soon as possible.**

    Hypersensitivity to nitrofurantoin may cause severe pulmonary manifestations, such as cough and dyspnea, which will gradually go away after the medication is discontinued. Bruising and epistaxis may be signs of thrombocytopenia and the provider should be notified. Agranulocytosis, leukopenia, and megaloblastic anemia may occur and signs are fatigue and increased infections. Peripheral nerve damage is another potentially serious adverse effect, and the client should notify the provider as soon as possible for numbness or tingling of the extremities. The medication does not make the urine pale, but the client should know it may make the urine brownish rust in color, but this adverse effect does not cause harm to the client. Nitrofurantoin may cause nausea and should be taken with milk or meals to minimize this problem.

 NCLEX® Connection: Pharmacological Therapies, Adverse Effects/Contraindications/Side Effects/Interactions

4. A nurse is reinforcing teaching to an adult client about her prescription for ciprofloxacin (Cipro). Which of the following adverse reactions should the nurse tell the client to watch for? (Select all that apply.)

    __X__ **Jaundice**

    __X__ **Vaginal yeast infection**

    _____ Irregular pulse rate

    _____ Urinary hesitancy

    __X__ **Achilles tendon pain**

    The nurse should reinforce teaching to the client taking ciprofloxacin about adverse reactions including jaundice (a sign of liver damage), suprainfection, which may cause a vaginal yeast infection or yeast infection of the throat or mouth, and Achilles tendon pain, which can be a sign of impending tendon rupture. Cardiovascular symptoms, such as irregular pulse and urinary hesitancy, are not expected adverse reactions for a client taking ciprofloxacin.

 NCLEX® Connection: Pharmacological Therapies, Adverse Effects/Contraindications/Side Effects/Interactions

UNIT 11	MEDICATIONS AFFECTING THE IMMUNE SYSTEM AND FOR INFECTIOUS DISEASES

Chapter 43   Mycobacterial, Fungal, and Parasitic Infections

Overview

- Tuberculosis is caused by *mycobacterium tuberculosis*, a slow-growing pathogen. This infection necessitates long-term treatment. Long-term treatment increases the risk for toxicity, poor patient adherence, and development of medication-resistant strains. Treatment for tuberculosis requires the use of at least two medications to which the pathogen is susceptible.

  o   The initial phase (induction phase) focuses on irradiating the active tubercle bacilli, which will result in noninfectious sputum. The second phase (continuation phase) works toward eliminating any other pathogens in the body.

- Length of treatment varies and may be as short as 6 months for medication-sensitive tuberculosis or as long as 24 months for medication-resistant infections. The medications for the first 2 months of the initial phase include isoniazid (INH), rifampin (Rifadin), ethambutol (Myambutol), and pyrazinamide. The medications for the last 4 months of the continuation phase include isoniazid and rifampin.

- Metronidazole (Flagyl) is the medication of choice for parasitic infections.

- Antifungal medications belong to a variety of chemical families and are used to treat systemic and superficial mycoses.

MEDICATION CLASSIFICATION: ANTIMYCOBACTERIAL (ANTITUBERCULOSIS)

- Select Prototype Medication – Isoniazid (INH)

Purpose

- Expected Pharmacological Action

  o   This medication is highly specific for mycobacteria. Isoniazid inhibits growth of mycobacteria by preventing synthesis of mycolic acid in the cell wall.

- Therapeutic Uses

  o   Prophylaxis and treatment of active and latent tuberculosis

    ■   Latent: INH only – 6 to 9 months

    ■   Active: Multiple medication therapy including INH, for a minimum of 6 months

Complications

SIDE/ADVERSE EFFECTS	NURSING INTERVENTIONS/CLIENT EDUCATION
Peripheral neuropathy (tingling, numbness, burning, pain resulting from deficiency of pyridoxine, vitamin B_6)	• Instruct clients to observe for symptoms and to notify the provider if symptoms occur. • Administer 50 to 200 mg of vitamin B_6 daily.
Hepatotoxicity (anorexia, malaise, fatigue, nausea, yellowish discoloration of skin and eyes)	• Instruct clients to observe for symptoms and notify the provider if symptoms occur. • Monitor liver function tests. • Instruct clients to avoid consumption of alcohol. • The provider may discontinue the medication if liver function test results are elevated.

 Contraindications/Precautions

- INH is contraindicated for clients with liver disease.

Interactions

MEDICATION/FOOD INTERACTIONS	NURSING INTERVENTIONS/CLIENT EDUCATION
INH inhibits metabolism of phenytoin, leading to toxicity. Ataxia and incoordination may indicate toxicity.	• Monitor the client's levels of phenytoin. • Administer adjusted dosage based on phenytoin levels.
Concurrent use of alcohol, rifampin, and pyrazinamide increases the risk for hepatotoxicity.	• Instruct clients to avoid alcohol consumption. • Monitor liver function.

Nursing Administration

- Administer by oral route.

- For active tuberculosis, direct observation therapy (DOT) is done to ensure adherence.

- Advise clients to take INH 1 hr before or 2 hr after meals. If gastric discomfort occurs, clients may take INH with meals.

- Instruct clients to complete the prescribed course of antimicrobial therapy, even though symptoms may resolve before completing the full course.

MEDICATION CLASSIFICATION: ANTIMYCOBACTERIAL (ANTITUBERCULOSIS)

- Select Prototype Medication – Rifampin (Rifadin)

Purpose

- Expected Pharmacological Action

  ○ Rifampin is bactericidal as a result of inhibition of protein synthesis.

- Therapeutic Uses

  ○ Effective for most gram-positive and gram-negative bacteria, *M. tuberculosis*, and *M. Leprae*.

- Route of Administration – Oral, IV

Complications

SIDE/ADVERSE EFFECTS	NURSING INTERVENTIONS/CLIENT EDUCATION
Discoloration of body fluids	• Inform clients of expected orange color of urine, saliva, sweat, and tears.
Hepatotoxicity (jaundice, anorexia, and fatigue)	• Monitor the client's liver function. • Advise clients to observe for symptoms and to notify the provider. • Instruct clients to avoid alcohol.
Mild GI discomfort associated (anorexia, nausea, and abdominal discomfort	• Inform clients that abdominal discomfort is mild and usually does not require intervention.

 Contraindications/Precautions

- Use cautiously in clients who have liver dysfunction.

Interactions

MEDICATION/FOOD INTERACTIONS	NURSING INTERVENTIONS/CLIENT EDUCATION
Rifampin accelerates metabolism of warfarin (Coumadin), oral contraceptives, protease inhibitors, and NNRTIs (medications for HIV), resulting In diminished effectiveness.	• The provider may increase the dosage of HIV medications. • Monitor PT and INR. • Instruct clients to use alternative form of birth control.
Concurrent use with INH and pyrazinamide increases risk of hepatotoxicity.	• Instruct clients to avoid alcohol consumption. • Monitor liver function.

Nursing Evaluation of Medication Effectiveness

- Depending on therapeutic intent, effectiveness may be evidenced by:

  ○ Improvement of tuberculosis symptoms such as clear breath sounds, no night sweats, increased appetite, no afternoon rises of temperature

  ○ Three negative sputum cultures for tuberculosis, usually taking 3 to 6 months to achieve

MEDICATION CLASSIFICATION: ANTIPROTOZOALS

- Select Prototype Medication — Metronidazole (Flagyl)

Purpose

- Expected Pharmacological Action

  ○ Metronidazole is a broad-spectrum antimicrobial with bactericidal activity against anaerobic micro-organisms.

- Therapeutic Uses

  ○ Treat protozoal infections (intestinal amebiasis, giardiasis, trichomoniasis) and obligate anaerobic bacteria (*Bacteroides fragilis*, antibiotic-induced *Clostridium difficile*, *Gardnerella vaginalis*).

  ○ Prophylaxis for clients who will have surgical procedures and are high risk for anaerobic infection (vaginal, abdominal, colorectal surgery)

  ○ Treat *H. pylori* in clients who have peptic ulcer disease in combination with tetracycline and bismuth salicylate.

- Route of Administration — Oral, IV

Complications

SIDE/ADVERSE EFFECTS	NURSING INTERVENTIONS/CLIENT EDUCATION
GI discomfort (nausea, vomiting, dry mouth, metallic taste)	• Advise clients to observe for symptoms and to notify the provider.
Darkening of urine	• Advise clients that this is a harmless effect of metronidazole.
CNS symptoms (numbness of extremities, ataxia, seizures)	• Advise clients to stop the medication and notify the provider if symptoms occur.

Contraindications/Precautions

- Use cautiously in clients with renal dysfunction to prevent accumulation of toxic levels with prolonged use.

- Avoid use during the first trimester of pregnancy, and use with caution during the rest of pregnancy because metronidazole can pass through the placenta.

Interactions

MEDICATION/FOOD INTERACTIONS	NURSING INTERVENTIONS/CLIENT EDUCATION
Alcohol causes a disulfiram-like reaction.	• Advise clients to avoid alcohol consumption.
Metronidazole inhibits inactivation of warfarin.	• Monitor PT and INR, and administer adjusted warfarin dosage as prescribed.

Nursing Administration

- Instruct clients to complete the prescribed course of antimicrobial therapy, even though symptoms may resolve before completing the full course.

Nursing Evaluation of Medication Effectiveness

- Depending on therapeutic intent, effectiveness may be evidenced by:

    o Improvement of symptoms (resolution of bloody mucoid diarrhea, formed stools, negative stool results for ameba and *Giardia*, decrease or absence of watery vaginal/urethral discharge, negative blood cultures for anaerobic organisms in the CNS, blood, bones and joints, soft tissues)

MEDICATION CLASSIFICATION: ANTIFUNGALS

- Select Prototype Medications:

    o Ketoconazole (Nizoral) – An azole for treating both superficial and systemic mycoses

- Other Medications:

    o Flucytosine (Ancobon)

    o Nystatin (Mycostatin)

    o Miconazole (Monistat 3)

    o Clotrimazole (Lotrimin)

    o Terbinafine (Lamisil)

    o Fluconazole (Diflucan)

    o Griseofulvin (Grifulvin)

    o Amphotericin B deoxycholate (Fungizone)

Purpose

- Expected Pharmacological Action

  ○ Antifungal agents act on fungal cell membranes to cause cell death. Depending on concentration, these agents can be fungistatic (slows growth on the fungus) or fungicidal (destroys the fungus).

- Therapeutic Uses

  ○ Treat systemic fungal infection (*Candidiasis, Aspergillosis, Cryptococcosis, Mucormycosis*) and nonopportunistic mycoses (*Blastomycosis, Histoplasmosis, Coccidioidomycosis*).

  ○ Treat superficial fungal infections – Dermatophytic infections (tinea pedis [ringworm of the foot], tinea cruris [ringworm of the groin]); candida infections of the skin and mucous membranes; and fungal infections of the nails (*Onychomycosis*).

Complications

SIDE/ADVERSE EFFECTS	NURSING INTERVENTIONS/CLIENT EDUCATION
Ketoconazole	
Hepatotoxicity (anorexia, nausea, vomiting, jaundice, dark urine, clay-colored stools)	• Obtain baseline liver function studies and monitor liver function monthly. • Advise clients to stop the medication and notify the provider if symptoms occur.
Effects on sex hormones: • In males – Gynecomastia (enlargement of breast), decreased libido, erectile dysfunction • In females – Irregular menstrual flow	• Advise clients to observe for symptoms and to notify the provider.

 Contraindications/Precautions

- Amphotericin B is highly toxic and should be reserved for severe life-threatening fungal infections.

- Antifungals are contraindicated in clients who have renal dysfunction because of the risk for nephrotoxicity.

Interactions

MEDICATION/FOOD INTERACTIONS	NURSING INTERVENTIONS/CLIENT EDUCATION
H$_2$ receptor antagonists, proton pump inhibitors, and antacids all decrease absorption by decreasing gastric acidity.	• Instruct clients to wait 2 hr after taking ketoconazole before administering these medications.
Inhibition of hepatic enzymes may increase levels of rifampin, phenytoin (Dilantin), warfarin (Coumadin), cyclosporine (Sandimmune), and sulfonylurea oral hypoglycemics.	• Avoid concurrent use.

Nursing Administration

- Instruct clients to complete the prescribed course of antimicrobial therapy, even though symptoms may resolve before completing the full course.

- Instruct clients that antifungals for topical use to treat superficial vulvovaginal candidiasis may be applied as a vaginal suppository or cream.

Nursing Evaluation of Medication Effectiveness

- Depending on therapeutic intent, effectiveness may be evidenced by:

  o Improvement of findings of systemic fungal infections, such as clear breath sounds and negative chest x-rays

  o Improvement of findings of superficial infections such as clear mucus membranes, clear nails, intact skin

APPLICATION EXERCISES

1. A nurse is caring for a client who has diabetes mellitus and pulmonary tuberculosis. The client has a new prescription for isoniazid (INH). Which of the following supplements should the nurse expect to administer to prevent an adverse effect of isoniazid?

   A. Ascorbic acid

   B. Pyridoxine

   C. Folic acid

   D. Cyanocobalamin

2. A nurse is caring for a client who has a prescription for oral ketoconazole (Nizoral), which he will be taking for several months to treat a systemic fungal infection. Which of the following should the nurse plan to monitor?

   A. BUN and serum creatinine levels

   B. Hemoglobin and hematocrit levels

   C. Liver function tests

   D. Thyroid function tests

3. A nurse is caring for a client who has a positive tuberculin skin test and has been diagnosed with latent tuberculosis. What treatment should the nurse expect the client to receive?

4. A nurse is monitoring a client with latent tuberculosis who has been taking twice-weekly isoniazid (INH) for the past 3 months. For which of the following findings should the nurse monitor the client?

   A. Jaundice

   B. Renal impairment

   C. Hypotension

   D. Palpitations

APPLICATION EXERCISES ANSWER KEY

1. A nurse is caring for a client who has diabetes mellitus and pulmonary tuberculosis. The client has a new prescription for isoniazid (INH). Which of the following supplements should the nurse expect to administer to prevent an adverse effect of isoniazid?

    A. Ascorbic acid

    B. Pyridoxine

    C. Folic acid

    D. Cyanocobalamin

    Pyridoxine (Vitamin B_6) is frequently prescribed along with isoniazid to prevent peripheral neuropathy for clients at an increased risk for peripheral neuropathy, such as diabetes or alcoholism. Ascorbic acid (vitamin C), folic acid, and cyanocobalamin (vitamin B_{12}) do not have the same action and are not prescribed to prevent an adverse effect.

 NCLEX® Connection: Pharmacological Therapies, Adverse Effects/Contraindications/Side Effects/Interactions

2. A nurse is caring for a client who has a prescription for oral ketoconazole (Nizoral), which he will be taking for several months to treat a systemic fungal infection. Which of the following should the nurse plan to monitor?

    A. BUN and serum creatinine levels

    B. Hemoglobin and hematocrit levels

    C. Liver function tests

    D. Thyroid function tests

    The nurse should plan to monitor liver function tests for the client because ketoconazole may cause hepatotoxicity. It is not necessary to monitor BUN and serum creatinine, hemoglobin and hematocrit, and thyroid function tests while the client is taking the medication.

 NCLEX® Connection: Pharmacological Therapies, Adverse Effects/Contraindications/Side Effects/Interactions

3. A nurse is caring for a client who has a positive tuberculin skin test and has been diagnosed with latent tuberculosis. What treatment should the nurse expect the client to receive?

    The nurse should expect the client who has latent (not active) tuberculosis to receive a prescription for isoniazid (INH) for 6 to 9 months. The client may be monitored for adherence by having the medication administered under the direct observation of a health care provider.

 NCLEX® Connection: Pharmacological Therapies, Expected Actions/Outcomes

4. A nurse is monitoring a client with latent tuberculosis who has been taking twice-weekly isoniazid (INH) for the past 3 months. For which of the following findings should the nurse monitor the client?

   A. Jaundice

   B. Renal impairment

   C. Hypotension

   D. Palpitations

   The nurse should monitor the client for jaundice and other signs of hepatotoxicity. Renal impairment, hypotension, and palpitations are not adverse effects of isoniazid.

 NCLEX® Connection: Pharmacological Therapies, Adverse Effects/Contraindications/Side Effects/Interactions

UNIT 11	MEDICATIONS AFFECTING THE IMMUNE SYSTEM AND FOR INFECTIOUS DISEASES
Chapter 44	Viral Infections, HIV, and AIDS

◎ Overview

- Most antiviral medications act by altering viral reproduction. Antiviral medications are only effective during viral replication. Therefore, they are ineffective when the virus is dormant.

- The human immunodeficiency virus (HIV) is a retrovirus. A retrovirus must attach to a host cell in order to replicate. RNA is changed into DNA using the enzyme reverse transcriptase.

- Antiretroviral agents used to treat HIV infections include antiretroviral agents and biologic response modifiers.

  ○ Antiretroviral agents may act by preventing the virus from entering the cells (fusion inhibitors). Others may act by inhibiting enzymes needed for HIV replication (nucleoside reverse transcriptase inhibitors [NRTIs], nonnucleoside reverse transcriptase inhibitors [NNRTIs], the protease inhibitors).

  ○ Biologic response modifiers, such as interleukin-2 (Interferon), act as immunostimulants to enhance the immune response. Use in combination with antiretroviral agents to reduce the advancement of the virus.

- Highly active antiretroviral therapy (HAART) involves using 3 to 4 HIV medications in combination with other antiretroviral medications to reduce medication resistance, adverse effects, and dosages.

MEDICATION CLASSIFICATION: ANTIVIRAL

- Select Prototype Medications

  ○ Acyclovir (Zovirax) – Oral, topical and IV

  ○ Ganciclovir (Cytovene) – Oral, IV

- Other Medications:

  ○ Interferon alfa-2b

  ○ Lamivudine (Epivir)

  ○ Oseltamivir (Tamiflu)

  ○ Ribavirin (Rebetol)

  ○ Amantadine (Symmetrel)

Purpose

- Expected Pharmacological Action

  o Acyclovir and ganciclovir prevent the synthesis of viral DNA and thus interrupts cell replication.

- Therapeutic Uses

  o Use acyclovir to treat herpes simplex and varicella-zoster infections.

  o Use ganciclovir for treatment and prevention of cytomegalovirus (CMV). Prevention therapy using ganciclovir is for clients who have HIV/AIDS, organ transplants, and other immunocompromised states.

  o Use interferon alfa-2b and lamivudine to treat hepatitis.

  o Use oseltamivir for treatment and prevention of infections from types A and B influenza viruses.

  o Use ribavirin to treat respiratory syncytial virus (RSV).

  o Use amantadine for treatment and prevention of infections of type A influenza viruses.

Complications

SIDE/ADVERSE EFFECTS	NURSING INTERVENTIONS/CLIENT EDUCATION
Acyclovir	
Acyclovir – Phlebitis and inflammation at the site of infusion	• Monitor IV sites for swelling and redness.
Nephrotoxicity	• Provide adequate hydration during infusion and 2 hr after. Increase oral fluid intake as prescribed. • Should be infused slowly (over 1 hr) • Monitor BUN and serum creatinine.
Mild discomfort associated with oral therapy (nausea, headache, diarrhea). Transient burning and stinging with topical application.	• Instruct clients to observe for symptoms and notify the provider if unmanageable. Advise clients that symptoms are usually self-limiting.
Ganciclovir	
Granulocytopenia and thrombocytopenia	• Obtain baseline CBC and platelet count. • Administer granulocyte colony-stimulating factors. • Monitor WBC, absolute neutrophil, and platelet counts.

Contraindications/Precautions

- IV acyclovir should be used cautiously in clients with renal impairment or dehydration, and clients taking nephrotoxic medications.

- Ganciclovir is Pregnancy Risk Category C; contraindicated in clients with a neutrophil count below 500/mm^3 or platelet counts less than 25,000/mm^3, and should be used cautiously in clients with pre-existing low white and platelet counts.

Interactions

MEDICATION/FOOD INTERACTIONS	NURSING INTERVENTIONS/CLIENT EDUCATION
Acyclovir	
Probenecid may decrease elimination of acyclovir.	• Monitor for medication toxicity.
Concurrent use of zidovudine may cause drowsiness and lethargy.	• Use with caution.
Ganciclovir	
Cytotoxic medications may cause increased toxicity.	• Use together with caution.
Concurrent use of trimethoprim-sulfamethoxazole (TMP-SMZ), probenecid, and zidovudine may result in increased bone marrow suppression.	• Avoid concurrent use.

Nursing Administration

- Acyclovir

  o For topical administration, advise clients to put on rubber gloves to avoid transfer of virus to other areas of the body.

  o Ensure clients receive adequate hydration during IV infusion.

  o Inform clients to expect symptom relief, but not a cure.

  o Instruct clients to wash affected area with soap and water 3 to 4 times/day and to keep the lesions dry after washing.

  o Advise clients to refrain from sexual contact while lesions are present.

  o Advise clients with healed herpetic lesions to continue to use condoms to prevent transmission of the virus.

- Ganciclovir

  o Administer oral medication with food.

  o Administer intraocular for CMV retinitis.

- Instruct clients to complete the prescribed course of antimicrobial therapy, even though symptoms may resolve before completing the full course.

Nursing Evaluation of Medication Effectiveness

- Depending on therapeutic intent, effectiveness may be evidenced by:

    o Improvement of findings such as healed genital lesions, decreased inflammation and pain, and improvement in vision

---

MEDICATION CLASSIFICATION: ENTRY/INFUSION INHIBITORS

- Select Prototype Medication – Enfuvirtide (Fuzeon)

Purpose

- Expected Pharmacological Action

    o Decreases and limits the spread of HIV by blocking HIV from attaching to and entering CDC4 T cell.

- Therapeutic Uses

    o Treatment of HIV that is unresponsive to other antiretrovirals

- Route of Administration – Subcutaneous

Complications

SIDE/ADVERSE EFFECTS	NURSING INTERVENTIONS/CLIENT EDUCATION
Localized reaction at injection site.	• Rotate injection sites. Monitor for swelling and redness.
Bacterial pneumonia (fever, cough or shortness of breath)	• Monitor breath sounds prior to start of therapy. Monitor for signs of pneumonia.
Fever, chills, rash, hypotension	• Monitor for medication reaction. Discontinue and notify the provider.

 Contraindications/Precautions

- Enfuvirtide is contraindicated in clients with medication hypersensitivity

- This medication is Pregnancy Risk Category B.

Interactions

- None significant

Nursing Administration

- Rotate injection sites and avoid areas with scars or bruising.

- Monitor for bacterial pneumonia.

- Monitor for medication reaction.

- Advise clients to notify the provider if they are pregnant or planning to become pregnant.

Nursing Evaluation of Medication Effectiveness

- Depending on therapeutic intent, effectiveness may be evidenced by the following:

    o The client will have a reduction of symptoms and remain free of opportunistic infection.

MEDICATION CLASSIFICATION: NUCLEOSIDE REVERSE TRANSCRIPTASE INHIBITORS (NRTIS)

- Select Prototype Medication – Zidovudine (Retrovir)

- Other Medications:

    o Didanosine (Videx)

    o Stavudine (Zerit)

    o Lamivudine (Epivir)

    o Abacavir (Ziagen)

- Combination Medications:

    o Abacavir, lamivudine zidovudine (Trizivir)

    o Abacavir, lamivudine (Epzicom)

    o Lamivudine, zidovudine (Combivir)

Purpose

- Expected Pharmacological Action

    o Reduce HIV symptoms by inhibiting DNA synthesis and thus viral replication

- Therapeutic Uses

    o HIV infection

- Route of Administration – Oral, IV

Complications

SIDE/ADVERSE EFFECTS	NURSING INTERVENTIONS/CLIENT EDUCATION
Bone marrow suppression resulting in anemia, agranulocytosis (neutropenia) and thrombocytopenia	• Monitor CBC and platelets. Advise clients that transfusions may be needed.
Lactic acidosis (hyperventilation, nausea, and abdominal pain)	• Monitor for symptoms of lactic acidosis and report to provider.
Nausea, vomiting, diarrhea	• Instruct clients to take the medication with food to reduce gastric irritation. Monitor fluids and electrolytes.
Hepatomegaly/fatty liver	• Monitor liver enzymes.

 Contraindications/Precautions

- These medications are Pregnancy Risk Category C. Pregnancy increases risk for lactic acidosis, liver enlargement, and fatty liver.

- These medications are contraindicated in clients with medication hypersensitivity.

- Use with caution in clients who have liver disease and bone marrow suppression.

Interactions

MEDICATION/FOOD INTERACTIONS	NURSING INTERVENTIONS/CLIENT EDUCATION
Probenecid, valproic acid, and methadone may increase zidovudine.	• Administer reduced dosage as prescribed. Monitor for medication toxicity.
Ganciclovir or medications that decrease bone marrow production may further suppress bone marrow.	• Use together with caution.
Rifampin and ritonavir may reduce zidovudine levels.	• Administer adjusted dosage if needed.
Phenytoin may alter both medication levels.	• Monitor medication levels.

Nursing Administration

- Monitor for bone marrow suppression. Obtain baseline CBC and platelets at the start of therapy and every 4 weeks.

- Administer epoetin alfa for anemia; monitor transfusions if prescribed.

- Administer colony-stimulating factors to treat neutropenia.

- Advise clients to monitor for fever, sore throat, increased bleeding, bruising or fatigue.

Nursing Evaluation of Medication Effectiveness

- Depending on therapeut ic intent, effectiveness may be evidenced by the following:
  - ○ The client will have a reduction of symptoms and remain free of opportunistic infection.

MEDICATION CLASSIFICATION: NON-NUCLEOSIDE REVERSE TRANSCRIPTASE INHIBITORS (NNRTIS)

- Select Prototype Medications – Efavirenz (Sustiva)
- Other Medications – Nevirapine (Viramune), etravirine (Intelence), delavirdine (Rescriptor)

Purpose

- Expected Pharmacological Action
  - ○ NNRTIs act directly on reverse transcriptase to stop HIV replication.
- Therapeutic Uses
  - ○ Primary HIV-1 infection
  - ○ Use in combination with other antiretroviral agents to prevent medication resistance
- Route of administration– Oral

Complications

SIDE/ADVERSE EFFECTS	NURSING INTERVENTIONS/CLIENT EDUCATION
Rash, which may become serious and lead to Steven's-Johnson syndrome	• Monitor for rash. Treat with diphenhydramine (Benadryl), if prescribed. • Instruct clients to notify the provider in case of fever or blistering.
Flu-like symptoms, headache, fatigue	• Monitor for adverse reactions. • Encourage clients to rest and consume adequate oral fluid intake.

 Contraindications/Precautions

- NNRTIs are Pregnancy Risk Category C.
- These medications are contraindicated in clients with medication hypersensitivity.
- Use with caution in clients who have liver disease.
- Use cautiously with other medications that are metabolized by the liver enzyme P450.

Interactions

MEDICATION/FOOD INTERACTIONS	NURSING INTERVENTIONS/CLIENT EDUCATION
Efavirenz may compete for metabolism with midazolam, triazolam (Halcion), alprazolam (Xanax) and ergotamine (Ergostar) and can result in toxicity of these medications.	• Monitor for medication toxicity.
Efavirenz can promote metabolism of saquinavir and indinavir.	• Avoid concurrent use.
Concurrent use with St. John's wort may decrease levels of efavirenz and other NNRTIs.	• Avoid concurrent use.
Concurrent use of efavirenz with ritonavir can result in increased levels of both medications.	• Avoid concurrent use.

Nursing Administration

- Give with another antiretroviral to reduce risk of medication resistance.

- Monitor for rash.

- Give with a high-fat meal to increase absorption.

Nursing Evaluation of Medication Effectiveness

- Depending on therapeutic intent, effectiveness may be evidenced by the following:

  o The client will have a reduction of symptoms and remain free of any opportunistic infection.

MEDICATION CLASSIFICATION: PROTEASE INHIBITORS

- Select Prototype Medication – Ritonavir (Norvir)

- Other Medications:

  o Saquinavir (Invirase)

  o Indinavir (Crixivan)

  o Amprenavir (Agenerase)

  o Nelfinavir (Viracept)

Purpose

- Expected Pharmacological Action

  o Protease inhibitors act against HIV-1 and HIV-2 to alter and inactivate the virus by inhibiting enzymes needed for HIV replication.

- Therapeutic Uses

  o HIV infections

  o Use in combination with another antiretroviral medication to reduce medication resistance.

- Route of administration – Oral

Complications

SIDE/ADVERSE EFFECTS	NURSING INTERVENTIONS/CLIENT EDUCATION
Diabetes mellitus/hyperglycemia	• Monitor serum glucose. Adjust diet and administer hypoglycemic medications as prescribed. Advise clients to monitor for increased thirst and urine output.
Hypersensitivity reaction	• Monitor for rash. Notify the provider if rash develops.
Nausea and vomiting	• Instruct clients to take medication with food to reduce GI effects and increase absorption.
Elevated serum lipids	• Monitor for hyperlipidemia. Assist clients with diet modification.
Thrombocytopenia, leukopenia (fever, sore throat, bruising, blood in stools)	• Monitor CBC. Monitor for signs of infection. Monitor for bleeding.

 Contraindications/Precautions

- Protease inhibitors are Pregnancy Risk Category B.

- Use with caution in clients who have liver disease.

Interactions

MEDICATION/FOOD INTERACTIONS	NURSING INTERVENTIONS/CLIENT EDUCATION
Ritonavir may cause these medications to accumulate to toxic levels – Bupropion, carbamazepine (Tegretol), diazepam (Valium), lidocaine, prednisone (Deltasone), clozapine (Clozaril), lovastatin (Mevacor), simvastatin (Zocor), alprazolam, and ergotamine.	• Avoid concurrent use.
Ritonavir may increase medication levels of sildenafil, tadalafil, and vardenafil.	• Use with caution. Tell clients the provider may reduce the dosage.
Ritonavir decreases levels of ethynyl estradiol in oral contraceptives.	• Instruct clients to use an alternative form of birth control.

Nursing Administration

- Instruct clients to report all other medications, including over-the-counter and herbal medications, to the provider.

- Give with food to increase absorption.

- Give along with another antiretroviral to reduce risk of medication resistance.

Nursing Evaluation of Medication Effectiveness

- Depending on therapeutic intent, effectiveness may be evidenced by the following:

  o The client will have a reduction of symptoms and remain free of any opportunistic infection.

APPLICATION EXERCISES

1. A client who recently had a heart transplant is being treated with ganciclovir (Cytovene) intermittent IV bolus daily. The nurse should recognize that ganciclovir is prescribed to prevent which of the following?

    A. Rejection of the transplanted organ

    B. Granulocytopenia

    C. Cytomegalovirus infection

    D. Thrombocytopenia

2. A client who is HIV-positive is receiving combination medication therapy (HAART therapy) of abacavir, zidovudine, and lamivudine to treat HIV. The nurse should recognize that the client is receiving HAART to do which of the following? (Select all that apply.)

    _____ Decrease medication resistance.

    _____ Reduce adverse medication effects.

    _____ Block antiretroviral agents from entering healthy cells.

    _____ Stimulate the immune system.

    _____ Reduce the medication dosages.

3. A nurse is reinforcing teaching to a client who is HIV-positive and has a new prescription for efavirenz (Sustiva), an NNRTI medication. Which of the following adverse effects should the nurse teach the client to watch for?

    A. A rash, which may begin within 2 weeks

    B. Orthostatic hypotension, which may occur following the first dose

    C. Hair loss, which may start after 2 to 3 days

    D. Ankle edema, which may occur after several months of therapy

4. A nurse is monitoring a client who has a prescription for zidovudine (Retrovir), a nucleotide reverse transcriptase inhibitor (NRTI), to treat HIV infection. Which of the following laboratory values indicate that the client may be experiencing a serious adverse effect to NRIT medications?

    A. BUN 14 mg/dL

    B. Hemoglobin 9 g/dL

    C. Fasting glucose 74 mg/dL

    D. Serum potassium 3.7 mEq/L

5. A nurse is reinforcing teaching to a client who is prescribed ritonavir (Norvir) twice daily to treat HIV. Which of the following should the nurse include in the instructions? (Select all that apply.)

    _____ Change positions slowly to prevent dizziness.

    _____ Take with food to minimize GI effects.

    _____ Report polydipsia or polyuria to the provider.

    _____ Avoid sun exposure as much as possible.

    _____ Have serum lipid levels checked every few months.

APPLICATION EXERCISES ANSWER KEY

1. A client who recently had a heart transplant is being treated with ganciclovir (Cytovene) intermittent IV bolus daily. The nurse should recognize that ganciclovir is prescribed to prevent which of the following?

    A. Rejection of the transplanted organ

    B. Granulocytopenia

    C. Cytomegalovirus infection

    D. Thrombocytopenia

    Use ganciclovir to prevent and treat cytomegalovirus (CMV) infection in clients who are immunocompromised due to an organ transplant, HIV infection, or clients who are receiving immunosuppressive medications. Ganciclovir does not prevent rejection of the transplant. It is an anti-viral agent and will not prevent bacterial infection. Granulocytopenia and thrombocytopenia are serious adverse effects of ganciclovir, and the medication does not prevent these problems from occurring.

     NCLEX® Connection: Pharmacological Therapies, Expected Actions/Outcomes

2. A client who is HIV-positive is receiving combination medication therapy (HAART therapy) of abacavir, zidovudine, and lamivudine to treat HIV. The nurse should recognize that the client is receiving HAART to do which of the following? (Select all that apply.)

__X__	**Decrease medication resistance.**
__X__	**Reduce adverse medication effects.**
_____	Block antiretroviral agents from entering healthy cells.
_____	Stimulate the immune system.
__X__	**Reduce the medication dosages.**

    HAART involves using 3 to 4 HIV medications in combination with other antiretroviral medications to reduce medication resistance, adverse effects, and dosages. Some of these agents are available together in one pill to reduce the amount of pills the client must take. HAART does not block antiretroviral agents from entering healthy cells. Biologic response modifiers stimulate the immune system.

     NCLEX® Connection: Pharmacological Therapies, Adverse Effects/Contraindications/Side Effects/Interactions

3. A nurse is reinforcing teaching to a client who is HIV-positive and has a new prescription for efavirenz (Sustiva), an NNRTI medication. Which of the following adverse effects should the nurse teach the client to watch for?

   A. A rash, which may begin within 2 weeks

   B. Orthostatic hypotension, which may occur following the first dose

   C. Hair loss, which may start after 2 to 3 days

   D. Ankle edema, which may occur after several months of therapy

   A rash may begin in many clients after 10 to 14 days of taking efavirenz. If the rash is severe, Stevens-Johnson syndrome may develop. The provider will discontinue the medication for a severe rash. Orthostatic hypotension, hair loss, and ankle edema are not expected adverse effects of efavirenz.

 NCLEX® Connection: Pharmacological Therapies, Adverse Effects/Contraindications/Side Effects/Interactions

4. A nurse is monitoring a client who has a prescription for zidovudine (Retrovir), a nucleotide reverse transcriptase inhibitor (NRTI), to treat HIV infection. Which of the following laboratory values indicate that the client may be experiencing a serious adverse effect to NRIT medications?

   A. BUN 14 mg/dL

   B. Hemoglobin 9 g/dL

   C. Fasting glucose 74 mg/dL

   D. Serum potassium 3.7 mEq/L

   Two serious adverse effects of NRTI medications include anemia and neutropenia from bone marrow suppression. A hemoglobin of 9 g/dL is of concern and may be caused by the medication. A BUN of 14 mg/dL is within the expected reference range, and changes in BUN are not expected adverse effects of NRTI medications. A fasting glucose of 74 mg/dL is within the expected reference range. Changes in blood glucose are not expected adverse effects of NRTI medications. A serum potassium of 3.7 mEq/L is within the expected reference range, and changes in potassium levels are not expected adverse effects of NRTI medications.

 NCLEX® Connection: Pharmacological Therapies, Adverse Effects/Contraindications/Side Effects/Interactions

5. A nurse is reinforcing teaching to a client who is prescribed ritonavir (Norvir) twice daily to treat HIV. Which of the following should the nurse include in the instructions? (Select all that apply.)

    _____ Change positions slowly to prevent dizziness.

    __X__ **Take with food to minimize GI effects.**

    __X__ **Report polydipsia or polyuria to the provider.**

    _____ Avoid sun exposure as much as possible.

    __X__ **Have serum lipid levels checked every few months.**

    Ritonavir should be taken with food to minimize GI adverse effects. Protease inhibitors, such as ritonavir, may cause hyperglycemia and diabetes, and the client should report polydipsia or polyuria to the provider. Monitor the client's lipid level every 3 to 4 months, because hyperlipidemia is a potential adverse effect. Orthostatic hypotension and photosensitivity are not expected adverse effects of protease inhibitors, so changing positions slowly and avoiding sun exposure are not necessary instructions for the client.

NCLEX® Connection: Pharmacological Therapies, Adverse Effects/Contraindications/Side Effects/Interactions

References

Berman, A., Snyder, S. J. (2012). *Kozier and Erb's fundamentals of nursing: Concepts, process, and practice* (9th ed.). Upper Saddle River, NJ: Pearson.

Curren, A. (2008). *Math for meds: Dosages and solutions* (10th ed). Cliften Park, NY: Delmar.

Dudek, S. G. (2010). *Nutrition essentials for nursing practice* (6th ed.). Philadelphia, PA: Lippincott Williams & Wilkins.

Ignatavicius, D. D., & Workman, M. L. (2010). *Medical-surgical nursing* (6th ed.). St. Louis, MO: Saunders.

Lehne, R. A. (2010). Pharmacology for nursing care (7th ed.). St. Louis: Saunders.

Lilley, L. L., Collins, S., Harrington, S., & Snyder, J. S. (2010). *Pharmacology and the nursing process* (6th Ed.). St. Louis, MO: Mosby.

Potter, P. A., & Perry, A. G. (2009). *Fundamentuls of nursing* (7th ed.). St. Louis, MO: Mosby.

Roach, S. S., & Ford, S. M. (2008). *Introductory clinical pharmacology*. Philadelphia, PA: Lippincott Williams & Wilkins.

Smeltzer, S. C., Bare, B. G., Hinklc, J. L., & Cheever, K. H. (2010). *Brunner and Suddarth's textbook of medical-surgical nursing* (12th ed.). Philadelphia, PA: Lippincott Williams & Wilkins.

Wilson, B. A., Shannon, M. T., & Shields, K. M. (2011). *Pearson nurse's drug guide 2011*. Upper Saddle River, NJ: Pearson.